BTEC Level 3 National Sport

Development, Coaching & Fitness

Second Edition

endorsed by edexcel

BTEC Level 3 National Sport

Development, Coaching & Fitness

Second Edition

Jennifer Stafford-Brown
and Simon Rea

DYNAMIC LEARNING

HODDER EDUCATION

Orders: please contact Bookpoint Ltd, 130 Milton Park, Abingdon, Oxon OX14 4SB. Telephone: (44) 01235 827720. Fax: (44) 01235 400454. Lines are open from 9.00 – 5.00, Monday to Saturday, with a 24-hour message answering service. You can also order through our website www.hoddereducation.co.uk.

British Library Cataloguing in Publication Data
A catalogue record for this title is available from the British Library

ISBN: 978 1 444 111 965

First Published 2010
Impression number 10 9 8 7 6 5 4 3 2 1
Year 2016 2015 2014 2013 2012 2011 2010

Cover photo © Stockbyte/Getty Images
Typeset by Fakenham Photosetting, Fakenham, Norfolk

Printed in Italy for Hodder Education, an Hachette UK Company, 338 Euston Road, London NW1 3BH
by **[printer to add]**

Contents

If you see this icon next to a unit, you will be able to access it by logging onto Dynamic Learning Student Online.

Acknowledgements

I would like to thank a number of people who have provided me with help in various different ways in researching and writing this textbook.

First of all, my thanks go out to my husband Matt and children Ellie and Alex for their patience and encouragement throughout the writing process, and to my parents, Ann and Brian, for all of their support and help over the years.

A big 'thank you!' to my friend and co-author, Simon, for all of his hard work, expertise and enthusiasm.

I would also like to thank a number of subject specialists including Paul Butler, David Pryce and Ian Gittens, for their contributions in writing or updating two units available within this textbook (**Unit 12** *Current Issues in Sport* and **Unit 24** *Physical Education & the Care of Young Children & Young People*) and a unit that is available via Dynamic Learning—**Unit 20** *Talent Identification and Development in Sport.*

Finally, I would also like to thank Lavinia Porter and Alison Walters and all of the people who have helped with the publication of this text book.

JENNIFER STAFFORD-BROWN

Thank you to all the people who made these books possible: Lavinia Porter and Alison Walters at Hodder; my co-author, Jenny, for her continual support and enthusiasm; and to the additional authors for sharing their expertise.

Thank you to my parents, Tony and Pam, the Sewells and the Samways, for their interest, support and understanding and continuing the family's love of sport.

Above all, to Tanya, who gave me the time and space to get the writing done and who brought love, fun and happiness to my life.

SIMON REA

The authors and publishers wish to thank the following for their permission to reproduce their images:

Unit 1 introduction	Warren Little/Getty Images
1.29	David Rogers/Getty Images
Unit 2 introduction	© Wolf/Corbis
2.1	www.purestockX.com
2.4	Jon Buckle/EMPICS Sport/Press Association Images
2.13	Bill Frakes/Sports Illustrated/Getty Images
Unit 3 introduction	Aflo Photo Agency/Photolibrary Group
3.4	Hamish Blair/Getty Images
3.6	© imagebroker/Alamy
3.7	STEVE ALLEN/SCIENCE PHOTOLIBRARY
Unit 4 introduction	Vincent Thian/AP Photo/Press Association Images
4.3	Bongarts/Getty Images
Unit 5 introduction	PA Wire/Press Association Images
5.1	Clive Brunskill/Getty Images
5.4	© Adrian Sherratt/Alamy
Unit 6 introduction	Gideon Hart/Photographer's Choice/Getty Images
6.1	© Roy Morsch/Corbis
6.5	© www.purestockX.com
6.6	© Caroline Cortizo/Alamy

Unit 7 introduction	Comstock Images/Getty Images
7.5	Glyn Kirk/Action Plus
7.7	© Shelley Gazin/The Image Works/www.topfoto.co.uk
Unit 8 & 9 introduction	Tom Dulat/Getty Images
8.1	Peter Spurrier/Action Plus
8.2	ANTONY DICKSON/AFP/Getty Images
8.3	Neil Tingle/Action Plus
8.4	Heinz Kluetmeier/Sports Illustrated/Getty Images
Unit 11 introduction	© Comstock/Corbis
11.3	Philip Wilkins/Photolibrary Group
11.4	© Comstock Select/Corbis
11.5	Photolibrary.com
11.6	© Maximilian Stock Ltd/Photolibrary Group
11.11	Neil Tingle/Action Plus
11.15	Maria Zarnayova/Isifa/Getty Images
Unit 12 introduction	PATRICK KOVARIK/AFP/Getty Images
Unit 13 introduction	Tom Dulat/Getty Images
13.1	© John Norris/Corbis
13.2	© Anderson Ross/Blend Images/Corbis
13.3	Gabriel Piko/EMPICS/Press Association Images
13.5	Simon Dawson/AP Photo/Press Association Images
13.6	© John Elk III/Alamy
13.7	Glyn Kirk/Action Plus
13.9	Sparky/The Image Bank/Getty Images
13.10	iStockPhoto.com/Simon Podgorek
Unit 14 introduction	© Roy Morsch/Corbis
14.1	ARTHUR GLAUBERMAN/SCIENCE PHOTOLIBRARY
14.2	MARTIN M. ROTKER/SCIENCE PHOTOLIBRARY
14.3	CNRI/SCIENCE PHOTOLIBRARY
14.6	iStockPhotos.com/Oleg Kozlov
16.1	Clive Brunskill/Getty Images
Units 17 introduction	Claudio Villa/Getty Images
Unit 19 introduction	Sipa Press/Rex Features
Unit 24 introduction	Sherman Ken/Photolibrary Group
24.1	© ACE STOCK LIMITED/Alamy
24.3	Donna Day/Workbook Stock/Getty Images
Unit 25 introduction	© Rick Becker-Leckrone/Corbis
Unit 26 introduction	Sipa Press/Rex Features
26.4	JOHN THYS/AFP/Getty Images
26.5	© Shepic/Alamy
Unit 42 introduction	GIANLUIGI GUERCIA/AFP/Getty Images
42.1	Asia Images RF/Photolibrary Group
42.2	Jim Olive/Peter Arnold Images/Photolibrary.com
42.3	Uppercrust Images/Getty Images
42.5	Tom Merton/OJO Images/Getty Images
42.6	Patrik Giardino/Photolibrary Group

Introduction

BTEC National Sport (Development, Coaching and Fitness) for the Edexcel examination boards is a subject that helps to prepare you for work in the sports industry or for higher education within the fields of sport science and sport.

BTEC Level 3 National Sport: Development, Coaching & Fitness Second Edition is a comprehensive textbook that covers all mandatory units in the BTEC National Sport (Development, Coaching and Fitness) qualifications that include:

- National Certificate in Sport
- National Subsidiary Diploma in Sport
- National Diploma in Sport (Development, Coaching and Fitness)
- National Extended Diploma in Sport (Development, Coaching and Fitness)

To ensure that you are following the correct pathway for your chosen qualification, please see the table in 'Pathways for BTEC National Sport (Development, Coaching and Fitness) Qualifications'.

As well as all mandatory units, ***BTEC Level 3 National Sport: Development, Coaching & Fitness Second Edition*** contains many of the more popular optional units that you can take. Some optional units have been provided as PDFs for you to read online or download via Dynamic Learning. For details of these, look for the Dynamic Learning icon on the Contents page. For details about Dynamic Learning and how to access these online units, see the inside front cover of this book.

The BTEC National Sports and BTEC National Sport (Development, Coaching and Fitness) qualifications are all assessed through coursework. You will be given assignments that cover all of the grading criteria for each unit that you are studying. ***BTEC Level 3 National Sport: Development, Coaching & Fitness Second Edition*** will help to show you where you can find the information related to the grading criteria that you are working on, which will help to ensure that you are including the appropriate subject content in your coursework.

Success in this qualification is a combination of your teacher's expertise, your own motivation and ability as a student, and accessibility to the appropriate resources – including a relevant textbook! Written by senior external verifiers and experienced BTEC National Sport teachers, ***BTEC Level 3 National Sport: Development, Coaching & Fitness Second Edition*** is highly relevant to your qualification and provides you with resources that will not only support and help you prepare for your assessments, but will also stretch and challenge you.

Within ***BTEC Level 3 National Sport: Development, Coaching & Fitness Second Edition*** you will find that each unit offers a wide range of learning resources, including:

- **Activities** related to each of the grading criteria to help you to practise assessment activities for your coursework. Each activity has a suggested time-frame so that you will have an idea of how long you need to spend on each.
- **Clear signposting throughout:** each section is clearly signposted with the relevant grading criteria
- **Quick quizzes:** at the end of each learning outcome are a number of short questions to help consolidate your knowledge before you move on to the next section.
- **Learning goals** are placed at the start of each unit to keep you on track with the requirements of the Edexcel BTEC National Sport (Development, Coaching and Fitness)
- **Definition boxes** are provided throughout, giving you clear definitions of complex physiological and technical phrases without you having to look these up in a separate glossary section
- **Useful websites** are suggested at the end of each unit so that you can access these directly to top up your knowledge in important areas of unit content
- **Figures:** Lots of sports photographs and clear illustrations to help bring your learning to life.

BTEC Level 3 National Sport: Development, Coaching & Fitness Second Edition is written in a clear, highly readable way that will help you to understand and learn about Sport and prepare you and provide information for your assessments in this course.

Pathways for BTEC National Sport (Development, Coaching and Fitness) Qualifications

To ensure that you are following the correct pathway for the **Certificate**, **Subsidiary Diploma** or **Diploma** in BTEC Sport (Development, Coaching and Fitness), please see the table below.

Unit	Certificate	Subsidiary Diploma	Diploma
1 Principles of Anatomy & Physiology in Sport	✓	✓	✓
2 The Physiology of Fitness	✓	✓	✓
3 Assessing Risk in Sport	✓	✓	✓
		Selection of one unit from 7 and 29, then selection of three of the remaining units	
4 Fitness Training & Programming		✓	✓
5 Sports Coaching		✓	✓
6 Sports Development		✓	✓
7 Fitness Testing for Sport & Exercise	✓	✓	✓
8 & **9** Practical Team & Individual Sports		✓	✓
			Selection of four units from below
10 Outdoor & Adventurous Activities		✓	✓
11 Sports Nutrition		✓	✓
12 Current Issues in Sport		✓	✓
13 Leadership in Sport		✓	✓
14 Exercise, Health & Lifestyle		✓	✓
15 Instructing Physical Activity & Exercise		✓	✓
16 Exercise for Specific Groups			
17 Psychology for Sports Performance		✓	✓
18 Sports Injuries			✓
19 Analysis of Sports Performance			

Unit	Certificate	Subsidiary Diploma	Diploma
20 Talent Identification & Development in Sport			
21 Sport & Exercise Massage			✓
22 Rules, Regulations & Officiating in Sport			✓
23 Organising Sports Events			✓
24 Physical Education & the Care of Children & Young People		✓	✓
25 Sport as a Business			✓
26 Work Experience in Sport		✓	✓
27 Technical & Tactical Skills in Sport		✓	
28 The Athlete's Lifestyle		✓	
29 Principles & Practice in Outdoor Adventure	✓	✓	
39 Sports Facilities & Operational Management		✓	✓
40 Sports Legacy Development			✓
41 Profiling Sports Performance			✓
42 Research Investigation in Sport & Exercise Sciences			✓
43 Laboratory & Experimental Methods in Sport & Exercise Sciences			✓

Note: Units 8 & 9 are combined within the Edexcel specification

To ensure that you are following the correct pathway for the **Extended Diploma** in BTEC Sport (Development, Coaching and Fitness), please see the table below.

Unit	Extended Diploma
1 Principles of Anatomy & Physiology in Sport	✓
2 The Physiology of Fitness	✓
3 Assessing Risk in Sport	✓
4 Fitness Training & Programming	✓
5 Sports Coaching	✓
6 Sports Development	✓
7 Fitness Testing for Sport & Exercise	✓
8 & 9 Practical Team & Individual Sports	✓
	Selection of 10 units from choices below
10 Outdoor & Adventurous Activities	✓
11 Sports Nutrition	✓
12 Current Issues in Sport	✓

Unit	Extended Diploma
13 Leadership in Sport	✓
14 Exercise, Health & Lifestyle	✓
15 Instructing Physical Activity & Exercise	✓
16 Exercise for Specific Groups	✓
17 Psychology for Sports Performance	✓
18 Sports Injuries	✓
19 Analysis of Sports Performance	✓
20 Talent Identification & Development in Sport	✓
21 Sport & Exercise Massage	✓
22 Rules, Regulations & Officiating in Sport	✓
23 Organising Sports Events	✓
24 Physical Education & the Care of Children & Young People	✓
25 Sport as a Business	✓
26 Work Experience in Sport	✓
27 Technical & Tactical Skills in Sport	
28 The Athlete's Lifestyle	
29 Principles & Practice in Outdoor Adventure	
39 Sports Facilities & Operational Management	✓
40 Sports Legacy Development	✓
41 Profiling Sports Performance	✓
42 Research Investigation in Sport & Exercise Sciences	✓
43 Laboratory & Experimental Methods in Sport & Exercise Sciences	✓

Note: Units 8 & 9 are combined for the Edexcel specification

1: Principles of Anatomy & Physiology in Sport

1.1 Introduction

In order for us to take part in sport and exercise, our body has to be able to produce energy and movement. Our body is made up of many different systems that work together to allow us to take part in physical activity, such as sprinting over a short distance or running continually for many miles.

This unit explores the structure and function of the main body systems involved in human movement – these include the skeletal, the muscular, the cardiovascular, the respiratory and the energy systems. These systems are all very different; however, they all work together to produce movement.

By the end of this unit you should know the:

- structure and function of the skeletal system
- structure and function of the muscular system
- structure and function of the cardiovascular system
- structure and function of the respiratory system
- different types of energy systems.

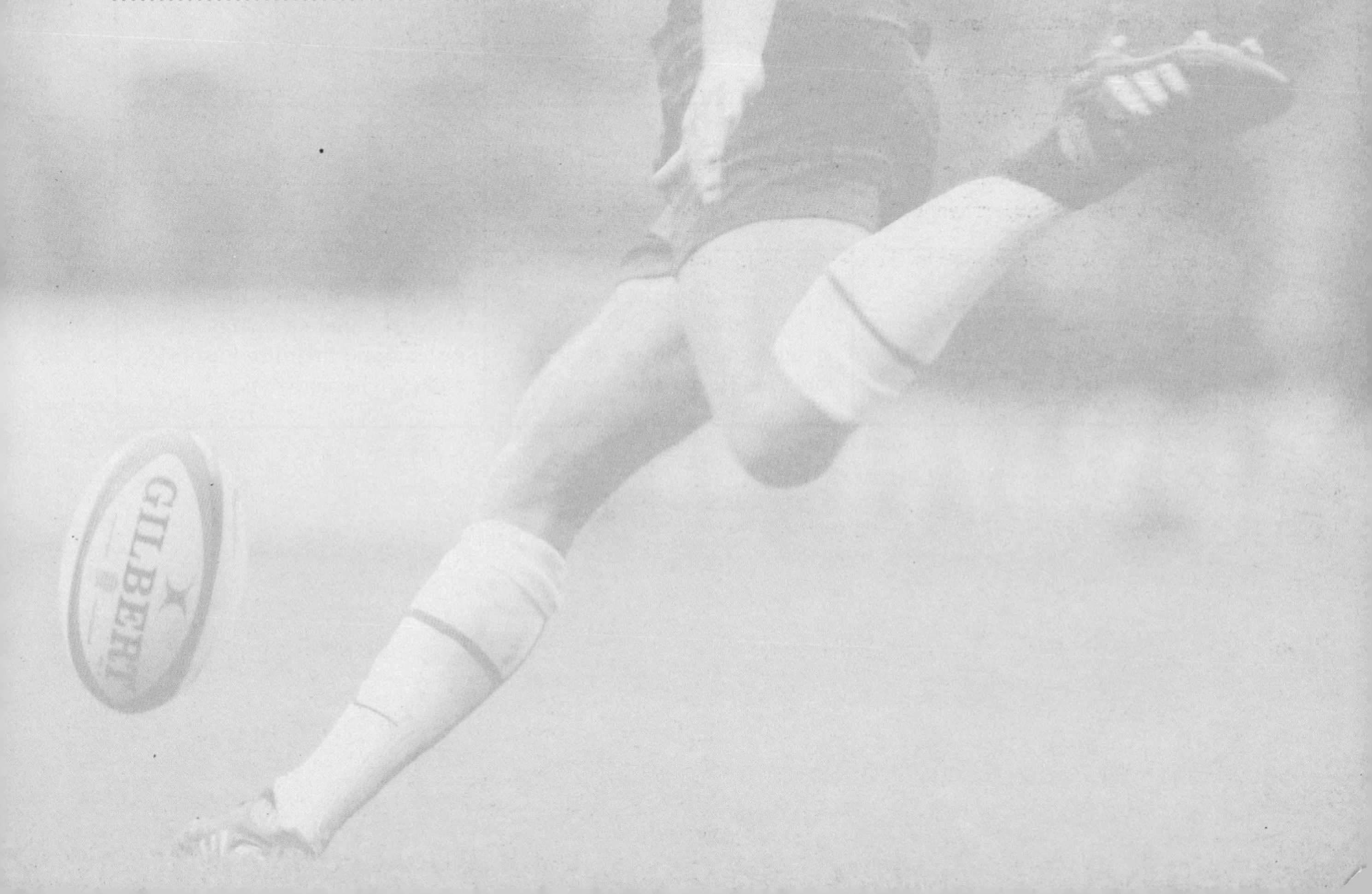

Assessment and grading criteria

To achieve a PASS grade the evidence must show that the learner is able to:	To achieve a MERIT grade the evidence must show that, in addition to the pass criteria, the learner is able to:	To achieve a DISTINCTION grade the evidence must show that, in addition to the pass and merit criteria, the learner is able to:
P1 describe the structure and function of the skeletal system		
P2 describe the different classifications of joints		
P3 identify the location of the major muscles in the human body		
P4 describe the function of the muscular system and the different fibre types	**M1** explain the function of the muscular system and the different fibre types	**D1** analyse the function of the muscular system and the different fibre types
P5 describe the structure and function of the cardiovascular system	**M2** explain the function of the cardiovascular system	
P6 describe the structure and function of the respiratory system	**M3** explain the function of the respiratory system	
P7 describe the three different energy systems and their use in sport and exercise activities.	**M4** explain the three different energy systems and their use in sport and exercise activities.	**D2** analyse the three different energy systems and their use in sport and exercise activities.

1.2 The Structure and Function of the Skeletal System

P1

The skeleton is the central structure of the body and provides the framework for all the soft tissue to attach to, giving the body its defined shape. The skeleton is made up of bones, joints and cartilage and enables us to perform simple and complex movements such as walking and running.

Axial and Appendicular Skeleton

The axial skeleton (Fig 1.1) is the central core of the body or its axis. It consists of the skull, the vertebrae, the sternum and the ribs. It provides the core that the limbs hang from.

The appendicular skeleton (Fig 1.2) comprises the parts hanging off the axial skeleton. It consists of the shoulder girdle (scapula and clavicle), the pelvic girdle, upper and lower limbs.

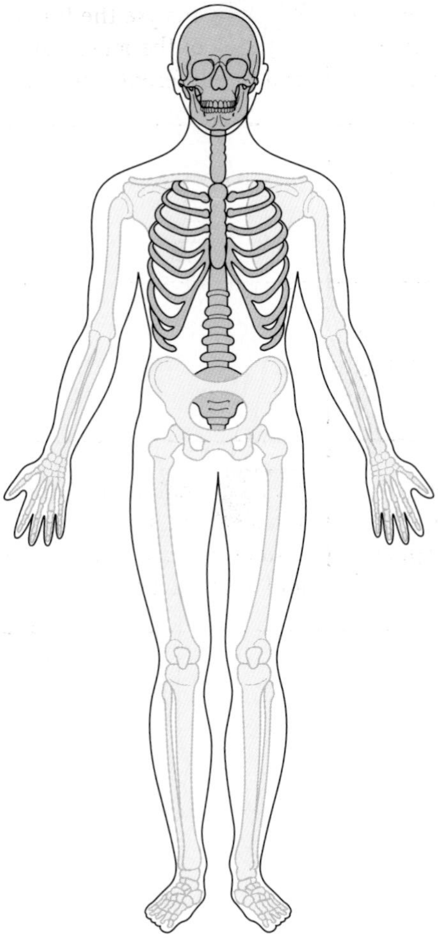

Fig 1.1 Axial skeleton

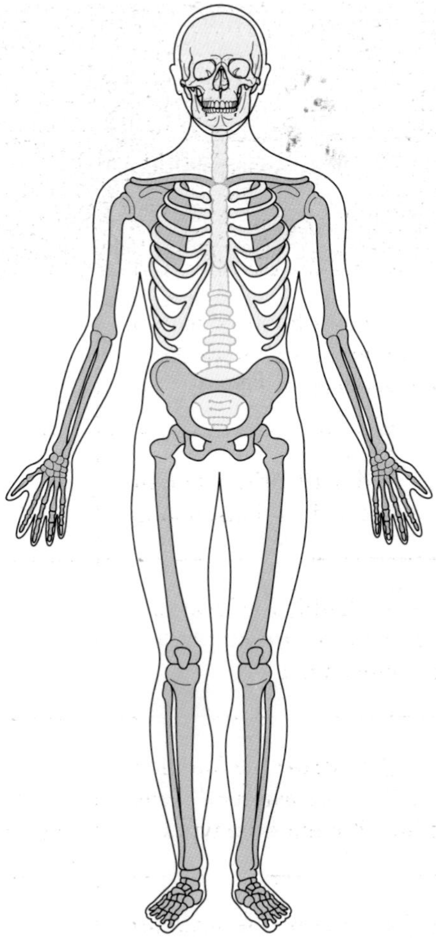

Fig 1.2 Appendicular skeleton

Types of Bone

The bones of the body fall into five general categories based on their shape.

- Long
- Short
- Flat
- Irregular
- Sesamoid.

Type of bone	Example in body	Description
Long	Femur, tibia, humerus	Cylindrical in shape and found in the limbs. Main function is to act as a lever
Short	Carpals, calcaneum	Small and compact, often equal in length and width. Designed for strength and weight bearing
Flat	Sternum, cranium, pelvis	Protection for the internal organs of the body
Irregular bones	Vertebrae, face	Complex individual shapes. Variety of functions, including protection and muscle attachment
Sesamoid	Patella	Found in a tendon. Eases joint movement and resists friction and compression

Table 1.1 Different types of joint

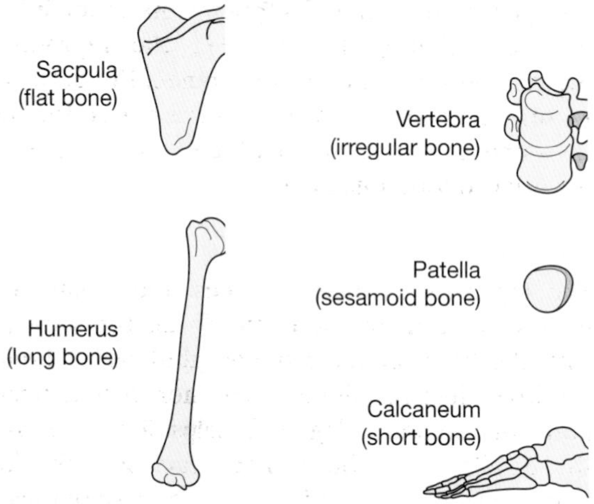

Fig 1.3 Five types of bone

Major Bones of the Body

The skeleton consists of 206 bones, over half of which are in the upper and lower limbs. Babies are born with around 300 bones and over time these fuse together to reduce the number.

Cranium

The cranium consists of eight bones fused together that act to protect your brain. There are 14 other facial bones, which form the face and jaw.

Sternum

This is the flat bone in the middle of the chest that is shaped like a dagger. It protects the heart and gives an attachment point for the ribs and the clavicles.

Ribs or Costals

Adults have 12 pairs of ribs, which run between the sternum and the thoracic vertebrae. The ribs are flat bones that form a protective cage around the heart and lungs. An individual will have seven pairs of ribs that attach to both the sternum and vertebrae

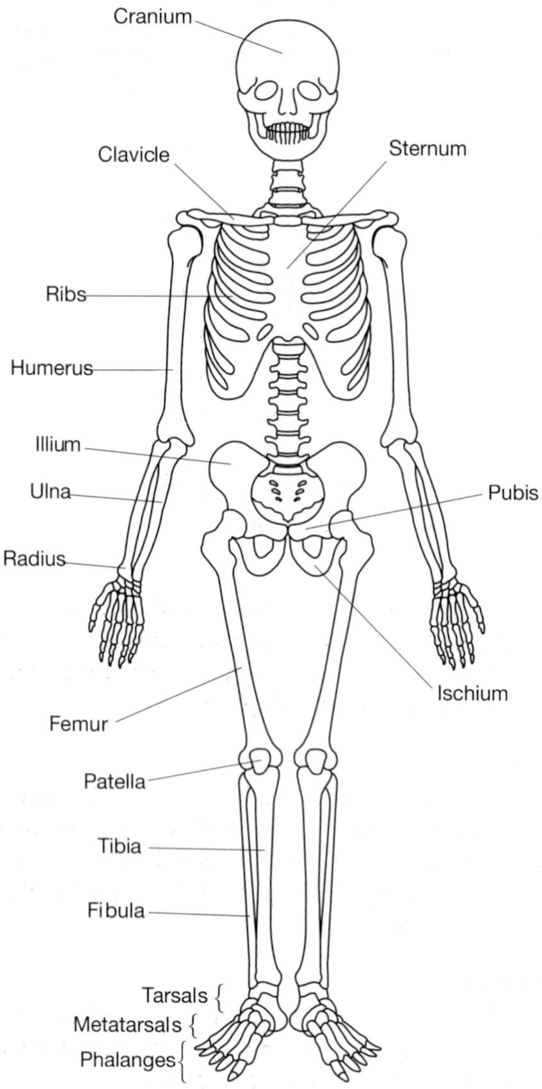

Fig 1.4 Anterior view of a skeleton

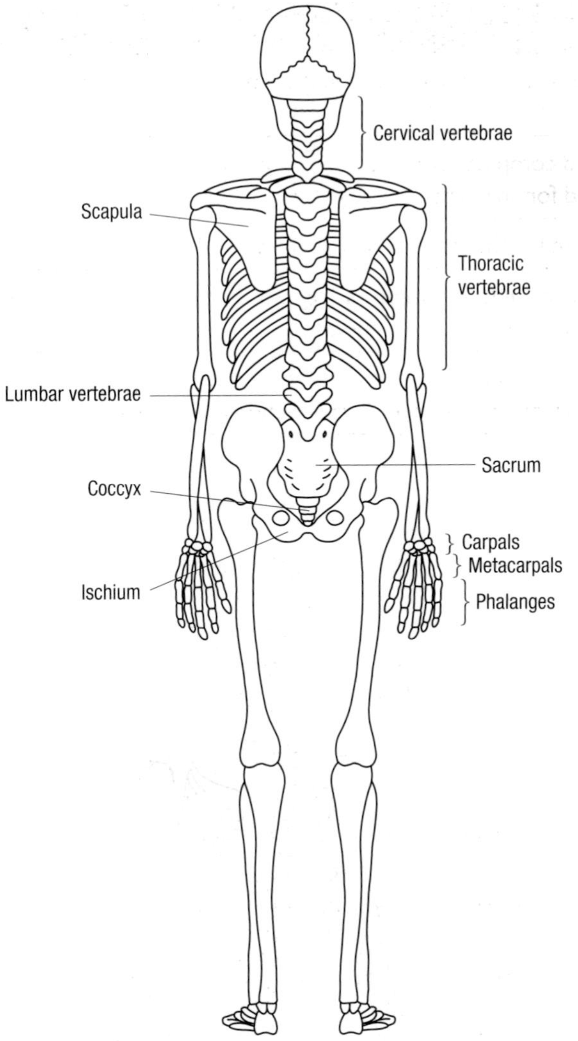

Fig 1.5 Posterior view of skeleton

(true ribs), three that attach from the vertebrae to a cartilage attachment on the sternum, and two that attach on the vertebrae but are free as they have no second attachment (floating ribs).

Clavicle

This bone connects the upper arm to the trunk of the body. One end is connected to the sternum and the other is connected to the scapula. The role of the clavicle is to keep the scapula at the correct distance from the sternum.

Scapula

This bone is situated on the back of the body. The scapula provides points of attachment for many muscles of the upper back and arms.

Arm

This consists of three bones: the humerus (upper arm), the radius and the ulna (lower arm). The ulna forms the elbow joint with the humerus and runs in line with the little finger. The radius is positioned beside the ulna and runs in line with the thumb side. When the hand turns, the radius turns across the ulna.

Hand

The hand has three areas made up of different types of bones. First, the wrist is made up of eight carpals, which are small bones arranged in two rows of four; the five long bones between the wrist and fingers are the metacarpals and the bones of the fingers are called phalanges. There are 14 phalanges altogether with three in each finger and two in the thumb. There are a total of 30 bones in the upper limb.

Pelvis

The pelvis protects and supports the lower internal organs, including the bladder, the reproductive organs and also, in pregnant women, the developing foetus. The pelvis consists of three bones, the ilium, the pubis and the ischium, which have become fused together to form one area.

The Leg

The leg consists of four bones: the femur is the longest bone in the body and forms the knee joint with the tibia, which is the weight-bearing bone of the lower leg; the fibula is the non-weight bearing bone of the lower leg and helps form the ankle; the patella is the bone that floats over the knee, it lies within the patella tendon and smoothes the movement of the tendons over the knee joint.

Foot

Like the hand, the foot has three areas: the seven tarsals, which form the ankle; the five metatarsals, which travel from the ankle to the toes; and the 14 phalanges, which make up the toes. There are three phalanges in each toe, with only two in the big toe. Again, the lower limb has 30 bones; it has one less tarsal but makes up for it with the patella.

Vertebrae

The spine is made up of five areas:

- cervical – 7
- thoracic – 12
- lumbar – 5
- sacrum – 5
- coccyx – 4.

The seven cervical vertebrae make up the neck and run to the shoulders. The twelve thoracic vertebrae make up the chest area, and the five lumbar vertebrae make up the lower back. The sacrum consists of five vertebrae, which are fixed together and form joints with the pelvis, and the coccyx, which is four bones joined together – the remnants of when we had a tail.

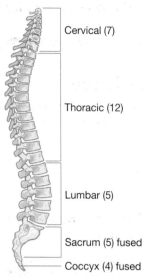

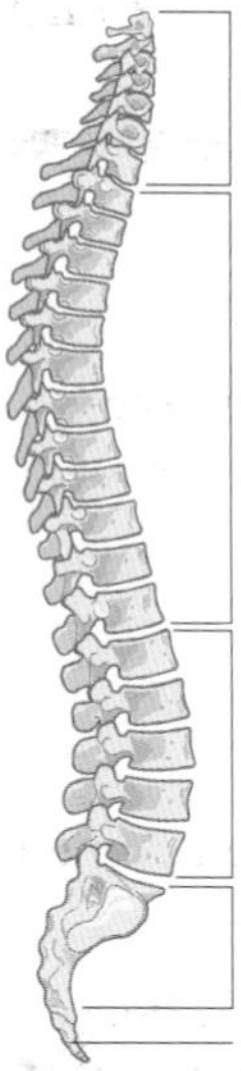

Fig 1.6 Structure of the vertebral column

Functions of the Skeleton

P1

The skeleton performs the following functions.

- Provides a bony framework for the body – the bones give the body a distinctive shape and a framework to which muscles and other soft tissue can attach. Without bones we would just be a big sac of muscles and fluids.
- Allows movement of the body as a whole and its individual parts – the bones act as levers, and by forming joints they allow muscles to pull on them and produce joint movements. This enables us to move in all directions and perform the functions we need on a daily basis.
- Offers protection to the organs found within the skeleton – the bones support and protect the vital organs they contain. For example, the skull protects the brain; the ribs offer protection to the heart and lungs; the vertebrae protect the spinal cord; and the pelvis offers protection to the sensitive reproductive organs.
- Production of blood cells – certain bones contain red bone marrow, and the bone marrow produces red blood cells, white blood cells and platelets. The bones that contain marrow are the pelvis, sternum, vertebrae, costals, cranial bones and clavicle.
- Storage of minerals and fats – the bones themselves are made of minerals stored within cartilage; therefore, they act as a mineral store for calcium, magnesium and phosphorous, which can be given up if the body requires the minerals for other functions. The bones also store dietary fats (triglycerides) within the yellow bone marrow.
- Attachment of soft tissue – bones provide surfaces for the attachment of soft tissue such as muscles, tendons and ligaments. This is why they are often irregular shapes and have bony points and grooves to provide attachment points.

Structure of a Long Bone

- Epiphysis – this is the ends of the bone.
- Diaphysis – this is the long shaft of the bone.
- Hyaline cartilage – this is the thin layer of bluish cartilage covering each end of the bone.
- Periosteum – this is the thin outer layer of the bone. It contains nerves and blood vessels that feed the bone.
- Compact bone – this is hard and resistant to bending.
- Cancellous bone – this lies in layers within the compact bone. It has a honeycomb appearance and gives the bones their elastic strength.

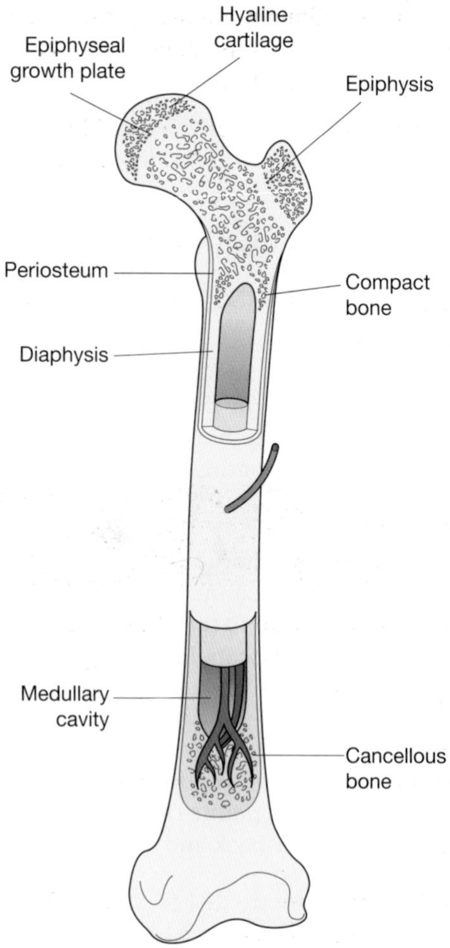

Fig 1.7 Long bone

- Medullary cavity – this is the hollow space down the middle of the compact bone and contains bone marrow. There are two types of bone marrow: red marrow, which produces blood cells, and yellow marrow, which stores fat.

Bone Growth

In a fetus, most of the skeleton consists of cartilage, which is a tough flexible tissue. As the fetus develops, minerals are laid down in the cartilage and the bones become harder and less flexible. This process is called ossification and it continues until we are adults. Bones keep growing until between the ages of 18 and 30, depending upon the bone and the body part. When a bone grows it occurs at the epiphyseal plate, which is an area just behind the head of the bone at each epiphysis; as a bone grows, its two ends are slowly pushed away from each other.

Bones are very much alive and full of activity. We know bones are living material because they can repair if they are damaged, grow when we are young and they produce blood cells. Bones contain blood vessels and nerves.

Bone is continually being broken down and replaced; this process is done by different cells, osteoblasts and osteoclasts:

- osteoblasts are cells that will build bone
- osteoclasts are cells that destroy or clean away old bone.

Osteoclasts and osteoblasts will replace around 10 per cent of bone every year; this means that no matter how old we are our skeleton is no older than ten years of age!

Key term

Ossification: The process of creating bone from cartilage.

Connective Tissue

There are connective tissues in the body to connect tissue and stabilise joints. There are three types of connective tissue:

- cartilage
- ligament
- tendon.

Cartilage is a dense and tough tissue that cushions joints. It comes in three types:

- hyaline (found at the ends of bones)
- fibro (thick chunks found in the knee and between vertebrae)
- elastic (gives shape to structures such as the ear and the nose).

Ligaments:

- attach bone to bone
- act to give stability to joints
- are tough, white and inelastic.

Tendons:

- attach muscle to bone
- carry the force from muscle contraction to the bone
- are tough, greyish and inelastic.

All these types of connective tissue have a very poor blood supply, hence their whitish colour, and will take a long time to repair if they become damaged.

Student activity 1.1 — 30 minutes — P1

Structure and function of the skeleton

Our skeleton is made up of 206 bones and has many different functions.

Task 1

Label a diagram of the skeleton to name all of the major bones.

Task 2

Draw a spider diagram that illustrates the different functions of the skeleton.

Task 3

Write a report that describes the structure and function of the different parts of the skeleton, including:

- the axial and appendicular skeletons
- the different types of bones
- the five main functions of the skeleton as a whole.

Joints

P2

The place where two or more bones meet is called a joint or an articulation. A joint is held together by ligaments, which give the joints their stability.

Key term

Joint: Where two or more bones meet

Joints are put into one of three categories depending upon the amount of movement available.

1 Fixed joints/fibrous – these joints allow no movement. These types of joints can be found between the plates in the skull.

2 Slightly moveable/cartilaginous – these joints allow a small amount of movement and are held in place by ligaments and cushioned by cartilage. These types of joints can be found between the vertebrae in the spine.

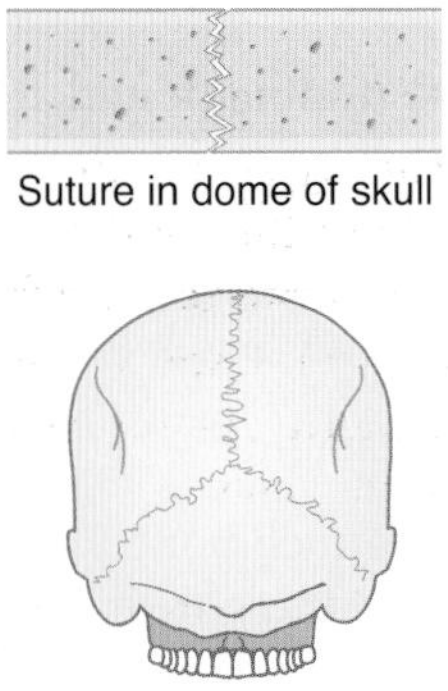

Fig 1.8 A fixed joint

3 Moveable/synovial – these joints allow a wide range of movement and all have a similar joint structure.

Figure 1.10 shows the structure of a synovial joint, which is made up of the following components.

- Synovial capsule – keeps the contents of the synovial joint in place.
- Synovial membrane – releases synovial fluid onto the joint.
- Synovial fluid – a thick 'oil like' solution that lubricates the joint and allows free movement.
- Articular cartilage – a bluish-white covering of cartilage that prevents wear and tear on the bones.

There are six types of synovial joints and all allow varying degrees of movement. The six types of synovial joint are: hinge, ball and socket, pivot, condyloid, sliding, and saddle.

Hinge joint

These can be found in the elbow (ulna and humerus) and knee (femur and tibia). They allow flexion and

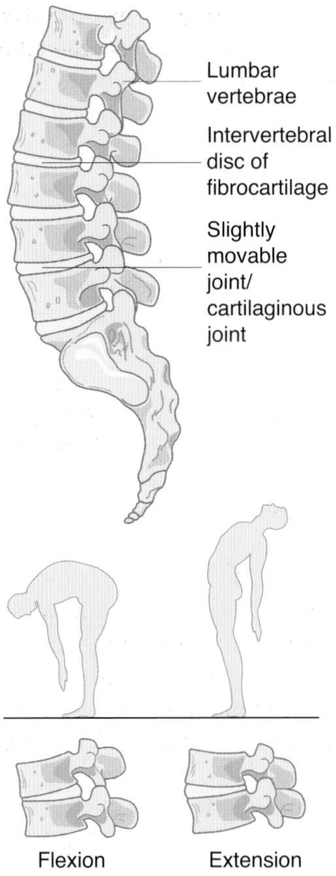

Fig 1.9 A cartilaginous joint

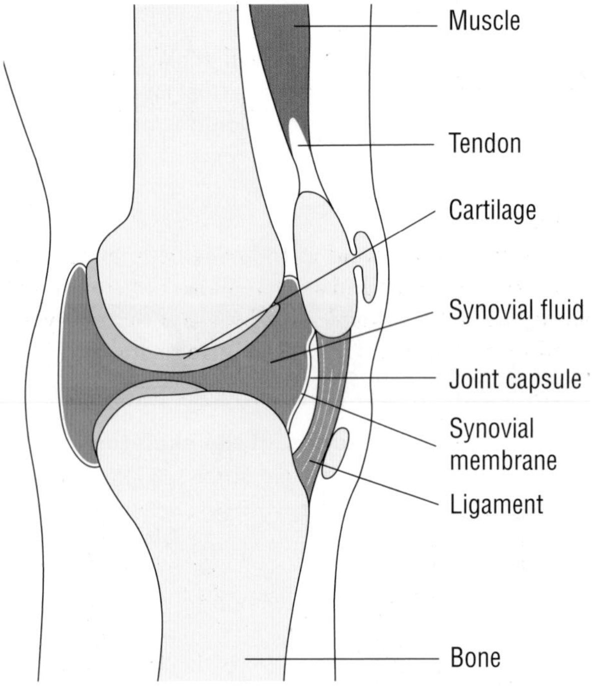

Fig 1.10 Structure of a synovial joint

extension of a joint. Hinge joints are like the hinges on a door, and allow you to move the elbow and knee in only one direction.

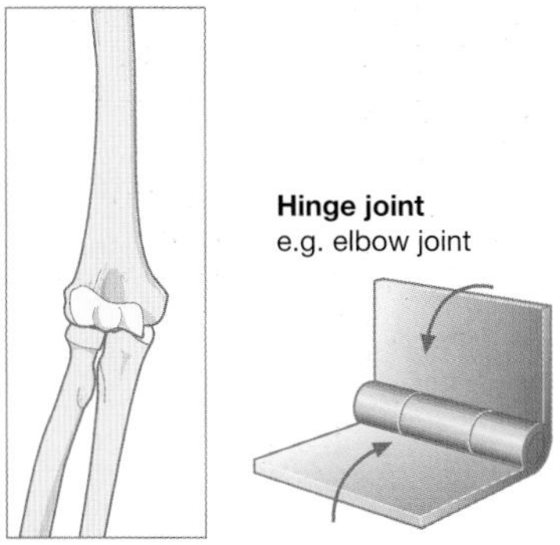

Fig 1.11 Hinge joint

Ball and Socket Joint

These types of joint can be found at the shoulder (scapula and humerus) and hip (pelvis and femur) and allow movement in almost every direction. A ball and socket joint is made up of a round end of one bone that fits into a small cup-like area of another bone.

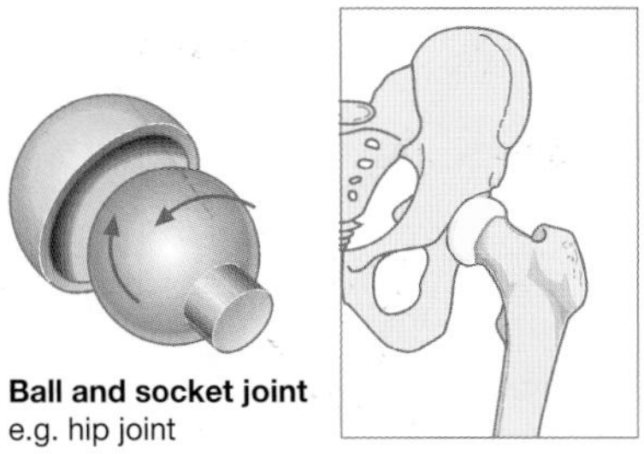

Fig 1.12 Ball and socket joint

Pivot Joint

This joint can be found in the neck between the top two vertebrae (atlas and axis). It allows only rotational movement – for example, it allows you to move your head from side to side as if you were saying 'no'.

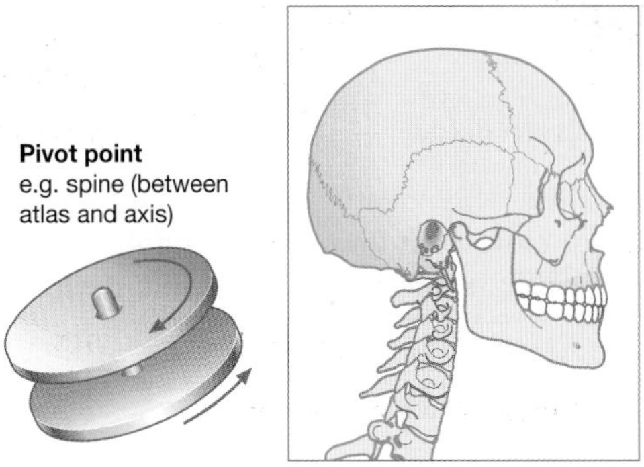

Fig 1.13 Pivot joint

Condyloid joint

This type of joint is found at the wrist. It allows movement in two planes; this is called biaxial. It allows you to bend and straighten the joint, and move it from side to side. The joints between the metacarpals and phalanges are also condyloid.

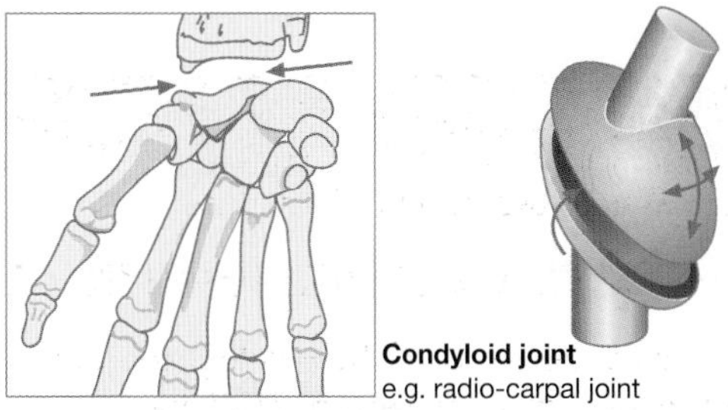

Fig 1.14 Condyloid joint

Saddle Joint

This type of joint is found only in the thumbs. It allows the joint to move in three planes: backwards and forwards, and from side to side, and across. This is a joint specific to primates and gives us 'manual dexterity', enabling us to hold a cup and write, among other skills.

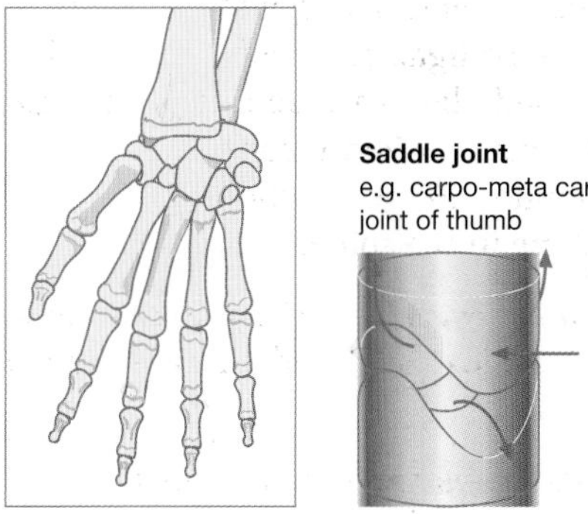

Fig 1.15 Saddle joint

Gliding Joint

This type of joint can be found in the carpal bones of the hand. These types of joint occur between the surfaces of two flat bones. They allow very limited movement in a range of directions.

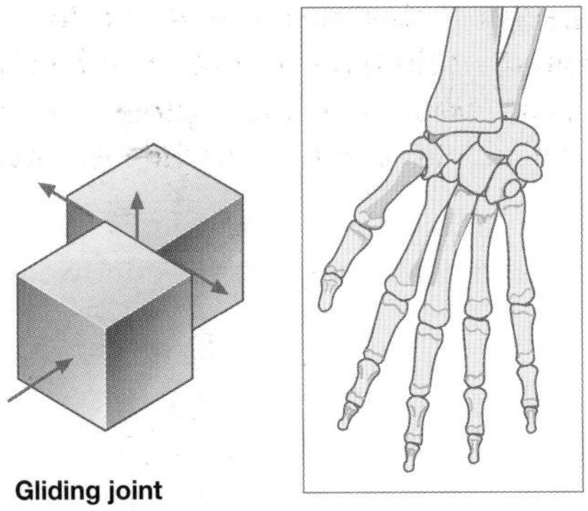

Fig 1.16 Gliding joint

Types of Joint Movement

To enable us to understand sporting movements we need to be able to describe or label joint movements. Joint movements are given specific terms (see below).

General Movements

General movements apply to more than one joint.

- Flexion – this occurs when the angle of a joint decreases. For example, when you bend the elbow it decreases from 180 degrees to around 30 degrees.

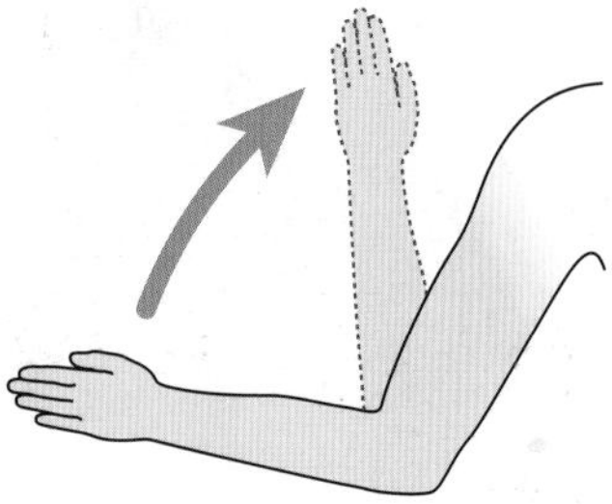

Fig 1.17 Flexion

- Extension – this occurs when the angle of a joint increases. For example, when you straighten the elbow it increases from 30 degrees to 180 degrees.

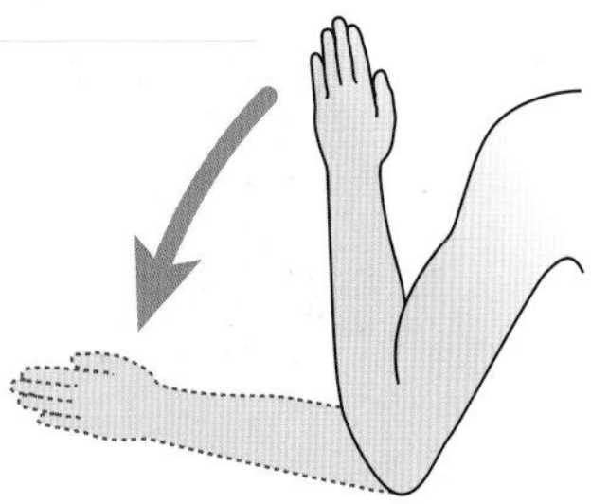

Fig 1.18 Extension

- Adduction – this means movement towards the midline of the body.

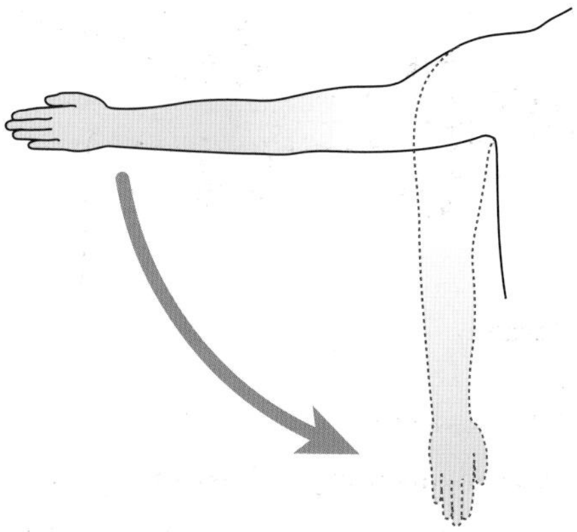

Fig 1.19 Adduction

- Abduction – this means movement away from the midline of the body. This occurs at the hip during a star jump.

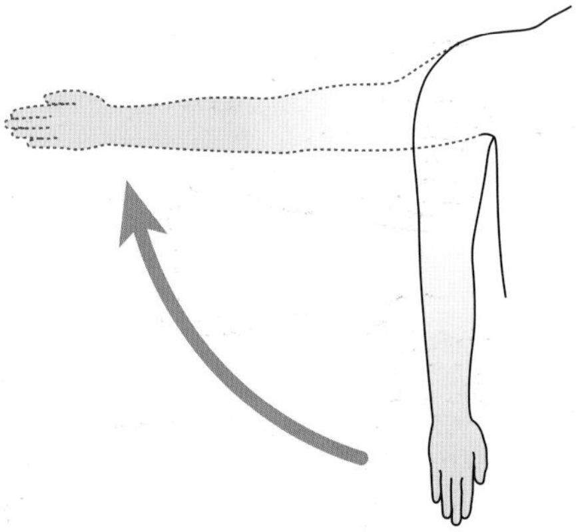

Fig 1.20 Abduction

- Circumduction – this means that the limb moves in a circle. This occurs at the shoulder joint during an overarm bowl in cricket.

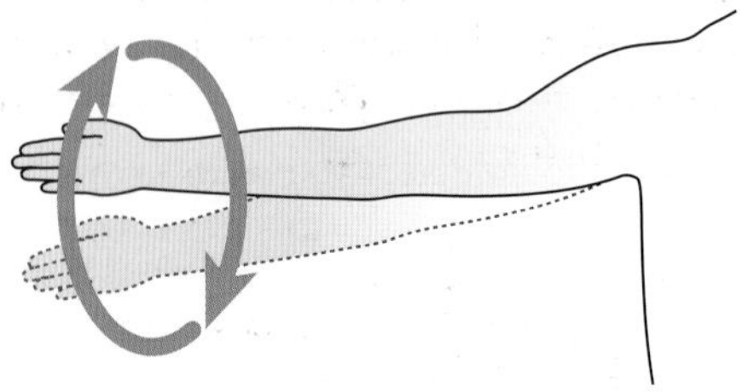

Fig 1.21 Circumduction

- Rotation – this means that the limb moves in a circular movement towards the middle of the body. This occurs in the hip in golf while performing a drive shot.

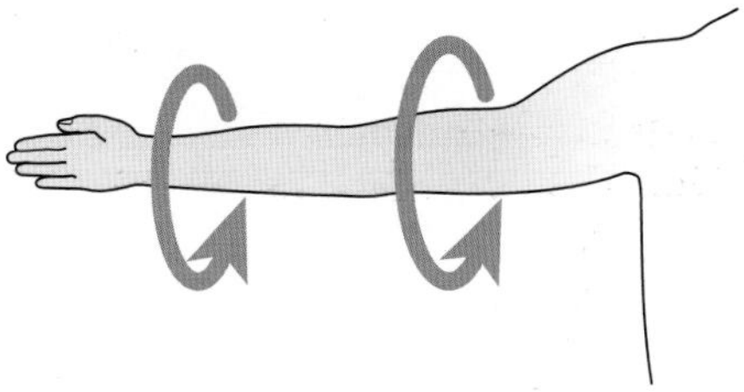

Fig 1.22 Rotation

Specific Movements

Specific movements apply to a specific joint.

- Pronation – this means when the hand is facing down while the elbow is flexed. Pronation occurs as the hand moves from facing up to facing down, and is the result of the movement of the pivot joint between the ulna and radius. This would happen when a spin bowler delivers the ball in cricket.

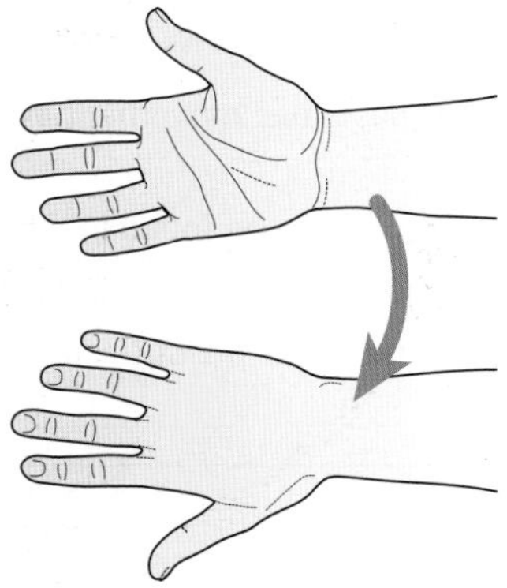

Fig 1.23 Pronation

- Supination – this means when the palm of the hand is facing up. Supination occurs as the hand moves from facing down to facing up, and is the result of the movement of the pivot joint between the ulna and radius. You can remember this by thinking that you carry a bowl of soup in a supinated position. Throwing a dart involves supination of the forearm.

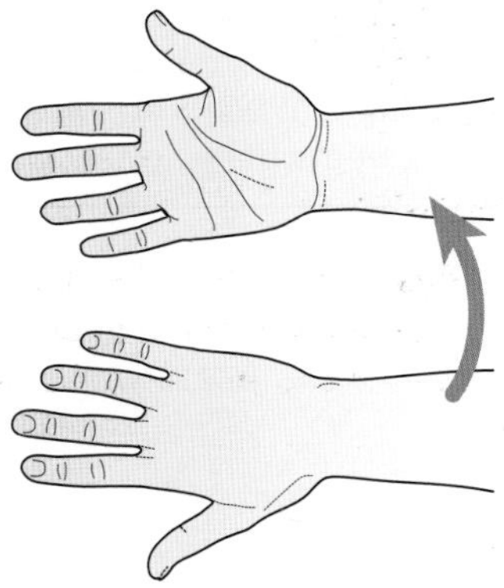

Fig 1.24 Supination

- Plantarflexion – this means that the foot moves away from the shin bone and you will be pointing your toes or raising onto your tiptoes. It is specific to your ankle joint and occurs when you walk.

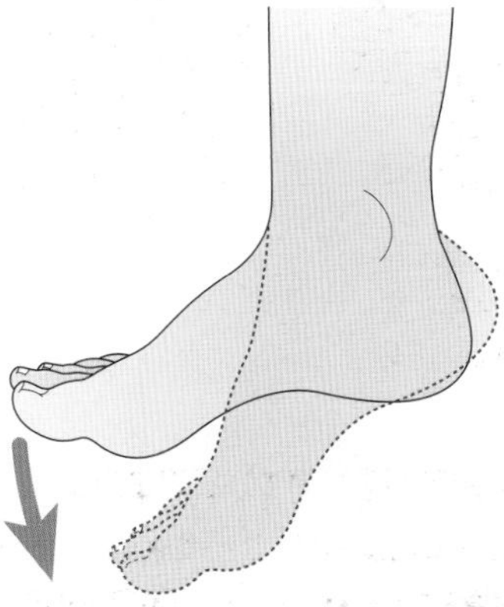

Fig 1.25 Plantarflexion

- Dorsiflexion – this means that the foot moves towards the shin as if you are pulling your toes up. It is specific to the ankle joint and occurs when you walk.

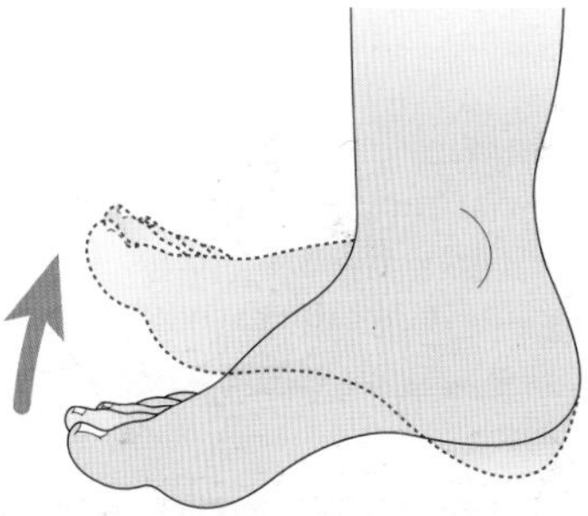

Fig 1.26 Dorsiflexion

- Inversion – this means that the soles of the feet are facing each other. It occurs at the gliding joints between the tarsals rather than at the ankle joint.

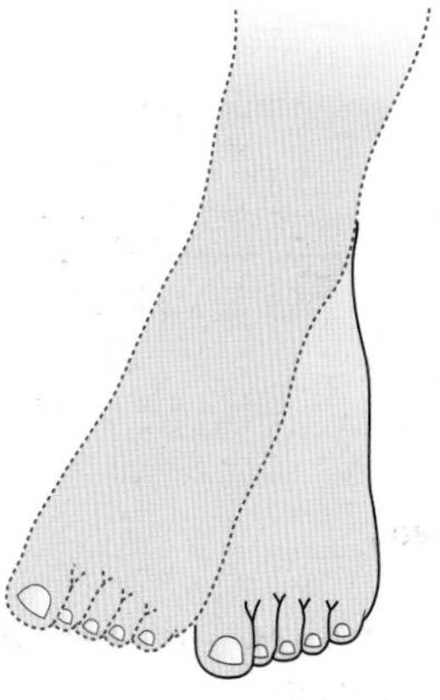

Fig 1.27 Inversion

- Eversion – this means that the soles of the feet are facing away from each other. It occurs at the gliding joints between the tarsals rather than at the ankle joint.

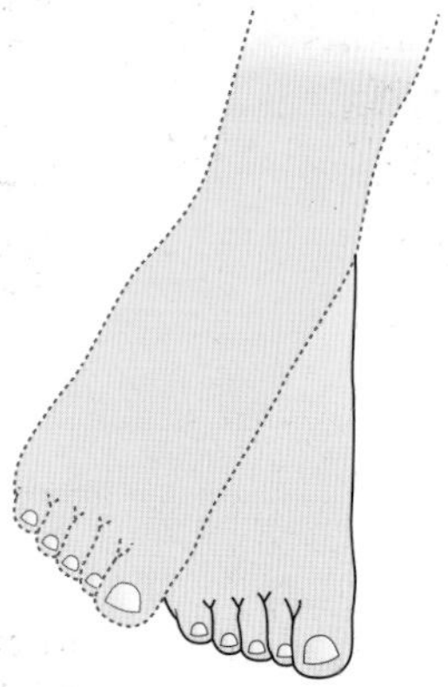

Fig 1.28 Eversion

- Hyperextension – this is the term given to an extreme or abnormal range of motion found within a joint – for example, at the knee or elbow.

Key learning points 1

- The functions of the skeleton are shape, movement, protection, blood production and mineral storage.
- Bones grow at their growth plates.
- There are three types of joint: fixed, slightly moveable and moveable/synovial.

Q Quick quiz 1

Ossification	Calcium	Flexion
Ribs	Abduction	Bone marrow
The leg	Bone marrow	
Immovable	Pivot	

Choose a word from the boxes above to answer each of the following questions.

1 What is the main mineral stored in bones?
2 Where are blood cells produced?
3 Which bones protect the heart and lungs?
4 Which limb consists of four bones?
5 What is the name given to the process of cartilage turning into bone?
6 The hinge joint allows only this type of movement and no other.
7 Which term describes movement away from the body?
8 This type of joint can be found in the neck.
9 This type of joint can be found in the skull.
10 This part of the bones produces new blood cells.

Student activity 1.2 — 30 minutes — P2

Different types of joints

The different joints in our body allow varying amounts of movement – some allow none, whereas others have a wide range of movement, which allows us to take part in sport and exercise activities.

Task 1

Describe the three different classifications of joints and give examples of each.

Task 2

Describe the six different types of synovial joint and the types of movements that they allow.

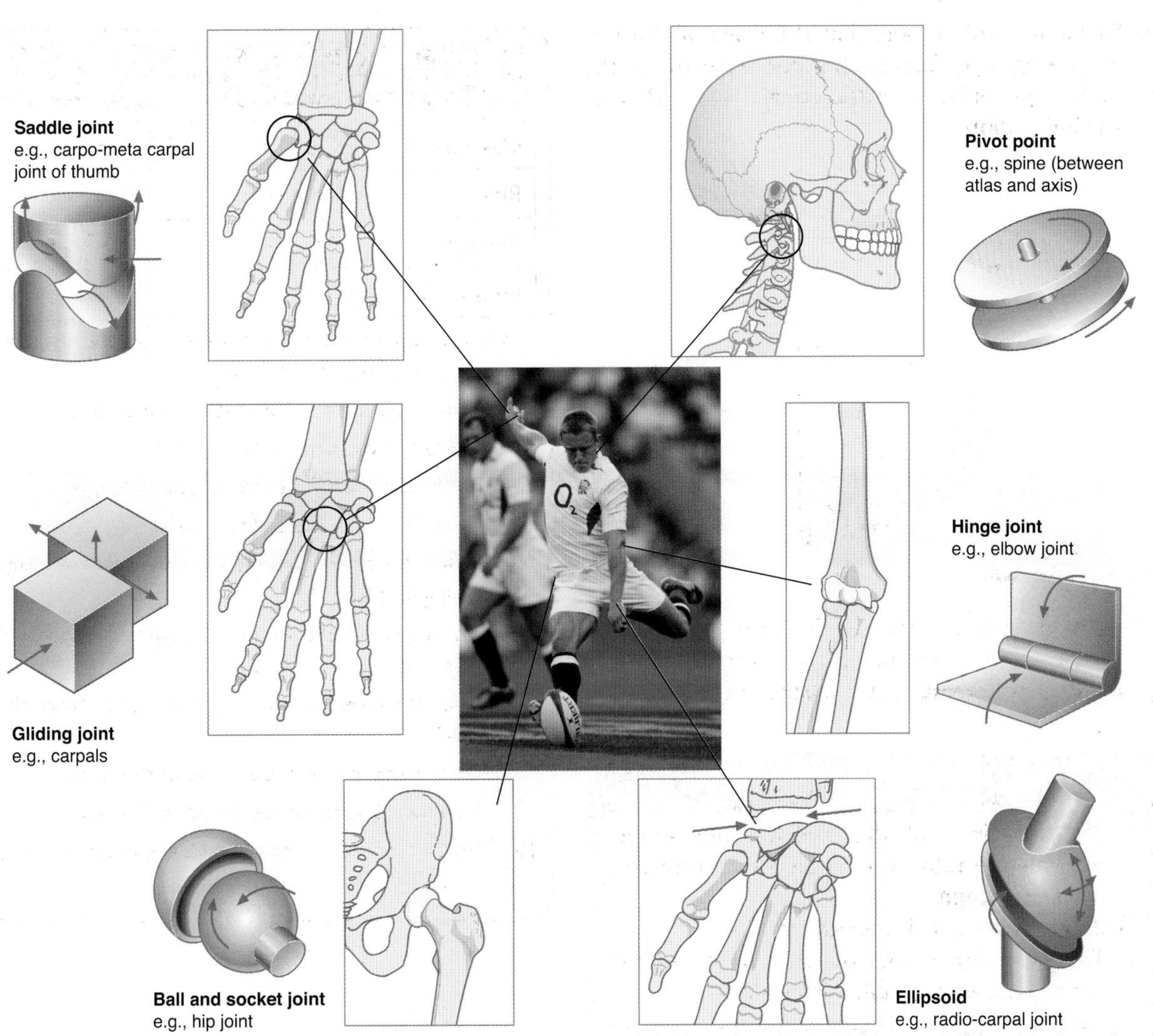

Fig 1.29 Synovial joints in action

1.3 The Structure and Function of the Muscular System

P3 P4 M1 D1

The muscular system will work in conjunction with the skeleton to produce movement of the limbs and body. The muscular system always has to work with the nervous system because it will produce a nervous impulse to initiate movement.

Major Muscles of the Body

P3

There are three types of muscle tissue: smooth, cardiac and skeletal.

1 **Smooth muscles** – smooth muscles are also called involuntary muscles because they are out of our conscious control. They can be found in the digestive system (large and small intestine), the circulatory system (artery and vein walls) and the urinary system. Smooth muscles contract with a peristaltic action in that the muscle fibres contract consecutively rather than at the same time, and this produces a wavelike effect. For example, when food is passed through the digestive system it is slowly squeezed through the intestines.
2 **Cardiac muscle** – the heart has its own specialist muscle tissue, which is cardiac muscle. Cardiac muscle is involuntary muscle. The heart has its own nerve supply via the sino-atrial node, and it works by sending a nervous impulse through consecutive cells. The heart will always contract fully – that is, all the fibres will contract – and contracts around 60–80 times a minute. The function of the myocardium is to pump blood around the body.

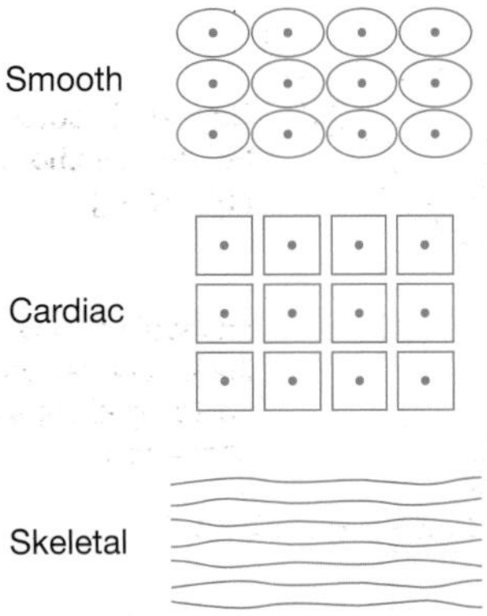

Fig 1.30 Types of muscle fibre under the microscope

3 Skeletal muscle – skeletal muscle is muscle that is attached to the skeleton across joints. It is under voluntary control as we decide when to contract muscles and produce movement. Skeletal muscle is arranged in rows of fibres, and it is also called striated, or striped, on account of its appearance. The coordinated contractions of skeletal muscle allow us to move smoothly and produce sports skills. There are over 700 skeletal muscles in the human body, and they make up around 40 per cent of our body weight (slightly less for a female).

Student activity 1.3 — 25 minutes — P3

Major muscles in the human body

There are lots of different muscles in the human body and you will need to know the names and locations of each so that you can go on to understand how they produced movements.

Task 1

Working in pairs, write the following muscle names on to some sticky labels:

- Biceps
- Biceps Brachii
- Biceps Femoris
- Deltoid
- Erector Spinae
- Gastrocnemius
- Gluteus Maximus
- Iliopsoas
- Latissimus Dorsi
- Obliques
- Pectoralis Major
- Rectus Abdominus
- Rectus Femoris
- Rhomboids
- Sartorius
- Semimembranosus
- Semitendinosus
- Soleus
- Teres Major
- Tibialis Anterior
- Trapezius
- Triceps
- Triceps Brachii
- Vastus Intermedius
- Vastus Lateralis
- Vastus Medialis

Task 2

One of you will be the anterior muscles and the other will be the posterior muscle groups. In your pairs, place the appropriate muscle labels over your partner's clothes to indicate where each major muscle is located.

Function of the Muscular System – Movement

Tendons are responsible for joining skeletal muscles to your skeleton. Skeletal muscles are held to the bones with the help of tendons.

Tendons are cords made of tough tissue; they work to connect muscle to bones. When the muscle contracts, it pulls on the tendon, which in turn pulls on the bone and makes the bone move.

When muscles contract they work as a group in that the muscle contracting is dependent on other muscles to enable it to do its job. A muscle can play one of four roles, as outlined below.

1 **Agonist (or prime mover)** – this muscle contracts to produce the desired movement.

2 **Antagonist** – this muscle relaxes to allow the agonist to contract.
3 **Synergist** – this muscle assists the agonist in producing the desired movement.
4 **Fixator** – these muscles will fix joints and the body in position to enable the desired movement to occur.

An antagonistic muscle pair comprises muscle that contracts to produce the movement and muscle that relaxes to produce the movement. For example, when you perform a bicep curl, the biceps brachii will be the agonist as it contracts to produce the movement, while the triceps brachii will be the antagonist as it relaxes to allow the movement to occur.

Types of Muscle Movement

Muscles can contract or develop tension in three different ways.

1 **Concentric contraction** – involves the muscle shortening and developing tension. The origin and insertion of the muscle move closer together and the muscle becomes fatter. To produce a concentric contraction, a movement must occur against gravity.
2 **Eccentric contraction** – an eccentric contraction involves the muscle lengthening to develop tension. The origin and the insertion of the muscle move further away from each other. An eccentric contraction provides the control of a movement on the downward phase, and it works to resist the force of gravity.

   If a person is performing a bench press, they will produce a concentric contraction to push the weight away from their body. However, on the downward phase they will produce an eccentric contraction to control the weight on the way down. If they did not, gravity would return their weight to the ground and they would be hurt in the process. The agonist muscle will produce concentric or eccentric contractions, while the antagonist muscle will always stay relaxed to allow the movement to occur.
3 **Isometric contraction** – if a muscle produces tension but stays the same length, then it will be an isometric contraction. This occurs when the body is fixed in one position; for example a gymnast on the rings in the crucifix position. Also, when we are standing up, our postural muscles produce isometric contractions

Muscle Fibre Types

Within our muscle we have two types of muscle fibre, which are called fast twitch and slow twitch fibres due

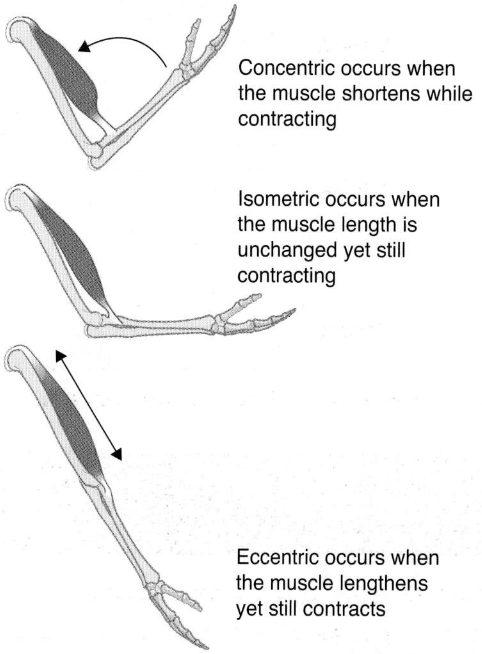

Concentric occurs when the muscle shortens while contracting
Isometric occurs when the muscle length is unchanged yet still contracting
Eccentric occurs when the muscle lengthens yet still contracts

Fig 1.31 Types of muscles contraction at the biceps brachii

to the speed at which they contract (see Table 1.2). If we look at the evolution of humans, we were originally hunters and gatherers; this meant that we had to walk long distances to find animals to eat and then, when we saw one, we would have to chase after it as fast as we could. Therefore, we adapted slow twitch muscle fibres to walk long distances and fast twitch muscle fibres to run quickly after our prey.

Slow Twitch Fibres (Type 1)

These will be red in colour as they have a good blood supply. They have a dense network of blood vessels, making them suited to endurance work and they are slow to fatigue. They also contain many mitochondria to make them more efficient at producing energy using oxygen.

> **Key term**
>
> **Mitochondria:** the energy-producing organelles within cells.

Fast Twitch Fibres (Type 2)

Fast twitch fibres will contract twice as quickly as slow twitch fibres and are thicker in size. They have a poor blood supply, are whiter in appearance and, due to the lack of oxygen, they will fatigue fairly quickly. Their faster, harder contractions make them suitable for producing fast, powerful actions such as sprinting and lifting heavy weights.

Within the group of fast twitch fibres there are two types: 2A and 2B. The type that is used depends upon the intensity of the chosen activity. Type 2B fibres work when a person is working very close to their maximum intensity, while type 2A work at slightly lower intensities but at higher intensities than slow twitch fibres are capable of. For example, a 100-m runner would be using type 2B fibres, while a 400-m runner would be using type 2A fibres.

Slow twitch (Type 1)	Fast twitch (Type 2)
Red	White
Contract slowly	Contract rapidly
Aerobic	Anaerobic
Endurance based	Speed/strength based
Can contract repeatedly	Easily exhausted
Exert less force	Exert great forces

Table 1.2 Basic characteristics of fast twitch and slow twitch

Key learning points 2

- There are three types of muscle: cardiac, smooth and skeletal.
- Cardiac and smooth muscle are involuntary and skeletal muscle is voluntary.
- Muscles work in antagonistic pairs where one muscle pulls (agonist) and the other muscle relaxes (antagonist).
- There are two types of muscle fibre – slow twitch and fast twitch,
- Slow twitch muscle fibres are used in endurance sports.
- There are two types of fast twitch muscle fibres: 2A and 2B. 2B are used in maximal intensity exercise, 2A during slightly lower intensity. Both are used for fast powerful actions such as sprinting or lifting weights.

Characteristics	Slow twitch (Type 1)	Fast oxidative glycolytic F.O.G. (Type 2A)	Fast twitch glycolytic F.T.G. (Type 2B)
Speed of contraction (ms)	Slow (110)	Fast (50)	Fast (50)
Force of contraction	Low	High	High
Size	Smaller	Large	Large
Mitochondrial density	High	Lower	Low
Myoglobin content	High	Lower	Low
Fatiguability	Fatigue resistant	Less resistant	Easily fatigued
Aerobic capacity	High	Medium	Low
Capillary density	High	High	Low
Anaerobic capacity	Low	Medium	High
Motor neuron size	Small	Large	Large
Fibres/motor neuron	10–180	300–800	300–800
Sarcoplasmic reticulum development	Low	High	High

Table 1.3 Structural characteristics of muscle fibres
Source: (Adapted from Sharkey *'Physiology of Fitness'*, Human Kinetics 1990).

Q Quick quiz 2

Answer the following questions about the muscular system.

1 Give three examples of where you may find smooth muscle.
2 Give five examples of skeletal muscles.
3 What is the name of the muscle that produces movement?
4 What is the name of the muscle that helps with the movement?
5 What is the name of the muscle that fixes the joint?
6 Look at the table below, then fill in the gaps:

Sporting action	Type of movement	Joint	Agonist	Antagonist	Fixator
Sit up – upwards phase	Flexion	Spine	Abdominals		
Press up – downwards phase	Flexion	Elbow		Triceps	
Football kick	Extension	Knee			
Chest press – upwards phase	Extension	Elbow			
Rugby conversion kick	Flexion	Hip			

(a) Name three athletes that would have mainly type I muscle fibres in their legs.
(b) Name three athletes that would have mainly type 2A muscle fibres in their legs.

Student activity 1.4 — 60 minutes — P4 M1 D1

The function of the muscular system

Our muscular system works to pull on our skeleton to produce movement.

Task 1

Using hand-drawn illustrations, describe, explain and analyse the function of the muscular system. Include in your answer:

- antagonistic muscle pairs
- fixator
- synergist
- different types of contraction.

Task 2

Describe, explain and analyse the different fibre types that can be found in muscle tissue, and give examples of the different sports in which they may be used.

1.4 The Cardiovascular System

P5 M2

The cardiovascular system is made up of three parts:

- heart
- blood vessels
- blood.

Close your hand into a fist and look at it. Your fist is approximately the same size as your heart, around 12 cm long, 9 cm wide and 6 cm thick. It is located behind the sternum and tilted to the left. The heart is made up mainly of cardiac muscle, which is also known as myocardium. The heart is a muscular pump that pumps the liquid, which is blood, through the pipes, which are the blood vessels.

The cardiovascular system is responsible for the following actions:

- delivering oxygen and nutrients to every part of the body
- carrying hormones to different parts of the body
- removing the waste products of energy production such as carbon dioxide and lactic acid
- maintaining body temperature by re-directing blood to the surface of the skin to dissipate heat.

Structure of the Heart

The heart is a large muscular pump that is made up of thick walls. The heart muscle is called the myocardium and is divided into two halves, which are separated by the septum. The right-hand side of the heart is responsible for pumping deoxygenated blood to the lungs, and the left-hand side pumps oxygenated blood around the body. Each side of the heart consists of two connected chambers. Each side will have an atrium and a ventricle. The top chambers – the atria (plural of atrium) – are where the blood collects when it enters the heart. The lower chambers are called the ventricles, and are the large pumps which send the blood up to the lungs or around the body. Once the blood has entered the heart from the veins it will be sucked into the ventricles as they relax, and there follows powerful contraction of the ventricles. The left ventricle is the largest and most muscular because it has to send the blood to the furthest destinations and thus has to produce the most pressure.

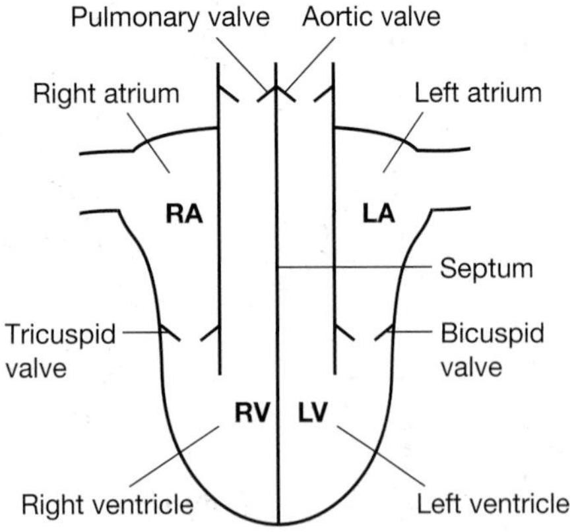

Fig 1.32 A simplified cross-section of the heart

Blood Flow through the Heart

Blood flows through the heart and around the body in one direction. This one-way 'street' is maintained due to special valves placed within the heart and within the blood vessels leading from the heart.

The heart is sometimes called a 'double pump' because the right-hand side of the heart pumps blood to the lungs and the left-hand side of the heart pumps blood to the body.

Right-hand side

1. When the heart is relaxed, deoxygenated blood from the body enters the heart via the venae cavae.
2. Blood enters the right atrium.
3. The right atrium contracts and pushes blood down through the tricuspid valve and into the right ventricle.
4. The right ventricle contracts, the tricuspid valve closes, and blood is pushed up and out of the heart through the semilunar valve and into the pulmonary artery, which takes the blood to the lungs.
5. The heart relaxes and the semilunar valves close to prevent blood flowing back into the heart.
6. The blood flows to the lungs where it becomes oxygenated and ready to be returned to the heart for distribution around the body.

Left-hand side

1. When the heart is relaxed, oxygenated blood from the lungs enters via the pulmonary vein.
2. Blood enters the left atria.
3. The left atria contracts and pushes blood down through the bicuspid valve and into the left ventricle.
4. The left ventricle contracts; the bicuspid valve closes to prevent blood flowing back into the heart. Blood is then pushed up and out of the heart through the semilunar valve and into the aorta, which is the large artery leaving the heart, taking blood to the rest of the body.
5. The heart relaxes and the semilunar valves close to prevent blood flowing back into the heart.

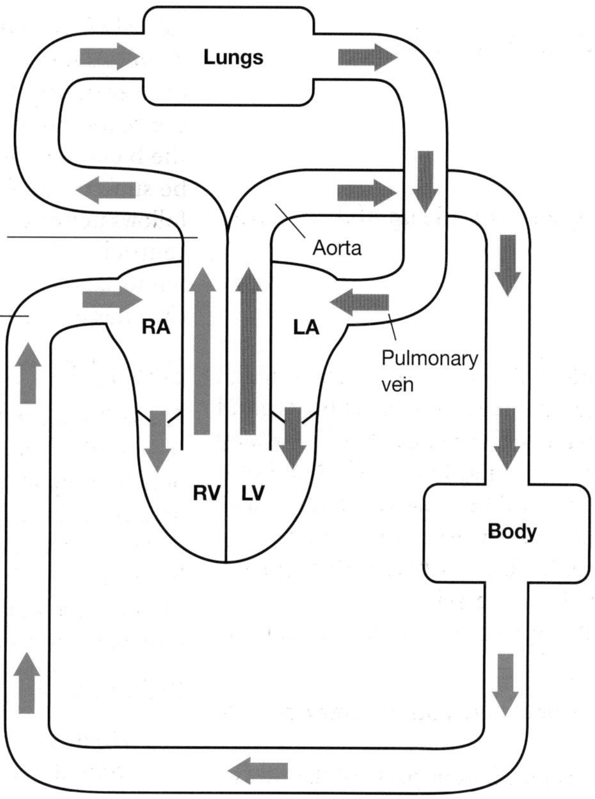

Fig 1.33 Blood flow through the heart

Blood Vessels

In order to make its journey around the body, blood is carried through five different types of blood vessels:

- arteries
- arterioles
- capillaries
- venules
- veins.

Arteries and Arterioles

Arteries are the large blood vessels that leave the heart. They have thick, muscular walls, which contract and relax to send blood to all parts of the body. The main artery leaving the heart is the aorta and it quickly splits up into smaller vessels, which are called the arterioles. Arterioles mean 'little arteries'. Artery walls contain elastic cartilage and smooth muscle. This flexible wall allows the vessels to expand and contract, which helps to push the blood along the length of the arteries. This action is called peristalsis and is how smooth muscle contracts.

Arteries do not contain any valves as they are not required and they predominantly carry oxygenated blood. The exception to this is the pulmonary artery, which carries deoxygenated blood away from the heart.

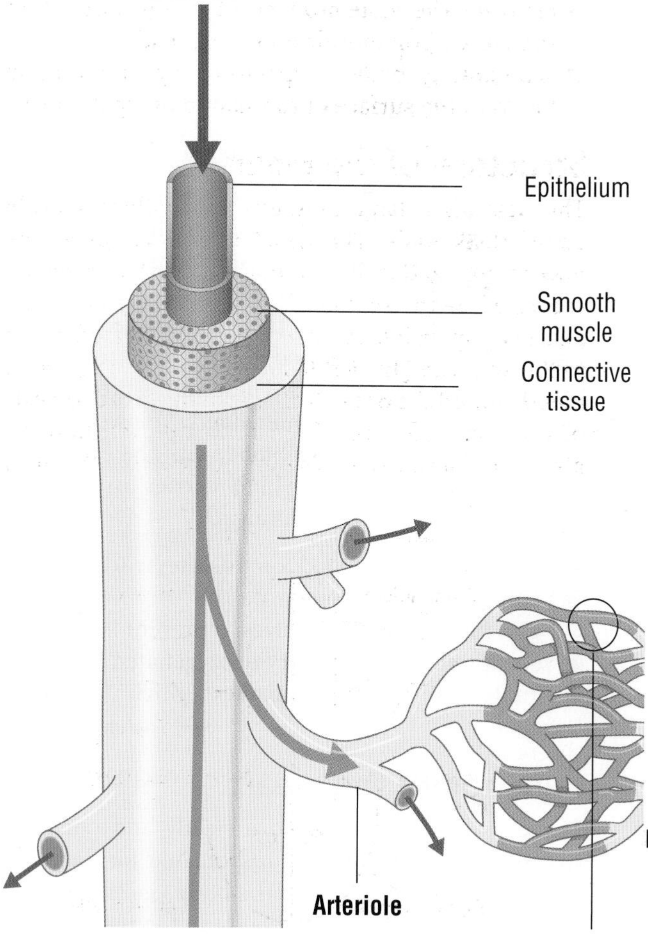

Fig 1.34 The five linked blood vessels

- Arteries carry blood away from the heart.
- Arteries have thick, muscular walls.
- Arteries carry predominantly oxygenated blood.
- Arterioles are the small branches of arteries.

Capillaries

Once the arteries and arterioles have divided, they will eventually feed blood into the smallest blood vessels, called capillaries. These are found in all parts of the body, especially the muscles, and are so tiny that their walls are only one cell thick. There are tiny spaces within these thin cell walls, which allow oxygen and other nutrients to pass through (a process called diffusion). The blood flows very slowly through the capillaries to allow for this process. In the capillaries the blood will also pick up the waste products of metabolism: carbon dioxide and lactic acid. There are more capillaries than any other type of blood vessel in the body.

- Capillaries are tiny blood vessels one cell thick.
- Small spaces in the thin walls of capillaries allow for diffusion.
- Oxygen and nutrients will diffuse into the cells.
- Carbon dioxide and lactic acid will flow from the cells into the capillaries.

Veins and Venules

The capillaries will eventually feed back into larger blood vessels called venules, which are the smallest veins, and they eventually become veins. The walls of these veins are thinner and less muscular than arteries, and they carry blood back to the heart. They also contain smooth muscle and contract to send the blood back to the heart. The veins are generally acting against gravity, so they contain non-return valves to prevent the blood flowing back once the smooth muscle has relaxed. These valves prevent the pooling of blood in the lower limbs. Veins predominantly carry deoxygenated blood, with the exception of the pulmonary vein, which carries oxygenated blood to the heart from the lungs.

- Veins always take blood towards the heart.
- Veins have thin, muscular walls.
- Veins have non-return valves to prevent backflow.
- Veins predominantly carry deoxygenated blood.
- Venules are smaller branches, which feed into veins.

Function of the Heart

The cells of the body need a steady and constant supply of oxygen. Blood is responsible for carrying and delivering oxygen to all the body's cells, and this blood is pumped around the body and to the lungs by the heart. The left-hand side of your heart pumps the oxygenated blood to the cells of the muscles, brain, kidneys, liver and all the other organs. The cells then take the oxygen out of the blood and use it to produce energy. This is called metabolism and it produces waste products, such as carbon dioxide. The deoxygenated blood then continues its journey back to the heart, enters the right-hand side and is pumped out of the right ventricle to the lungs. At the lungs, the blood becomes oxygenated and the waste product carbon dioxide is 'unloaded' and breathed out.

Blood

Blood is the medium in which all the cells are carried to transport nutrients and oxygen to the cells of the body. Among other things, blood will transport the following: oxygen, glucose, proteins, fats, vitamins, hormones, enzymes, platelets, carbon dioxide and electrolytes.

Blood is made up of four components:

- red blood cells
- white blood cells
- platelets
- plasma.

Blood can be described as a thick, gloopy substance due to the high concentration of solids it carries. Blood is made up of 55 per cent plasma and 45 per cent solids, which is a very high concentration.

Red Blood Cells

Of the blood cells in the body, around 99 per cent of them are red blood cells or erythrocytes. They are red in colour due to the presence of a red-coloured protein called haemoglobin. Haemoglobin has a massive attraction for oxygen, and thus the main role of the red blood cells is to take on and transport oxygen to the cells. There are many millions of red blood cells in the body; for example, there are 5 million red blood cells for 1 mm^3 volume of blood.

White Blood Cells

White blood cells are colourless or transparent and are far fewer in number (1:700 ratio of white to red blood cells). The role of white blood cells, or leucocytes, is to fight infection; they are part of the body's immune system. They destroy bacteria and other dangerous organisms and thus remove disease from the body.

Platelets

Platelets are not full cells but rather parts of cells; they act by stopping blood loss through clotting. They become sticky when in contact with the air to form the initial stage of repair to damaged tissue. Platelets also need a substance called factor 8 to enable them to clot. A haemophiliac is a person whose blood does not clot; this is not because they are short of platelets but rather factor 8, which enables the platelets to become active.

Plasma

Plasma is the liquid part of the blood, which is straw-coloured in appearance. It is the solution in which all the solids are carried.

Key learning points 3

- The heart has four chambers, two atria and two ventricles.
- The ventricles pump blood to the body and lungs.
- Valves in the heart make sure blood flows in one direction.
- Blood travels through five different types of blood vessesls, arteries, arterioles, capillaries, venules and veins.
- The heart adapts to aerobic training by becoming bigger and stronger.

Q Quick quiz 3

Structure of the heart

Fill in the blanks.

The heart is split into ________ sides and has ______ chambers. The top two chambers are called ________ and the bottom two chambers are called ___________. The heart is split into two separate sides by the ___________.

There are _____ valves that allow the blood to pass through the heart in one direction. The valve between the atrium and ventricle on the right side of the heart is called the ___________ valve. The valve on the left side of the heart between the atrium and the ventricle is called the _________ valve. The valve between the pulmonary artery and right ventricle is called the ___________ valve. The valve between the left ventricle and the aorta is called the __________ valve.

Student activity 1.5

60 minutes | P5 | M2

Structure and function of the cardiovascular system

Our cardiovascular system is responsible for supplying our body with blood, which contain nutrients and oxygen that provide our muscles with energy for movement.

Task 1

By hand, draw:

(a) the structure of the heart

(b) a diagram to illustrate how blood circulates through the heart, to the lungs and to the body.

Task 2

Describe and explain the structure of the cardiovascular system including:

- the heart
- the blood vessels.

Task 3

Describe and explain the function of the cardiovascular system.

1.5 The Respiratory System

P6 **M3**

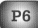

The respiratory system is responsible for transporting the oxygen from the air we breathe into our body. Our body then uses this oxygen in combination with the food we have eaten to produce energy. This energy is then used to keep us alive by supplying our heart with energy to keep beating and pumping blood around the body, which in turn allows us to move and take part in sports and many more different types of activities. Each person has two lungs running the length of the ribcage; the right lung is slightly larger than the left lung. The left lung has to make space for the heart in an area called the cardiac notch.

Structure of the Respiratory System

The aim of the respiratory system is to provide contact between the outside and internal environments so that oxygen can be absorbed by the blood and carbon dioxide can be given up. It is made up of a system of tubes and muscles, which deliver the air into two lungs. The average person takes around 26,000 breaths a day to deliver the required amount of oxygen to the cells of the body.

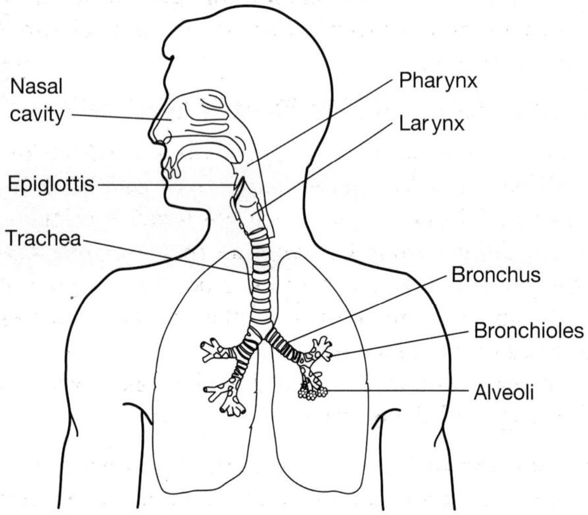

Fig 1.35 The respiratory system

Figure 1.35 shows the respiratory system in which the following processes occur.

1. Air enters the body through the mouth and nose.
2. It passes through the pharynx, which is the back of the throat area.
3. It then passes through the larynx, which is responsible for voice production.
4. Air passes over the epiglottis. The epiglottis closes over the trachea when we swallow food to stop the food going down 'the wrong way' into our trachea and down into our lungs.
5. The air enters the trachea, which is a membranous tube with horseshoe-shaped cartilage that keeps it open and delivers air to the lungs.
6. The trachea will divide into two bronchi, one into each lung.
7. The two main bronchi will divide into bronchioles, which will further subdivide 23 times and result in 8 million terminal bronchioles in each lung.
8. Around the bronchioles are groups of air sacs, called alveoli. There are around 600 million alveoli in each lung, and it is here that the exchange of gases (oxygen and carbon dioxide) occurs. Each alveolus is in contact with a capillary where the blood is present.

Respiratory Muscles

The respiratory system also includes two types of muscles that work to move air into and out of the lungs.

The diaphragm is a large dome-shaped muscle that covers the bottom of the ribcage. At rest it is dome-shaped, but when contracted it flattens and pushes the two sides of the ribcage away from each other.

The intercostal muscles attach between the ribs; when they contract they push the ribs up and out and increase the size of the chest cavity, drawing air in. If you put your hands on your ribs and breathe in, you will feel your ribs push up and out; this is the action of the intercostal muscles.

Mechanisms of Breathing

Breathing is the term given to inhaling air into the lungs and then exhaling air out. The process basically works on the principle of making the thoracic cavity (chest) larger, which decreases the pressure of air within the lungs. The surrounding air is then at a higher pressure, which means that air is forced into the lungs. Then the thoracic cavity is returned to its original size, which forces air out of the lungs.

Breathing In (Inhalation)

At rest

The diaphragm contracts and moves downwards; this results in an increase in the sise of the thoracic cavity and air is forced into the lungs.

Exercise

During exercise, the diaphragm and intercostal muscles contract, which makes the ribs move upwards and outwards, and results in more air being taken into the lungs.

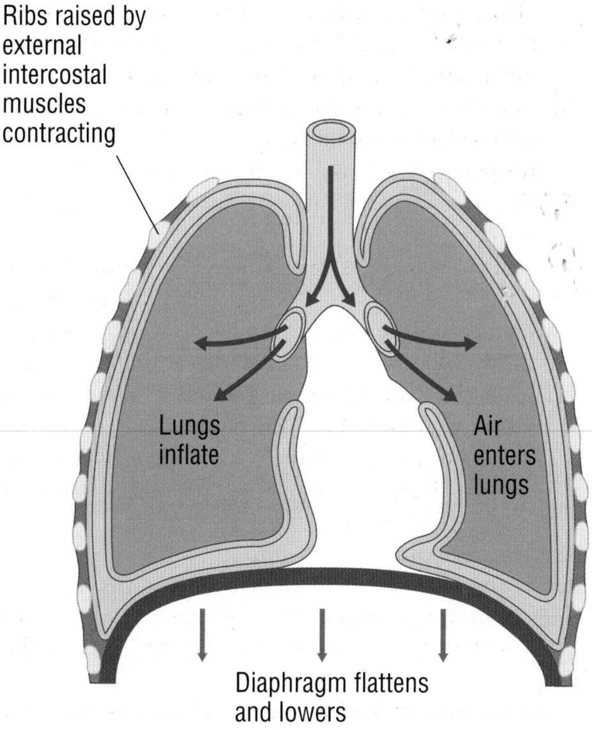

Fig 1.36 Inhalation, diaphragm and intercostal muscles

Breathing Out (Exhalation)

At rest

The diaphragm relaxes and returns upwards to a domed position. The thoracic cavity gets smaller, which results in an increase in air pressure within the lungs so that air is breathed out of the lungs.

Exercise

During exercise, the intercostal muscles contract to help decrease the size of the thoracic cavity, which results in a more forcible breath out.

Composition of Air

The air that is inspired is made up of a mixture of gasses; the air exhaled is different in its composition of gases (see Table 1.4).

Inhaled air	Gas	Exhaled air
79.04%	Nitrogen	79%
20.93%	Oxygen	17%
0.03%	Carbon dioxide	4%

Table 1.4 Composition of inhaled and exhaled air

Oxygen is extracted from the air and replaced by carbon dioxide. However, most of the oxygen stays in the air and this is why mouth-to-mouth resuscitation works, because there is still 17 per cent available to the casualty.

Functions of the Respiratory System

The aim of breathing is to get oxygen into the bloodstream where it can be delivered to the cells of the body. At the cells it enters the mitochondria where it combines with fats and carbohydrates to produce energy, with carbon dioxide and water produced as waste products. This energy is used to produce muscular contractions, among other things.

Fats/carbohydrates + oxygen = energy + carbon dioxide + water

It is important to say that when the body produces more energy, the amount of carbon dioxide increases in the body and which dissolves in the water in the body so that it becomes a weak acid. The body does not like the acidity of the blood to increase, so the respiratory centre in the brain speeds up the rate of breathing to get rid of the excess carbon dioxide. Therefore, the breathing rate increases because carbon dioxide levels rise, rather than as a result of the cells demanding more oxygen.

Diffusion of Gases

Key term

Diffusion: the movement of gas from an area of high concentration to an area of low concentration.

Gases will move around through a process of diffusion.

Diffusion is how gases move from one place to another. For example, if a person is wearing perfume, it will diffuse around a room so that everyone can smell it. This is because the person is in an area of high concentration of the perfume and the gas moves to areas of low concentration.

In the respiratory system diffusion takes place in the lungs and the muscles.

- Diffusion in the lungs – in the lungs we have a high concentration of oxygen, and in the muscles we have a high concentration of carbon dioxide, and they will diffuse across the semi-permeable membrane. Oxygen is attracted into the blood by the haemoglobin, which is a protein in the red blood cells, and it attaches to this haemoglobin.
- Diffusion in the muscles – in the muscles we have a high concentration of carbon dioxide and a low concentration of oxygen due to the process of energy production. As a result the oxygen diffuses into the muscles and is attracted by the myoglobin in the muscles and the carbon dioxide diffuses

nto the bloodstream. It is then taken to the lungs to be breathed out.

Key term

Myoglobin: oxygen binds to myoglobin to be stored in the muscles

Respiratory Volumes

In order to assess an individual's lung function, we use a spirometer. An example of the readings given by a spirometer is shown in Fig 1.37.

An individual will have a lung capacity of around 5 litres, which is about the amount of air in a basketball. It will be slightly lower for a female and slightly higher for a male, due to the differing sizes of the male and female ribcages.

Tidal volume
This is the amount of air breathed in with each breath.

Inspiratory reserve volume
This is the amount of space that is available for air to be inhaled. If you breathe in and stop, and then try to breathe in more, this extra air inhaled is the inspiratory volume.

Expiratory reserve volume
This is the amount of air that could be exhaled after you have breathed out. If you exhale and then stop, and then try to exhale more, the air that comes out is the expiratory reserve volume.

Vital capacity
This is the maximum amount of air that can be breathed in and out during one breath. It is the tidal volume, plus the inspiratory reserve volume, plus the expiratory reserve volume.

Residual volume
This is the amount of air left in the lungs after a full exhalation. Around 1 litre will always remain, or else the lungs would deflate and breathing would stop.

Total lung volume
This is the vital capacity plus the residual volume, and measures the maximum amount of air that can be present in the lungs at any moment.

Breathing rate
This is the number of breaths taken per minute.

Respiratory volume
This is the amount of air that is moving through the lungs every minute:

Respiratory volume = breathing rate × tidal volume

For example, at rest a person may have a tidal volume of 0.5 litres per minute and a breathing rate of 12 breaths per minute. But during exercise both of these will rise, and at high exercise intensities tidal volume may rise to 3 litres per minute and breathing rate to 35 breaths per minute.

At rest respiratory volume:

$$0.5 \text{ litres} \times 12 = 6 \text{ litres/minute}$$

During exercise respiratory volume:

$$3 \text{ litres} \times 35 = 105 \text{ litres/minute}$$

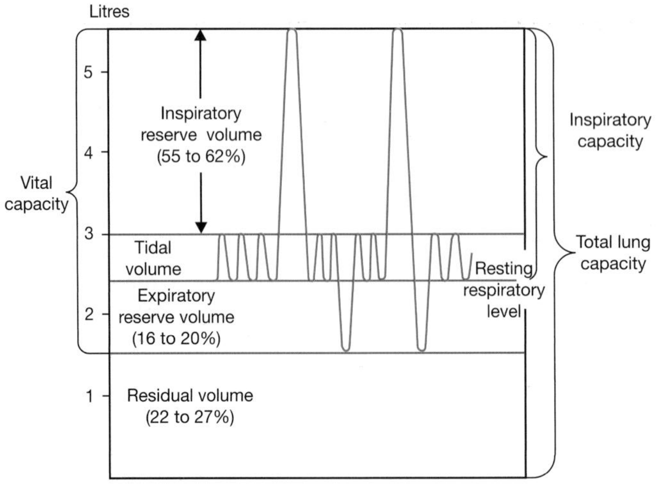

Fig 1.37 Lung volumes as shown on a spirometer trace

Key learning points 4

- Air travels into the body through the mouth and nose, down the trachea and into the bronchus. It then passes into the bronchioles and down into the alveoli. In the alveoli gaseous exchange takes place, which takes oxygen into the body and passes carbon dioxide out of the body.
- The diaphragm and intercostal muscles contract to allow you to breathe in and out.

Q Quick quiz 4

1 Describe which structures air flows through on its way from the mouth to the alveoli.

2 Explain the mechanics of breathing in and out.

3 What happens to tidal volume during exercise? Explain why this occurs.

Epiglottis	Diffusion	Trachea	Flattens	Inhalation
Carbon dioxide	Diaphragm	Oxygen	Gaseous exchange	Alveoli

4 Choose a word from the boxes above to answer the following.

(a) This gas passes out of the blood stream and into the lungs.

(b) When a person swallows, this closes over the trachea to prevent food going into the lungs.

(c) This has horseshoe-shaped cartilage to help to keep it open.

(d) The diaphragm does this during breathing in.

(e) This is the process where gases move from a high to a low concentration.

(f) This is the area in the lungs where gaseous exchange takes place.

(g) When exhaling, this muscle relaxes and moves upwards into a domed position.

(h) This is the name of the process in the lungs where oxygen is taken into the blood and carbon dioxide is breathed out.

(i) All of our body cells need this gas to survive.

(k) The name of the process for breathing in.

Student activity 1.6 — 45 minutes — P6 M3

The structure and function of the respiratory system

Task 1

By hand draw the structure of the respiratory system. Include in your diagram the following structures:

- nasal cavity
- epiglottis
- pharynx
- larynx
- trachea
- bronchus
- bronchioles
- lungs
- pleural membrane
- thoracic cavity
- visceral pleura
- pleural fluid
- alveoli
- diaphragm
- intercostals muscle – internal and external.

Task 2

Write a report that:

(a) Describes and explains the structure of each part of the respiratory system.

(b) Describes and explains the function of the respiratory system.

1.6 Energy Systems

P7 M4 D2

The body needs a steady supply of energy to enable it to perform the functions it needs to stay alive:

- muscular contractions and movement
- circulation
- transmission of nerve impulses
- digestion of foods
- repairing and replacing tissue.

ATP

The only form of energy that the body can use is called ATP, or adenosine triphosphate. In the muscles ATP will provide the energy to enable the muscle fibres to shorten and develop tension. As long as there is a supply of ATP then the muscles will be able to contract. To supply this energy the body has three different energy systems:

- creatine phosphate system
- lactic acid system
- aerobic system.

ATP is produced by breaking down the foods that we eat in our diet. The food types that contain energy in the form of kilocalories (kcals) are:

carbohydrate	1 g gives 4 kcals
fat	1 g gives 9 kcals
protein	1 g gives 4 kcals

ATP is a high-energy compound made up of one adenosine molecule attached to three phosphate molecules. These molecules are bound together by high-energy bonds.

The adenosine and phosphate molecules do not contain any energy; the energy is stored in the high-energy bonds and therefore to liberate energy we need to break down the bonds attaching the molecules. To break one of the bonds we need an enzyme called ATPase. When ATP has been broken down we are left with a second compound called adenosine di phosphate (ADP). A loose phosphate will also be created by the reaction.

Unfortunately, we have very limited stores of ATP in the muscles and ADP cannot be broken down any further. To allow further production of energy we need to remake or resynthesise ATP. We have the ingredients in ADP and the spare phosphate, and what is needed is energy to reattach the phosphate to the ADP. It is the three-energy system that provides the energy for this reaction to happen.

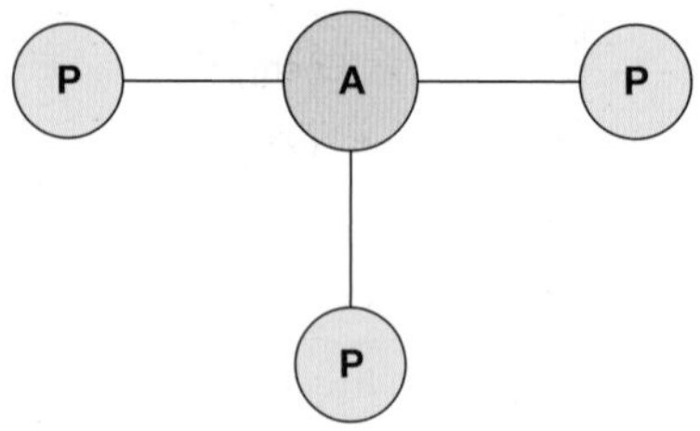

Fig 1.38 ATP

Creatine Phosphate System

If energy is needed for an activity of high intensity and low duration, such as 100-m sprinting, or jumping in basketball, it will be needed very rapidly to produce a muscular contraction. The cells contain a small amount of ATP (about 3 seconds' worth) and a small amount of a second high-energy compound called creatine phosphate (CP). There is enough CP to provide a further 5 to 7 seconds' worth of energy. The CP will be broken down to provide the energy to resynthesise the ATP.

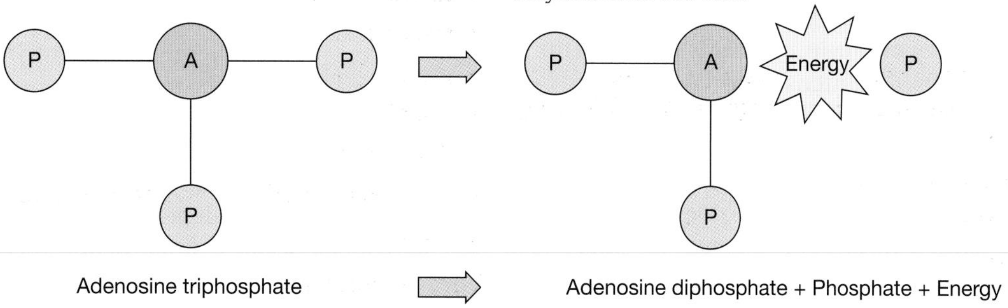

Fig 1.39 Breakdown of ATP to ADP

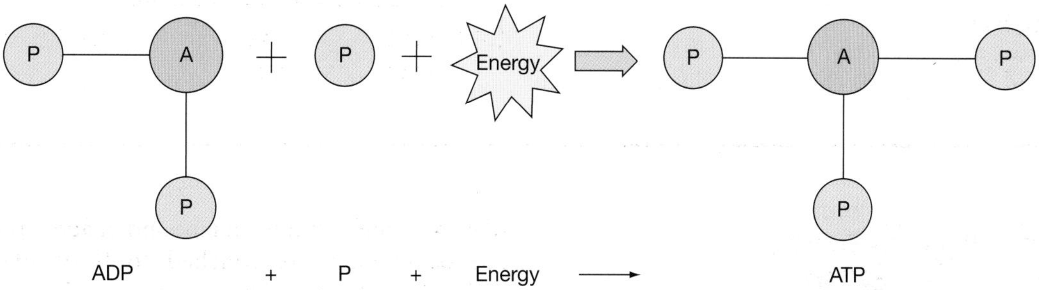

Fig 1.40 Resynthesis of ATP

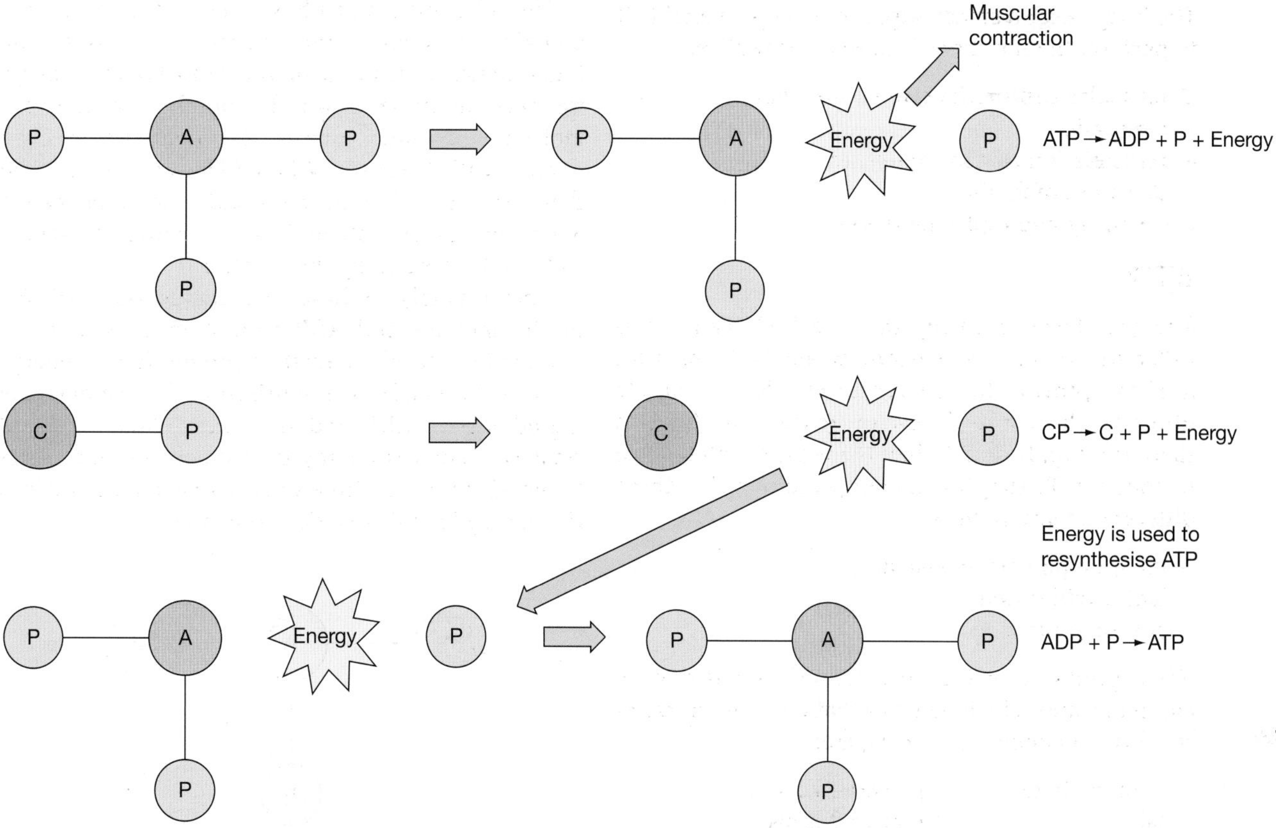

Fig 1.41 Creatine phosphate resynthesises ATP

This system will last until the stored CP has run out. Along with breaking down the stores of ATP in the muscles this system will last for around 8 to 10 seconds and is used for high-intensity activities.

Lactic Acid System

When stores of ATP and PC have run out, the body has a second way of providing energy quickly. This is used when activity is intense and lasts around 1 to 3 minutes. This system relies upon the breakdown of glucose that has been stored in the muscles (this is called glycogen). Energy for muscular contraction is still needed rapidly and the body does not have time to deliver oxygen to the working muscles; therefore, the glucose has to be broken down without oxygen. This is called anaerobic (absence of oxygen) and is referred to as anaerobic glycolysis.

As glucose is broken down in the muscles to provide the energy to resynthesise ATP, a by-product, lactic acid, is produced. This lactic acid can produce a burning, uncomfortable feeling in the muscles and limit performance. In reality the glucose is first broken down into pyruvic acid and then into lactic acid. This process will produce three ATP per glucose molecule.

Glucose → Pyruvic acid = no oxygen → Energy = Lactic acid

Aerobic System

This system differs from the other two because it requires oxygen to break down glucose or fat and produce energy for the resynthesis of ATP. It will be used when the intensity of an activity is lower and the duration longer. It tends to be used during rhythmical, repetitive activities such as long-distance running, cycling and swimming.

The aerobic system will produce carbon dioxide, water and heat as waste products of the aerobic breakdown of glucose and fats. Carbon dioxide is breathed out with some of the water, which can also be lost as sweat when the heat is dissipated from the body.

The aerobic system can produce energy by breaking down glucose (from carbohydrates) or fat. Fat is a much richer store of energy for ATP resynthesis, but can be used only in low-intensity exercise because it is a lengthy process. At the higher intensities fuel is needed more quickly and glucose will be used to provide this energy.

The fuel used also depends upon the fitness of the individual because fitter people become more effective at burning fats. The result of this is that their glycogen stores will go further and last longer. For example, Paula Radcliffe can run a marathon without any discernible loss of performance towards the end of the race.

The aerobic system provides the most plentiful supply of oxygen in that if one molecule of glycogen is broken down aerobically it will provide 38 ATP; while one molecule of fat will provide 128 ATP.

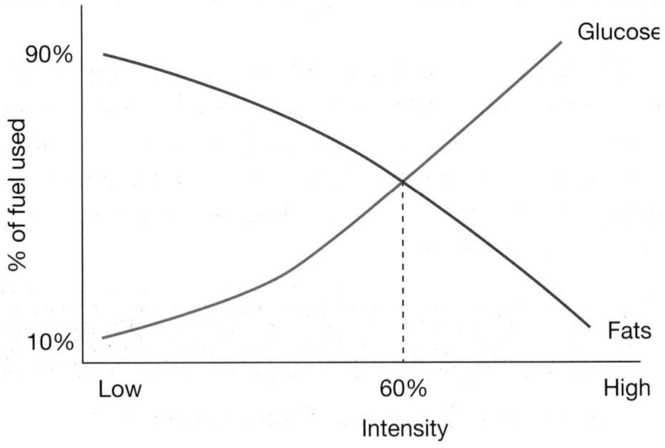

Fig 1.42 Fuel used for the aerobic system depends upon the intensity of the activity

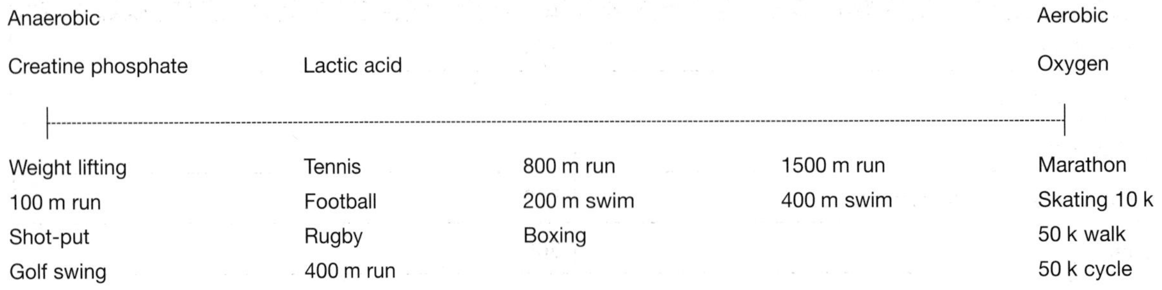

Fig 1.43 Energy continuum

Criteria	Creatine phosphate	Lactic acid	Aerobic
Speed of energy production	Very fast	Fast	Slow
Energy source	Creatine phosphate	Glycogen	Glycogen and fat
Amount of ATP produced	Very limited	Limited	Unlimited
Production of waste products	None	Lactic acid is produced as a by-product	Carbon dioxide and water which are eliminated
Duration of energy production	8–10 seconds	1–3 minutes	Up to 2 hours
Intensity used as % of maximum intensity	High intensity (95–100%)	Moderate to high intensity (60–95%)	Low intensity (<60%)
Length of time to recover	30 seconds to 4 minutes	20 minutes to 2 hours	Time to rest and replace glycogen stores

Table 1.5 Summary of energy systems

Application to Sport

Different sports will utilise different energy systems depending upon the demands of the sport and the speed at which energy is required (see Table 1.5 and Fig 1.43).

The sports of football and tennis may appear to use the aerobic system because they last for a long time; however, they predominantly use the anaerobic system due to the fact that they involve bursts of energy followed by periods of recovery, rather than consistent movement.

Key learning points 5

- ATP is used by muscles to produce movement.
- ATP is produced through three energy systems – creatine phosphate, lactic acid and the aerobic energy system.
- The creatine phosphate and lacitc acid energy systems do not use oxygen and are classes as anearobic energy systems.

Q Quick quiz 5

Energy requirements of physical activity

In order to take part in sports, our bodies use the food we have eaten to go through the energy systems to produce energy. Different sports have different energy requirements:

Type of exercise	Kilocalories used per hour
Aerobics	450
Aqua aerobics	400
Bicycling	450
Cross-country ski machine	500
Hiking	500
Jogging, 5 mph	500
Rowing	550
Running	700
Skipping with rope	700

Type of exercise	Kilocalories used per hour
Spinning	650
Step aerobics	550
Squash	650
Swimming	500
Table tennis	290
Tennis	350
Walking, 3 mph	280

1 Look at the list of energy requirements for different sports in the table above. Note the four that require the most kcalories, and try to explain why you think they require the most energy.
2 Which activities would use the CP energy system?
3 Which activites would use the lactic acid energy system?
4 Which activities would use the aerobic energy system?

Student activity 1.7 — 60 minutes — P7 M4 D2

Energy Systems and sport and exercise

Task 1

Select different sport or exercise activities that uses the:

(a) the creatine phosphate energy sytem
(b) lactic acid energy sytem
(c) aerobic energy systems.

Task 2

Describe, explain and analyse the three different energy systems and how they are used in your selected sport and exercise activities.

Further reading

Kapit, W. and Elson, L. (2001) *The Anatomy Coloring Book*, Benjamin Cummings.

Wesson, K., Wiggins-James, N., Thompson, G. and Hartigan, S. (2005) *Sport and PE: A Complete Guide to Advanced Level Study*, Hodder Arnold.

Useful websites

www.bhf.org.uk/research_health_professionals/resources.aspx
Guidance, statistics and information about research publications from the British Heart Foundation.

www.bhf.org.uk/keeping_your_heart_healthy/Default.aspx
Information for the general public on how to keep your heart healthy.

www.getbodysmart.com
An online examination of human anatomy and physiology that will help you to see the structure of the different body systems.

www.innerbody.com
Good information and diagrams of the different body systems.

www.instantanatomy.net
Useful anatomy pictures and information.

www.medtropolis.com/VBody.asp
A very good interactive website for anatomy with quizzes and tutorials.

2: The Physiology of Fitness

2.1 Introduction

Our body allows us to take part in a huge variety of sports and exercises. In order for us to carry out these activities, the body has to undergo a series of changes that provide us with the ability and the energy to carry out these actions.

This unit starts by exploring the responses of the cardiovascular, respiratory and energy systems to the anticipation and initial stress of exercise. There then follows a study of the response of the body after a period of around 20 minutes' exercise, when a steady state has been achieved. The mechanisms of fatigue are then explored, followed by the methods by which we recover from sports and exercise. A look at the ways in which the body adapts to repeated bouts of aerobic and anaerobic exercise completes the unit.

By the end of this unit you should:

- be able to investigate the initial responses of the body to exercise
- be able to investigate how the body responds to steady-state exercise
- know about fatigue and how the body recovers from exercise
- know how the body adapts to long-term exercise.

Assessment and grading criteria		
To achieve a PASS grade the evidence must show that the learner is able to:	**To achieve a MERIT grade the evidence must show that, in addition to the pass criteria, the learner is able to:**	**To achieve a DISTINCTION grade the evidence must show that, in addition to the pass and merit criteria, the learner is able to:**
P1 investigate the initial responses of the cardiovascular and respiratory systems to exercise	**M1** explain the initial responses of the cardiovascular, respiratory, neuromuscular and energy systems to exercise	**D1** analyse the initial responses of the cardiovascular, respiratory, neuromuscular and energy systems to exercise
P2 describe the initial responses of the neuromuscular and energy systems to exercise		
P3 investigate how the cardiovascular and respiratory systems respond to steady-state exercise	**M2** explain how the cardiovascular, respiratory, neuromuscular and energy systems respond to steady-state exercise	**D2** analyse the responses of the cardiovascular, respiratory, neuromuscular and energy systems to steady-state exercise
P4 describe how the neuromuscular and energy systems respond to steady-state exercise		
P5 describe fatigue and how the body recovers from exercise	**M3** explain fatigue, and how the body recovers from exercise	
P6 describe how the cardiovascular and respiratory systems adapt to long-term exercise	**M4** explain how the cardiovascular, respiratory, neuromuscular, energy and skeletal systems adapt to long-term exercise.	**D3** analyse how the cardiovascular, respiratory, neuromuscular, energy and skeletal systems adapt to long-term exercise.
P7 describe how the neuromuscular, energy and skeletal systems adapt to long-term exercise.		

2.2 The Initial Responses of the Body to Exercise

P1 P2 M1 D1

Exercise

There are two main classifications of the types of exercise that we take part in: aerobic and anaerobic.

- Aerobic exercises use oxygen in the process of supplying energy to the body. These types of exercises are low-intensity and will usually allow us to talk while taking part in them – for example, walking, jogging, cycling and swimming.
- Anaerobic exercises do not use oxygen in the process of supplying energy to the body. These types of exercises are of a high intensity, so we do not have 'the breath' to talk while participating – for example, sprinting, high jump, speed swimming and 400-m running.

The Cardiovascular System's Initial Response to Exercise

The cardiovascular system consists of the heart and the blood vessels through which the heart pumps blood around the body. During exercise, a number of changes take place to the cardiovascular system to ensure that the muscles receive the required amounts of oxygen and nutrients. The structure of the cardiovascular system is discussed in more detail in Unit 1: Principles of Anatomy & Physiology in Sport.

During exercise, the heart rate needs to be increased in order to ensure that the working muscles receive adequate amounts of nutrients and oxygen, and that waste products are removed. Before you even start exercising there is an increase in your heart rate, called the 'anticipatory rise', which occurs because when you think about exercising it stimulates the sympathetic nervous system to release adrenaline.

> **Key term**
>
> **Adrenaline (also known as epinephrine):** a hormone released during times of stress which gets the body ready for action, increasing blood pressure, heart rate, and so on.

One of the effects of adrenaline is to make the heart beat faster. Once exercise has started, there is an increase in carbon dioxide and lactic acid in the body, which is detected by chemoreceptors.

The chemoreceptors trigger the sympathetic nervous system to increase the release of adrenaline, which further increases heart rate. In a trained athlete, the heart rate can increase by up to three times within one minute of starting exercise. As exercise continues, the body becomes warmer, which

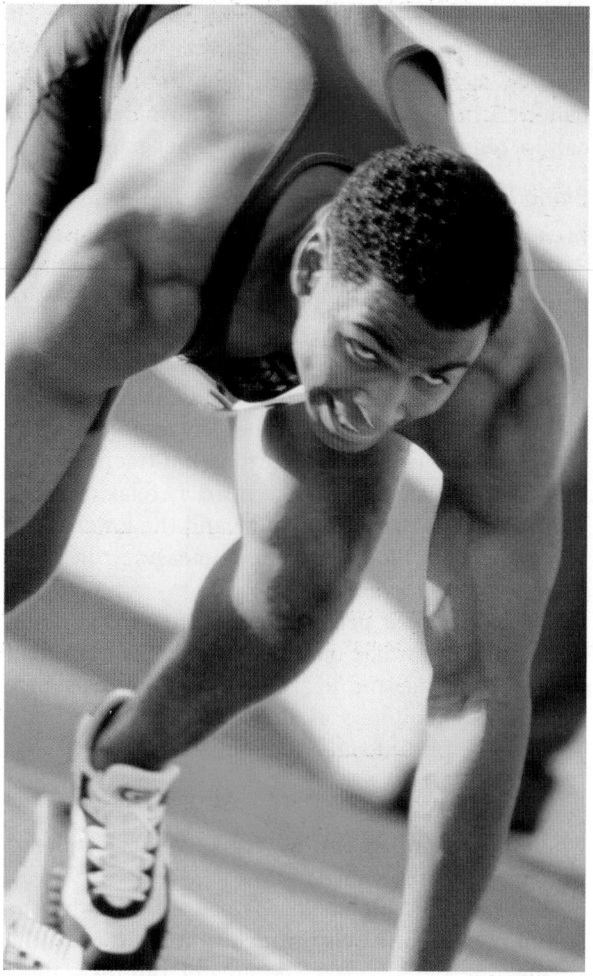

Fig 2.1 A runner at the outset of exercise

> **Key term**
>
> **Chemoreceptor:** a group of cells that detect changes in the chemical environment around them and transmit this message to the brain so that the body can respond accordingly.

will also help to increase the heart rate because it increases the speed of the conduction of nerve impulses across the heart.

Cardiac Output

Cardiac output is the amount of blood pumped from the heart every minute and is the product of heart rate and stroke volume.

Cardiac output (litres per minute) = heart rate (bpm) × Stroke volume (litres)

The shorthand for this equation is:

$$Q = HR \times SV$$

The stroke volume is around 70 to 90 millilitres. It varies depending on a variety of factors. Generally, the fitter you are, the larger your stroke volume is and males tend to have larger stroke volumes than females. At rest, a person's cardiac output is approximately 5 litres per minute, while during exercise it can increase to as much as 30 litres per minute.

Blood Pressure

Blood pressure is necessary in order for blood to flow around the body. The pressure is a result of the heart contracting and forcing blood into the blood vessels. Two values are given when a person has their blood pressure taken.

A typical blood pressure for the average adult male is 120/80. The two values correspond to the systolic value (when the heart is contracting) and the diastolic value (when the heart is relaxing). The higher value is the systolic value and the lower is the diastolic value. Blood pressure is measured in milligrams of mercury: mmHg.

The value for a person's blood pressure is determined by the cardiac output (Q), which is a product of stroke volume and heart rate, and the resistance the blood encounters as it flows around the body. This can be put into an equation:

$$\text{Blood pressure} = Q \times R$$

where Q = cardiac output (stroke volume × heart rate) and R = resistance to flow.

Resistance to blood flow is caused both by the size of the blood vessels through which it travels (the smaller the blood vessel, the greater the resistance) and by the thickness of the blood (the thicker the blood, the greater the resistance).

Changing the resistance to blood flow can alter blood pressure. This is done by involuntary smooth muscles in the arterioles relaxing or contracting in order to alter the diameter of the arterioles. As the smooth muscle contracts, the diameter of the blood vessel gets smaller, so blood pressure is increased. As the smooth muscle relaxes, the diameter of the blood vessel is increased, which decreases the pressure of the blood flowing through it. The same principle can be applied to altering the diameter of water flow through a hose. If you place your finger over part of the opening of the hose, making the diameter smaller, the water will flow out quite forcibly because it is under higher pressure. However, if the water is left to flow unhindered through the end of the hose, it is under lower pressure, and will therefore not 'spurt' so far because there is less resistance.

A reduction in blood pressure is detected by baroreceptors in the aorta and the carotid artery.

> **Key term**
>
> **Baroreceptor:** a collection of cells that detect a change in blood pressure. They send signals to the brain so that the body can respond appropriately.

This detection is passed to the central nervous system (CNS), which then sends a nervous impulse to the arterioles to constrict. This increases the blood pressure and also has the effect of increasing the heart rate.

When blood pressure is increased, the baroreceptors detect this and signal the CNS, which makes the arterioles dilate and reduces blood pressure.

Changes to Blood Pressure During the Onset of Exercise

Exercise has the effect of increasing heart rate, which will result in an increased cardiac output, which will have the effect of increasing blood pressure. This can be seen from the equation:

$$BP = Q \times R$$

If cardiac output is increased and the resistance to blood flow does not change, then blood pressure will also automatically increase.

A typical blood pressure reading for a person at the onset of exercise would be around 120/80 mmHg.

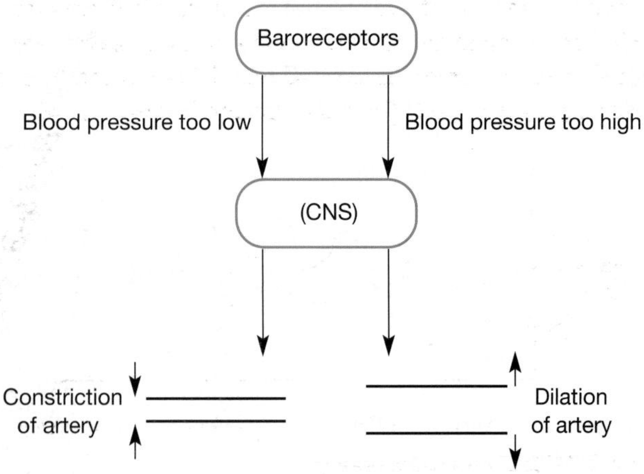

Fig 2.2 How baroreceptors initiate response to high blood pressure and low blood pressure

The Respiratory System's Initial Response to Exercise

The respiratory system is responsible for getting oxygen into the body and getting carbon dioxide out of the body. It is described in detail in Unit 1: Anatomy for Sport and Exercise. The oxygen is used to help produce energy while we take part in sporting activities. The process of creating energy also produces a waste product called carbon dioxide, which needs to be removed from the body.

Pulmonary Ventilation and Breathing Rate

The amount of air we breathe in and out per minute is called pulmonary ventilation and is given the symbol V_E.

Pulmonary ventilation can be worked out using the following equation:

$$V_E = \text{Frequency} \times \text{Tidal volume}$$

Frequency is the number of breaths per minute.

Tidal volume is the volume of air breathed in and out during one breath. At rest, the average breathing rate is around 12 breaths per minute. The average tidal volume is 0.5 litres (this will vary depending on the age, gender and size of a person).

Therefore, the average pulmonary ventilation at rest is:

$$V_E = 12 \times 0.5$$

$$V_E = 6 \text{ litres}$$

When you start to exercise, you need to take more oxygen into your body for it to be used to help produce energy. At the start of exercise, this increased oxygen demand occurs by breathing at a faster rate and breathing in more air and breathing out more air during each breath (i.e. tidal volume increases).

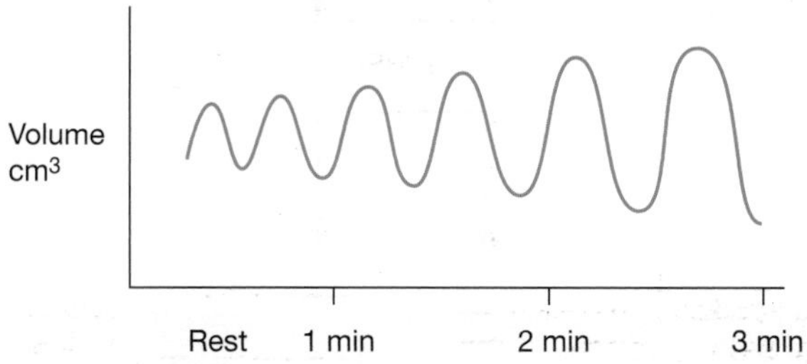

Fig 2.3 Tidal volume increasing

The intercostal muscles are used to aid breathing during exercise.

> **Key term**
>
> **Intercostal muscles:** located between the ribs, there are two types of intercostal muscle – internal and external. They help with inspiration and expiration during exercise.

The external intercostal muscles help with inspiration and the internal intercostal muscles help with expiration. As exercise becomes more strenuous, the abdominal muscles will also help aid expiration.

During anaerobic exercises, such as weightlifting, it is not uncommon for people to perform a Valsalva manoeuvre. This is basically the process of breathing out against a closed glottis or against a closed mouth and nose.

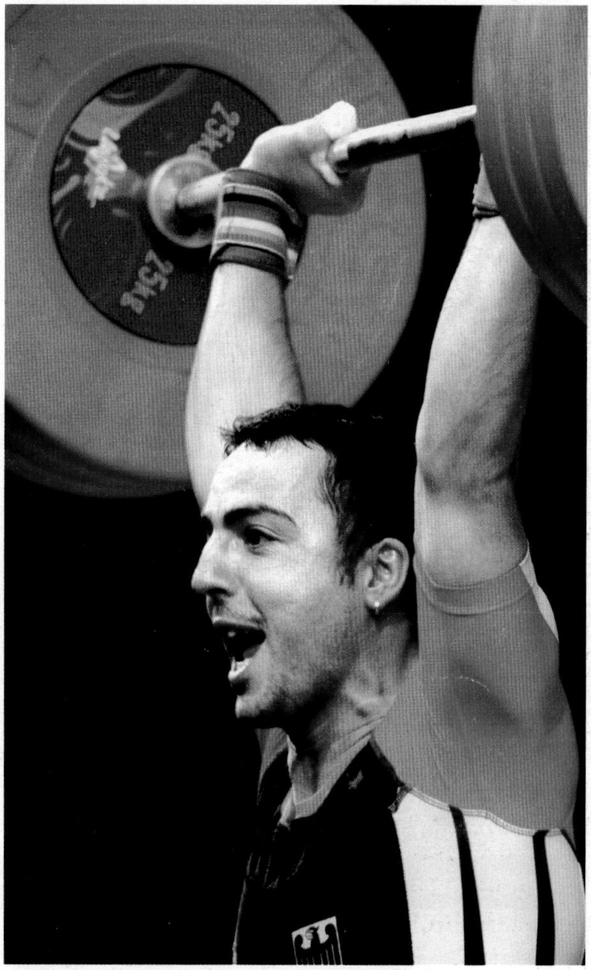

Fig 2.4 Weight lifting uses the Valsalva manoeuvre

The process of performing the Valsalva manoeuvre while lifting heavy weights helps to stabilise the shoulder girdle and torso. This helps the lifter to move the weight more efficiently. This process produces a marked increase in blood pressure and reduces blood flow to the thoracic cavity. Therefore, any person suffering with high blood pressure or heart problems should avoid this move.

Key term

Thoracic cavity: the part of the body that is enclosed by the ribcage and the diaphragm, containing the heart and the lungs.

Student activity 2.1

90–120 mins P1 M1 D1

In order to find out what happens to the cardio-vascular and respiratory systems during the initial stages of exercise, it is necessary to observe someone or take part in exercise and monitor the response of these systems.

Task 1

The aim of this activity is to examine what happens to heart rate before and during the onset of exercise. You will need the following equipment:

- Stopwatch or heart rate monitor
- Skipping rope
- Sports clothes
- Bench
- Pen and paper.

Follow the method set out below and record your results in the table; then answer the questions that follow.

- If you have a heart-rate monitor, place it around your chest. If not, find your pulse point, either on your neck or at your wrist.
- Sit quietly for five minutes, then take your resting heart rate. If you have a heart-rate monitor, write down the heart rate that appears on the monitor. If not, feel for your pulse point, then count your heart rate for 30 seconds. Double this figure and write it down.
- Think about what exercise you are about to perform for one minute.
- Record your heart rate after having thought about your exercise.
- Perform step-ups on to a bench for two minutes or skip for two minutes with a skipping rope.
- Immediately after you have finished your exercise, record your heart rate.

1. What happened to your heart rate immediately before you started exercising?
2. What caused this change in your heart rate and why is it necessary?
3. Explain and analyse why there is a difference between your resting heart rate, your pre-exercise heart rate and your post-exercise heart rate.

Task 2

- While sitting or lying down, count the number of breaths you breathe in during one minute – try to breathe as normally as possible. Write this number down and then work out your pulmonary ventilation using the equation: **VE = Frequency × Tidal volume**.
- Now take part in some form of exercise, such as skipping or step-ups, for three minutes.
- Immediately after completing your exercise, count the number of breaths you breathe in during one minute, then record your pulmonary ventilation.
- Explain and analyse why there is a difference between your resting pulmonary ventilation rate and your post-exercise pulmonary ventilation rate.

Resting heart rate (bpm)	Pre-exercise heart rate (bpm)	Post-exercise heart rate (bpm)

Initial Response of the Neuromuscular System

When we want to produce muscle movement, we have to get the message from our brain to our muscles. This communication between the brain and muscle is achieved through nerve impulses. A nerve impulse is an electrical current that runs from the central nervous system (CNS) through nerves and then to the muscle tissue, and results in muscle contraction. The term used to describe the signal travelling from the CNS to the muscle is called an action potential. Nerves that signal muscles to contract are called motor neurones.

> **Key terms**
>
> **Central nervous system:** consists of the brain and the spinal cord.
>
> **Motor** neurone: a nerve that signals a muscle to contract.

The neuromuscular junction is the place at which the nerve and muscle meet. The nerve transmits its signal to make the muscle contract in the following manner:

- The pre-synaptic membrane reacts to the signal by its vesicles releasing acetylcholine.
- Acetylcholine diffuses across the gap between the nerve and the muscle (the synaptic cleft) and produces an electrical signal called the excitatory post-synaptic action potential.
- If the excitatory post-synaptic potential is big enough, it will make the muscle tissue contract.
- Once the muscle has carried out its desired movement, the enzyme cholinesterase breaks down the acetylcholine to leave the muscle ready to receive its next signal.

Motor Units

> **Key term**
>
> **Motor unit:** group of muscle fibres stimulated by one nerve.

As there are so many muscle fibres, a nerve stimulates more than just one fibre. In fact, it has a group of between 15 and 2000 muscle fibres, depending on the muscle it is connected to. This group of muscle fibres is called a motor unit.

When we want to produce muscle movements, we send signals from our CNS to the motor neurones. The strength of the signal determines whether the signal will reach the motor unit. This is called the all-or-nothing principle, which means that if the strength of the nerve signal is large enough, all of the motor unit will contract. And if the strength of the signal is not big enough, no part of the motor unit will contract. When we exercise, especially when we want to exert high levels of force, our motor units produce muscle contraction at different rates. Therefore, you will find that different parts of the muscle are contracting at slightly different times. This has the effect of producing smooth muscle contractions.

Muscle Spindles

A muscle spindle is an organ placed within the muscle which communicates with the CNS. The purpose of the muscle spindle is to detect when the muscle is in a state of contraction. When a muscle is contracted it changes the tension on the muscle spindle. This is relayed to the CNS and the CNS can deal with this information accordingly, by either increasing the contraction of the muscle or relaxing the muscle.

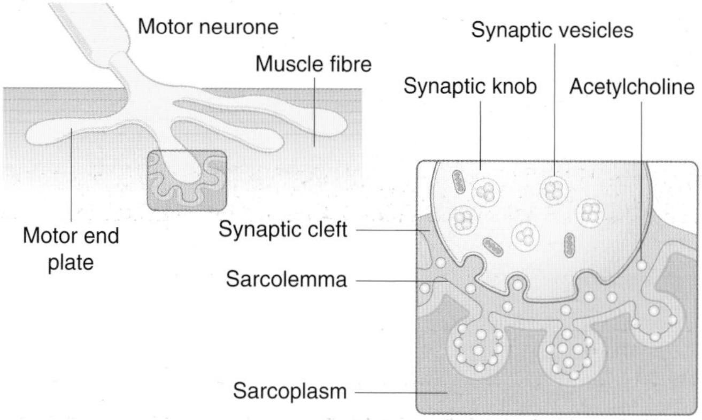

Fig 2.5 The neural transmission process

Initial Response of the Energy Systems

The function of energy systems is to produce adenosine triphosphate (ATP). ATP is used to make our muscles contract and therefore allows us to take part in exercise. It is basically a protein (adenosine) with three (tri) phosphates (phosphate) attached to it.

When chemical bonds are broken, energy is released. Therefore, when a phosphate is broken off the ATP to make ADP (adenosine diphosphate – di = two) energy is released, which is used to make the muscles contract.

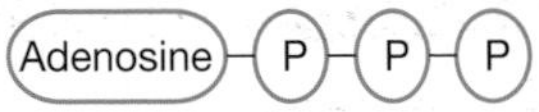

Fig 2.6 Adenosine triphosphate (ATP)

ATP is not stored in large amounts in skeletal muscle and therefore has to be continually made from ADP for our muscles to continue contracting. There are three energy systems that the body uses to make ATP. They differ in the rate at which they make ATP. At the onset of exercise we will want ATP supplied very quickly. However, if we are on a long walk we do not need such a fast production of ATP, so the body uses a different energy system to make it.

Phosphocreatine Energy System

At the onset of exercise, the energy system that supplies the majority of ATP is the phosphocreatine system (also known as the creatine phosphate system). It supplies ATP much quicker than any other energy system. It produces ATP in the absence of oxygen, and is therefore an anaerobic energy system.

Phosphocreatine (PC) is made up of a phosphate and a creatine molecule. When the bond between the phosphate and the creatine is broken, energy is released which is then used to make the bond between ADP and a phosphate.

PC stores are used for rapid, high-intensity contractions, such as in sprinting or jumping. These stores only last for about ten seconds.

Lactic Acid Energy System

Once our PC stores have run out, we use the lactic acid system. This is also known as anaerobic glycolysis, which literally means the breakdown of glucose in the absence of oxygen. When glucose is broken down it is converted into a substance called pyruvate. When there is no oxygen present, the pyruvate is converted into lactic acid. This system produces ATP very quickly, but not as quickly as the PC system:

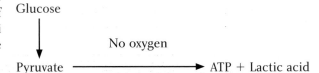

Glucose
↓
Pyruvate —— No oxygen ——→ ATP + Lactic acid

The lactic acid energy system is the one that is producing the majority of the ATP during high-intensity exercise lasting between 30 seconds and three minutes, such as an 800 m race.

> **Key learning points 1**
>
> - At the onset of exercise, the various systems respond to try to increase oxygen delivery, energy production and carbon dioxide removal.
> - Cardiovascular system: increased heart rate, increased blood pressure, increased cardiac output.
> - Respiratory system: increased pulmonary ventilation, increased breathing rate, increased tidal volume.
> - Neuromuscular system: increased number of nerve transmissions, skeletal muscular contraction.
> - Energy system: ATP production through phosphocreatine energy system and lactic acid energy system.

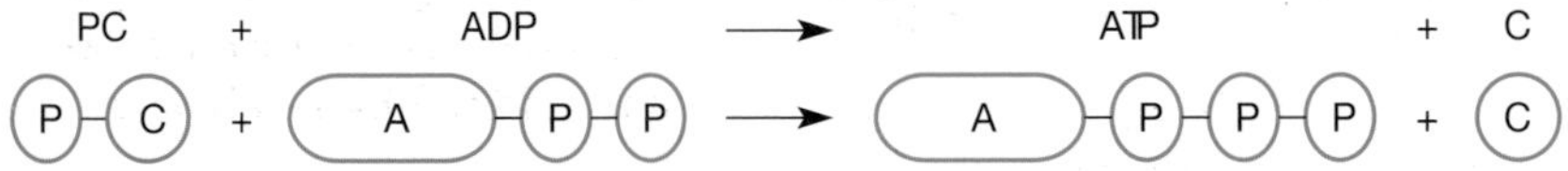

Fig 2.7 Phosphocreatine energy system

Student activity 2.2

60–90 mins

P2 M1 D1

Task 1

Draw a spider diagram that illustrates the initial responses of the neuromuscular system and energy systems to exercise.

Task 2

Write a report that describes, explains and analyses the initial responses of the neuromuscular system to exercise.

Task 3

Write a report that describes, explains and analyses the initial responses of the energy systems to exercise.

Quick quiz 1

Choose the appropriate term from the following list to answer the questions below:

- Adrenaline
- Synovial fluid
- Pulmonary ventilation
- 12
- Electric current
- Micro-tears
- 120/80
- Valsalva manoeuvre
- Tidal volume
- Skeletal muscle.

1. This is the average number of breaths in and out for a person at rest.
2. This hormone is released before exercise to increase the heart rate.
3. A nerve impulse is an ________?
4. This is the technical term for breaths per minute.
5. This is released into the joints during a warm-up to help increase their range of movement.
6. This is an adult's average resting blood pressure.
7. The amount of air breathed in and out in one breath.
8. This is performed to help to stabilise the shoulder girdle and torso.
9. These occur in muscle tissue during resistance exercises.
10. Blood is directed here during exercise.

2.3 How the Body Responds to Steady-State Exercise

P3 P4 M2 D2

Once we have been performing continuous exercise for a period of around 20 minutes, our body reaches a 'steady state'. Continuous exercise includes all forms of exercise that have no stopping periods, such as jogging, swimming or cycling. Examples of non-continuous exercise would be weightlifting, interval training and boxing.

Key term

Steady state: when the body is working at a steady state it means that lactic acid removal is occurring at the same pace as lactic acid production.

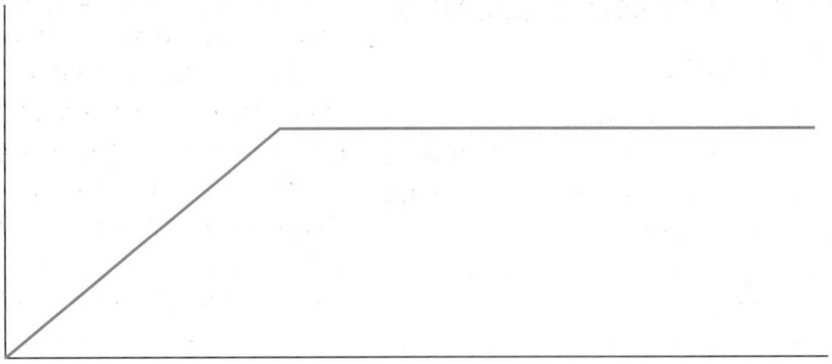

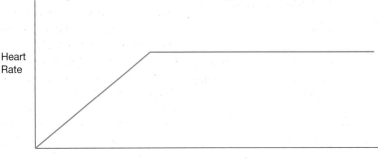

Fig 2.8 Heart rate response during continuous exercise

Various changes will have occurred in the body to allow this steady state to occur.

Cardiovascular:

- Heart rate levels off
- Increased stroke volume
- Vasodilation of blood vessels leading to working muscles
- Blood pressure levels off
- Thermoregulation.

Respiratory:

- Tidal volume levels off
- Breathing rate levels off
- Oxygen is unloaded from haemoglobin much more readily.

Neuromuscular:

- Increased pliability of muscles
- Increased speed of neural transmissions.

Energy:

- Aerobic ATP production.

Cardiovascular Response to Steady-state Exercise

Heart rate peaks during the first few minutes of exercise and then levels off.

Stroke Volume

While exercising, there is an increase in venous return.

> **Key term**
>
> **Venous return:** the amount of blood returned to the heart after circulating around the body.

This increased volume of blood has the effect of stretching the cardiac muscle to a greater degree than normal. This stretching has the effect of making the heart contract much more forcibly and thereby pumping out more blood during each contraction, so stroke volume is increased during exercise. This effect is known as Starling's law.

Blood Flow

The average cardiac output is around 5 litres per minute. When this blood is circulated around the body, some organs receive more blood than others. However, during exercise, the working muscles need a greater proportion of blood in order to supply them with energy. The body is able to redirect blood flow by constricting the blood vessels leading to organs that do not require such a large blood flow, and dilating the blood vessels feeding the muscles that do. The process of blood vessels constricting is called vasoconstriction and the process of blood vessels dilating is called vasodilation.

> **Key term**
>
> **Constriction:** becoming smaller.

> **Key term**
>
> **Dilation:** becoming larger.

Changes to Blood Pressure During Steady-state Exercise

Dilation of the blood vessels feeding the working muscle acts to reduce blood pressure, but this is counteracted by the increase in blood pressure caused by increased cardiac output.

Exercise raises systolic pressure, but there is only a slight change in diastolic pressure.

Immediately after exercise there is a fall in systolic pressure, as the skeletal muscular pump is no longer pumping blood from the muscles to the heart. This can lead to blood pooling in the muscles and cause the athlete to faint, as not enough blood is being pumped to the brain.

Thermoregulation

Thermoregulation is the process of maintaining a constant body core temperature. In humans this temperature is 37 °C. The skin temperature of the body can vary a great deal. If the core temperature is increased or decreased by 1 °C or more, this will affect an athlete's physical and mental performance. When exercising, we produce a great deal of excess heat. The cardiovascular system is vitally important in ensuring that we are able to lose this excess heat so that our core temperature does not increase. Excess heat is lost through sweating and dilatation of peripheral blood vessels, so that blood passes close to the surface of the skin. As the sweat evaporates, it cools down the skin surface. This has the effect of cooling the blood as it travels through the blood vessels that are close to the skin surface. When we are exercising at a high intensity in hot conditions, between 15 and 25 per cent of the cardiac output is directed to the skin.

Respiratory Responses

After having peaked in the first few minutes, if exercise remains at the same intensity, tidal volume and breathing rate level off and remain the same until exercise is terminated.

Oxygen Dissociation Curve

Only 1.5 per cent of oxygen is carried in the blood plasma. The majority of oxygen is transported in the blood by haemoglobin. Oxygen reacts with haemoglobin to make oxyhaemoglobin. The reaction of oxygen with haemoglobin is temporary and completely reversible. This means that oxygen can be unloaded from haemoglobin. The binding of oxygen to haemoglobin is dependent on the partial pressure of oxygen. Oxygen combines with haemoglobin in oxygen-rich situations, such as in the lungs.

Oxygen is released by haemoglobin in places where there is little oxygen, such as in exercising muscle.

The oxygen dissociation curve is an S-shaped curve that represents the ease with which haemoglobin releases oxygen when it is exposed to tissues of different concentrations of oxygen. The curve starts with a steep rise because haemoglobin has a high affinity for oxygen. This means that when there is a small rise in the partial pressure of oxygen, haemoglobin picks up and binds oxygen to it easily. Thus, in the lungs, the blood is rapidly saturated with oxygen. However, only a small drop in the partial pressure of oxygen results in a large drop in the percentage saturation of haemoglobin. Thus, in exercising muscles, where there is a low partial pressure of oxygen, the haemoglobin readily unloads the oxygen for use by the tissues.

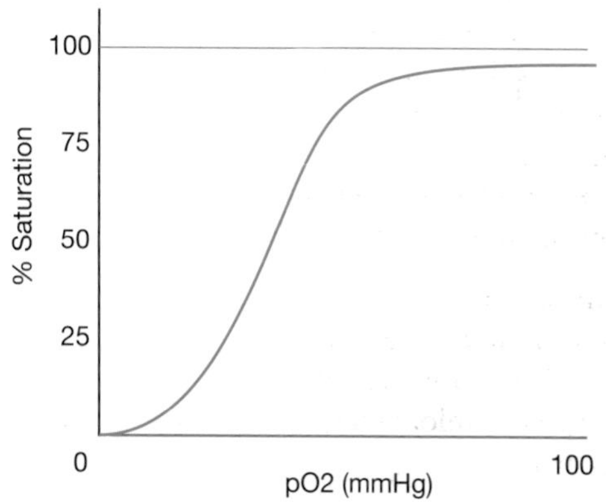

Fig 2.9 Oxygen dissociation curve

Changes in blood carbon dioxide level and hydrogen ion concentration (pH) cause shifts in the oxygen dissociation curve. These shifts enhance oxygen release in tissues and increase oxygen uptake in the lungs. This is known as the Bohr effect, named after the Danish physiologist, Christian Bohr, who discovered it. During exercise, the blood becomes more acidic because of the increased production of carbon dioxide.

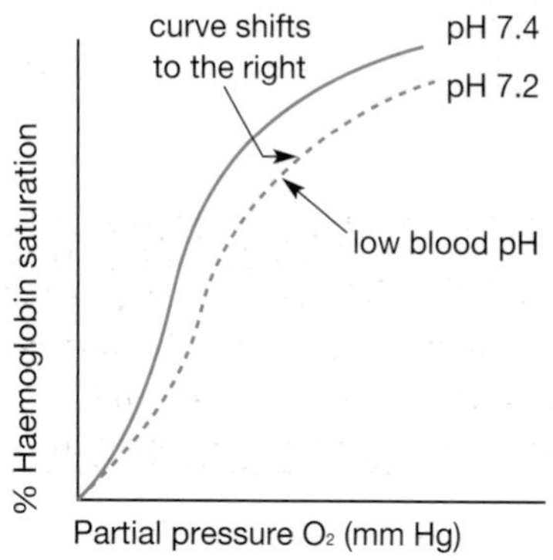

Fig 2.10 Shift in oxygen dissociation curve

This increase in carbon dioxide and decrease in pH shifts the dissociation curve to the right for a given partial pressure of oxygen, releasing more oxygen to the tissues.

In the lungs, there is a low partial pressure of carbon dioxide and low hydrogen ion concentration, which shifts the dissociation curve to the left for a given partial pressure of oxygen, and therefore enhances oxygen uptake.

As muscles exercise, they also increase in temperature. This has the effect of shifting the curve to the right, which means oxygen is released much more readily. Conversely, a decreased temperature shifts the curve to the left, which increases oxygen uptake.

Student activity 2.3

90–120 mins

P3 M2 D2

During steady-state exercise, the cardiovascular and respiratory systems adapt to the exercise and respond in order to allow us to continue exercising for sustained periods of time.

Work in groups of three or four. You will need the following equipment:

- Electrical sphygmomanometer
- Treadmill or cycle ergometer
- Pen and paper
- Heart-rate monitor
- Stopwatch
- Sports clothes.

Follow the method set out below and record your results in the table; then answer the questions that follow.

- Choose a continuous exercise, such as jogging on a treadmill or cycling on an ergometer.
- Attach the sphygmomanometer and heart-rate monitor to the exercising person and record their resting heart rate and blood pressure.
- Record the subject's resting pulmonary ventilation.
- Your subject should perform aerobic exercise. Try to ensure that they are exercising at the same intensity throughout the duration of the exercise.
- At regular 5-minute intervals, take your subject's blood pressure, heart rate and pulmonary ventilation (ensuring that they continue to exercise throughout).
- After 25 minutes of exercise, and when the last readings have been taken, your subject can stop exercising.
- After a break of at least 10 minutes, record your subject's blood pressure, heart rate and pulmonary ventilation.

1. Plot these results on a graph.
2. Examine these results, then write a report that explains and analyses how the cardiovascular and respiratory systems respond to steady-state exercise.

	Resting	5 mins exercise	10 mins exercise	15 mins exercise	20 mins exercise	25 mins exercise	10 mins recovery
Blood pressure (mmHg)							
Heart rate (bpm)							
Pulmonary ventilation (VE)							

Neuromuscular Response

As more blood is pumped through the muscles and excess heat is generated through exercising, muscle tissue warms up. The warmer the muscle tissue becomes, the more pliable it is.

> **Key term**
>
> **Pliable:** able to be stretched, shaped or bent.

This means that the muscle tissue is able to stretch to greater lengths without tearing. You can apply this principle to plasticine. If you take a piece of plasticine out of its container and pull it outwards with two hands, the plasticine will quickly break in two. But if you were to warm up the plasticine by rolling it in your hands, and then pull it apart, you would find that it is able to stretch much further without breaking.

As the muscle tissue warms up, the rate at which nervous impulses are sent and received is increased as the heat increases the speed of transmission.

Energy System's Response

The aerobic energy system provides ATP at a slower rate than the previous two energy systems discussed. It is responsible for producing the majority of our energy while our bodies are at rest or taking part in low-intensity exercise such as jogging. It uses a series of reactions, the first being aerobic glycolysis, as it occurs when oxygen is available to break down glucose. As in the anaerobic energy system, glucose is broken down into pyruvate. Because oxygen is present, pyruvate is not turned into lactic acid, but continues to be broken down through a series of chemical reactions, which include:

- The Krebs Cycle – pyruvate from aerobic glycolysis combines with Coenzyme A (CoA) to form acetyl CoA, which combines and reacts with a number of different compounds to produce ATP, hydrogen and carbon dioxide
- The Electron Transport Chain – the hydrogen atoms produced from the Krebs Cycle enter this chain and are passed along a chain of electron carriers, eventually combining with oxygen to form ATP and water.

Both the Krebs Cycle and the Electron Transport Chain take place in organelles called mitochondria.

The majority of ATP is produced in these organelles, so they are very important for energy production. They are rod-shaped and have an inner and outer membrane. The inner membrane is arranged into many folds that project inwards. These folds are called cristae and provide a large surface area for energy production to take place.

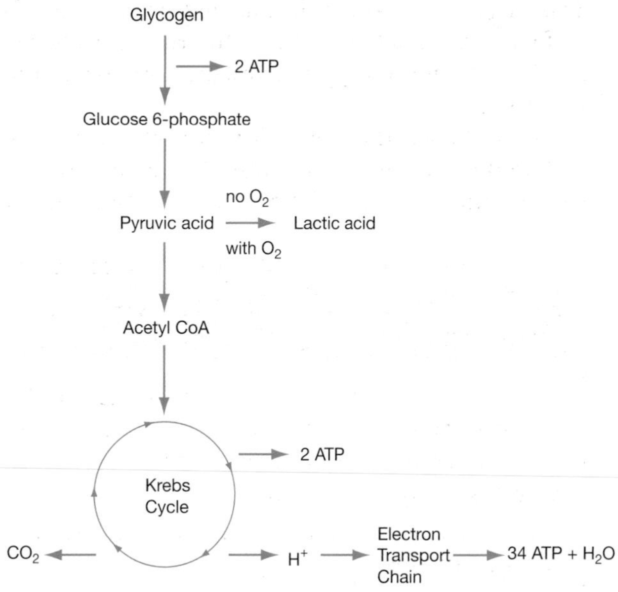

Fig 2.11 Aerobic energy system

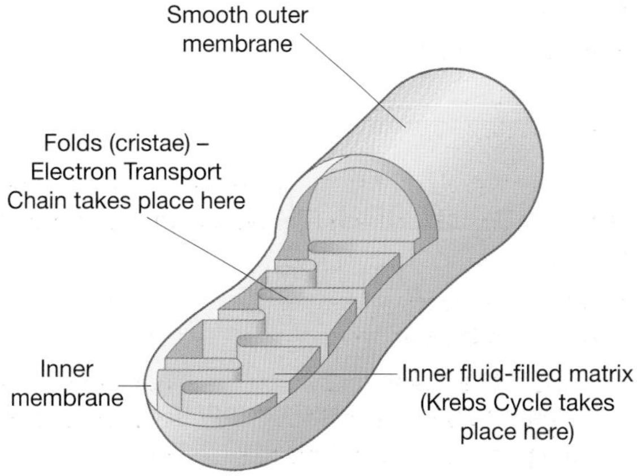

Fig 2.12 Mitochondrion

> **Key learning points 2**
>
> When exercising at a steady state, the body undergoes the following responses:
>
> - Cardiovascular responses: HR levels off, increased stroke volume, vasodilation of blood vessels leading to working muscles, BP levels off.
> - Respiratory responses: tidal volume levels off, breathing rate levels off, oxygen is unloaded from haemoglobin much more readily.
> - Neuromuscular responses: increased pliability of muscles, increased speed of neural transmissions.
> - Energy system responses: aerobic ATP production.

Student activity 2.4 60–90 mins P4 M2 D2

Write a report that describes, explains and analyses the responses of the neuromuscular and energy systems to steady-state exercise.

Quick quiz 2

1. Give three examples of steady-state exercise.
2. Give two responses from the following body systems to show how they adapt to steady-state exercise:
3. (a) Cardiovascular system.
   (b) Respiratory system.
   (c) Neuromuscular system.
4. Draw a graph to illustrate how heart rate responds to steady-state exercise.
5. Describe Starling's law.
6. Explain the oxygen dissociation curve.
7. Which energy system is used during steady-state exercise?
8. In which organelle is the majority of ATP produced during steady-state exercise?

2.4 Fatigue and How the Body Recovers from Exercise

P5 M3

We cannot continue to exercise indefinitely because we will eventually fatigue.

Key term

Fatigue: tiredness from physical exertion.

Fatigue occurs as a result of a number of factors, including:

- Depletion of energy sources, such as reduced quantities of phosphocreatine, glucose and glycogen
- Effects of waste products, such as increased production of lactic acid and carbon dioxide
- Neuromuscular fatigue, such as depletion of acetylcholine and reduced calcium ion release.

As a result, it is necessary to rest in order to recover and return the body to its pre-exercise state.

Depletion of Energy Sources

In order to exercise, we must break down the energy stored in our body and turn it into ATP. Sources of energy include phosphocreatine, glucose and glycogen. We have only enough phosphocreatine to last us for ten seconds of maximal exercise. We then switch to glucose for energy production. We have around 15 to 20 g of glucose in our bloodstream, around 345 g of glycogen in our muscles, and 90 to 110 g of glycogen stored in our liver. When our blood sugar levels are low, the liver converts either its store of glycogen into glucose or the skeletal muscles' store of glycogen into glucose. We have only enough glycogen stores to last us for around two hours. So once the body's stores of glucose and glycogen are used up, we become fatigued and/or have to exercise at a lower intensity.

Effects of Waste Products

Lactic acid is the main by-product of anaerobic glycolysis. Blood always contains a small amount of lactic acid, and during high-intensity exercise this increases greatly. The increased production of lactic acid results in the pH of the blood decreasing. A blood pH of 6.4 or lower affects muscle and neural function and eventually prevents continued exercise.

Onset of blood lactate accumulation (OBLA) is the point at which lactic acid begins to accumulate in the muscles. It is also known as the anaerobic threshold. OBLA is considered to occur at somewhere between 85 and 90 per cent of your maximum heart rate.

Neuromuscular Fatigue

Neuromuscular fatigue means that the muscles are either not able to receive signals from the CNS that stimulate the muscle to contract or that the muscle tissue is unable to function properly.

High-intensity exercise or exercise for long periods of time can eventually interfere with calcium release, which is required for muscle contraction. If no calcium ions are available, the muscle is unable to contract.

Alternatively, transmission of nerve impulses can be affected, as the availability of acetylcholine can be decreased, which prevents the nervous stimulation reaching the muscle tissue/motor unit.

Recovery Process

After taking part in any type of exercise, the body has to recover and return to its pre-exercise state.

Excess post-exercise oxygen consumption (EPOC) is also referred to as oxygen debt. EPOC is the total oxygen consumed after exercise in excess of pre-exercise levels. It occurs when the exercise performed is totally or partially anaerobic. As a result, energy is supplied by the anaerobic energy systems, which results in lactic acid production. When the person stops exercising, breathing rate remains elevated so that extra oxygen is breathed in to:

- Break down lactic acid to carbon dioxide and water
- Replenish ATP, phosphocreatine and glycogen
- Pay back any oxygen that has been borrowed from haemoglobin and myoglobin.

After a bout of vigorous exercise, five events must take place before the muscle can operate again:

1. ATP must be replaced.
2. PC stores must be replenished.
3. Lactic acid must be removed.
4. Myoglobin must be replenished with oxygen.
5. Glycogen stores must be replenished.

The replacement of ATP and PC takes around three minutes and the removal of lactic acid takes around 20 minutes after stopping exercise, but the oxygen replenishment of myoglobin and refilling the glycogen stores take between 24 and 48 hours. If the exercise bout was of a very high intensity, it will take longer to recover. However, the fitter you are, the faster you will recover. The faster the debt can be repaid, the sooner the performer can exercise again.

The oxygen debt consists of two separate components:

- Alactacid debt (fast component)
- Lactacid debt (slow component).

Alactacid Debt

Alactacid oxygen debt is the process of recovery that does not involve lactic acid. The aerobic energy system is used to produce the ATP required to replenish the PC stores and ATP stores in the body:

$$\text{ADP} + \text{P} + \text{Oxygen} = \text{ATP}$$

$$\text{ATP} + \text{C} + \text{P} = \text{PC} + \text{ADP}$$

Around 50 per cent of the replenishment occurs during the first 30 seconds, while full recovery occurs at about three minutes.

The alactacid oxygen debt ranges between 2 and 3.5 litres of oxygen. The fitter you are, the greater the debt, because training increases the PC content within the muscle cells. However, the recovery time of a fitter person is reduced because they have enhanced methods of oxygen delivery, such as increased capillarisation and an improved cardiorespiratory system. These increase the rate of ATP production from the aerobic energy system.

Lactacid Debt

The lactacid oxygen debt takes much longer to complete and can last for minutes or hours, depending on the severity of the exercise. The process involves oxygen, which is required to break down the lactic acid produced during anaerobic glycolysis into pyruvate. Pyruvate can then enter the aerobic energy system and eventually be broken down into carbon dioxide and water.

$$\text{Lactic acid} + \text{Oxygen} = \text{Pyruvate}$$

Lactic acid can also be converted in the liver to glycogen and stored either in the liver or in muscle tissue. Research has shown that an active recovery increases the rate of removal of lactic acid, so walking or slow jogging after a bout of exercise will help to decrease the time it takes to rid the body of lactic acid. An active recovery keeps the heart rate and breathing rate up, which has the effect of increasing the rate of delivery of oxygen to the working muscles. This then helps to rid the body of the lactic acid.

Therefore, a cool-down is very important after any form of activity in order to maximise recovery. Failure to cool down adequately means that the levels of lactic acid will remain elevated. It is thought that this acidity level affects the pain receptors and contributes to the muscle soreness which people may feel some time after having exercised. This muscle soreness, termed delayed onset of muscle soreness (DOMS), is at its most uncomfortable 36 to 48 hours after exercise has ceased.

Muscle glycogen stores must also be restored. This is attained through a high carbohydrate diet and rest. It can take several days to recover muscle glycogen stores, depending on the intensity of the exercise.

Key learning points 3

- Fatigue occurs because of:
  - Depletion of energy sources
  - Accumulation of waste products
  - Lack of calcium ion availability
  - Decreased availability of acetylcholine.
- Recovery after exercise involves taking in excess oxygen in order to return the body to its pre-exercise state.
- Alactic phase of recovery: ATP and PC production takes place in the first few minutes of recovery.
- Lactic phase of recovery: lactic acid is removed and turned into pyruvate and myoglobin; stores of oxygen are repleted and glycogen stores are repleted.
- An active recovery increases the rate of lactic acid removal.

Student activity 2.5

60–90 mins **P5** **M3**

- Place a heart-rate monitor around your chest or take your heart rate by pressing on a pulse point and counting your pulse for one minute. Stand against a wall, then bend your knees and slide down the wall so that your knees are at right angles – you will be in a 'ski squat' position'.
- After 30 seconds or one minute, count your pulse and remain in the ski squat position.
- You will no doubt feel that your legs are very sore and you cannot maintain this position for very long, but your heart rate has not reached maximal values. You have had to stop this exercise because you have experienced neuromuscular fatigue in your quadriceps muscles!

Task 1

Describe and explain the process involved when a person becomes fatigued through taking part in exercise.

Task 2

You will need the following equipment:

- Stopwatch
- Running track/gym
- Sports clothes.

Follow the method set out below and record your results in the table; then answer the questions that follow.

- Take your resting pulse rate and make a note of it in the results table.
- Take part in some form of intense exercise that lasts at least five minutes.
- Find your pulse, then record your pulse for a ten-second count every minute after the exercise until your heart rate returns to its original level.
- Convert your heart rate into beats per minute by multiplying by six.

	Beats per minute
Resting pulse rate	
Immediately after exercise	
1 minute after exercise	
2 minutes after exercise	
3 minutes after exercise	
4 minutes after exercise	
5 minutes after exercise	

1. Explain why your heart rate was different from resting levels immediately after exercise had stopped.
2. Explain why your heart rate remained elevated after three minutes of rest.
3. Draw a graph to illustrate the fast and slow components of the recovery process.
4. Write a report that describes and explains the recovery process from exercise participation.

Quick quiz 3

1. List three reasons why fatigue can occur.
2. How much glucose do we have in our bloodstream?
3. What is the main by-product of anaerobic glycolysis?
4. At what blood pH is muscle and neural function affected?
5. Which ions are required for muscle contraction?
6. What does EPOC stand for?
7. After a bout of vigorous exercise, what five events must occur before a muscle can operate again?
8. What is alactacid debt?
9. What is lactacid debt?

2.5 How the Body Adapts to Long-Term Exercise

P6 P7 M4 D3

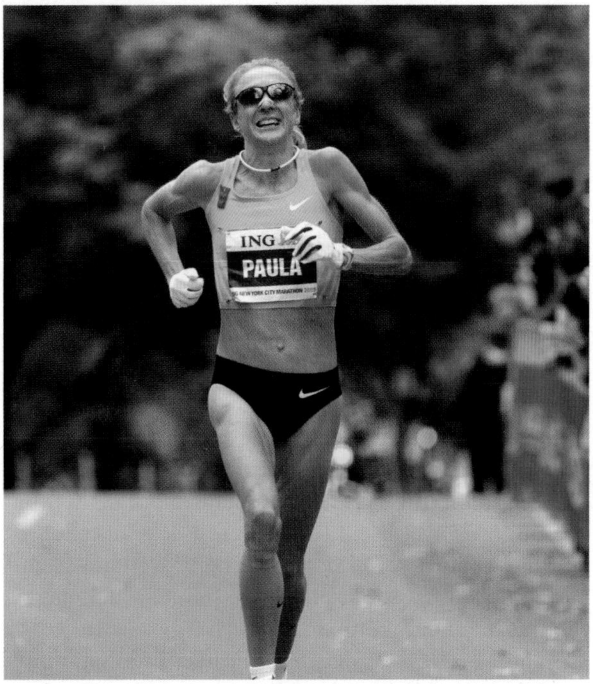

Fig 2.13 The athlete's body has adapted to strength training

Long-term exercise is also known as chronic exercise and means that a person has been participating in regular exercise for long periods of time (a minimum of eight weeks). This regular participation affects the body in a number of ways that make it more able to cope with the stresses of the exercise. This results in the person being able to exercise at higher intensities and/or for longer periods of time. This process is called adaptation.

Cardiovascular Adaptations

The main adaptations that occur to the cardiovascular system through endurance training are concerned with increasing the delivery of oxygen to the working muscles. If you were to dissect the heart of a top endurance athlete, you would find that the size of the walls of the left ventricle are markedly thicker than those of a person who does not perform endurance exercise. This adaptation is called cardiac hypertrophy.

Key term

Cardiac hypertrophy: the size of the heart wall becomes thicker and stronger.

Adaptation occurs in the same way that we increase the size of our skeletal muscles – the more we exercise our muscles, the larger or more toned they become. In the same way, the more we exercise our heart through aerobic training, the larger it will become. This will then have the effect of increasing the stroke volume, which is the amount of blood that the heart can pump out per beat. As the heart wall becomes bigger, it can pump more blood per beat, as the thicker wall can contract more forcibly. As the stroke volume is increased, the heart no longer needs to beat as often to get the same amount of blood around the body. This results in a decrease in heart rate which is known as bradycardia.

Key term

Bradycardia: decreased resting heart rate.

An average male adult's heart rate is 70 beats per minute (bpm). However, Lance Armstrong, a Tour de France champion, had a resting heart rate of 30 bpm! As stroke volume increases, cardiac output also increases, so an endurance athlete's heart can pump more blood per minute than other people's. However, resting values of cardiac output do not change. An endurance athlete has more capillaries, allowing more blood to travel through them. This process, called capillarisation, aids in the extraction of oxygen. An increase in haemoglobin due to an increase in the number of red blood cells (which contain the haemoglobin) further aids the transport of oxygen. Though haemoglobin content rises, the increase in blood plasma is greater, and consequently the blood haematocrit (ratio of red blood cell volume to total blood volume) is reduced, which lowers viscosity (thickness) and enables the blood to flow more easily.

Strength training produces very few adaptations to the cardiovascular system, as this training does not stress the heart or oxygen delivery and extraction systems for sustained periods of time.

Respiratory Adaptations

The respiratory system deals with taking oxygen into the body and also with helping to remove waste products associated with muscle metabolism. Training reduces the resting respiratory rate and the breathing rate during sub-maximal exercise. Endurance training can also provide a small increase in lung volumes: vital capacity increases slightly, as does tidal volume during maximal exercise. The increased strength of the respiratory muscles is partly responsible for this as it aids lung inflation.

Endurance training also increases the capillarisation around the alveoli in the lungs. This helps to increase the rate of gas exchange in the lungs and, therefore, increase the amount of oxygen entering the blood and the amount of carbon dioxide leaving the blood.

Strength training produces very few adaptations to the respiratory system, as this type of training uses the anaerobic energy systems, whereas the respiratory system is only really concerned with the aerobic energy system.

Neuromuscular and Energy Systems' adaptations

Endurance training results in an increase in the muscular stores of muscle glycogen. There is increased delivery of oxygen to the muscles through an increase in the concentration of myoglobin and increased capillary density through the muscle. The ability of skeletal muscle to consume oxygen is increased as a direct result of an increase in the number and size of the mitochondria and an increase in the activity and concentration of enzymes involved in the aerobic processes that take place in the mitochondria. As a result, there is greater scope to use glycogen and fat as fuels. Slow-twitch fibres can enlarge by up to 22 per cent, which gives greater potential for aerobic energy production. Hypertrophy of slow-twitch fibres means that there is a corresponding increase in the stores of glycogen and triglycerides. This ensures a continuous supply of energy, enabling exercise to be performed for longer.

These adaptations result in an increased maximal oxygen consumption (VO_2max) being obtained before the anaerobic threshold is reached and fatigue begins.

High-intensity training results in hypertrophy of fast-twitch fibres. There are increased levels of ATP and PC in the muscle and an increased capacity to generate ATP by the PC energy system. This is partly due to the increased activity of the enzymes which break down PC. ATP production by anaerobic glycolysis is increased as a result of enhanced activity of the glycolytic enzymes. There is also an increased ability to break down glycogen in the absence of oxygen.

As lactic acid accumulates, it decreases the pH levels of the blood, making it more acidic. This increased level of hydrogen ions will eventually prevent the glycolytic enzyme functioning. However, anaerobic training increases the buffering capacity of the body and enables it to work for longer in periods of high acidity.

Energy System Adaptation

Aerobic training will increase the number of mitochondria in slow-twitch muscle fibres. This will allow greater production of ATP through the aerobic energy system. Greater amounts of glycogen can be stored in the liver and skeletal muscle. Aerobic training results in an increase in the number of enzymes required for body fat to be broken down, and more body fat is stored in muscle tissue, which means that more fat can be used as an energy source.

Anaerobic or strength training predominantly uses the PC and lactic acid energy system. Chronic anaerobic/strength training increases the body's tolerance levels to low pH. This means more energy can be produced by the lactic acid energy system, and the increased production of lactic acid can be tolerated for longer.

Skeletal Adaptations

Our skeleton responds to aerobic weight-bearing exercise or resistance exercise by becoming stronger and more able to withstand impact, which means you are less likely to break a bone if you fall over.

Key term

Weight-bearing exercise: this is when we are using our body weight as a form of resistance (e.g. walking, running).

This occurs because the stimulation of exercise means the mineral content (calcium in particular) is increased, which makes bones harder and stronger. Exercise also has an effect on joints, by increasing the thickness of cartilage at the ends of the bones and increasing the production of synovial fluid. This will have the effect of making joints stronger and less prone to injury. Strength training increases the strength of muscle tendons, which again makes them less prone to injury. Lastly, the ligaments which hold our bones together are able to stretch to a greater degree, which helps to prevent injuries such as joint strains.

Key learning points 4

- Adaptations to aerobic exercise:
  - Cardiovascular system: cardiac hypertrophy, increased SV, decreased resting HR, increased number of capillaries, increased number of red blood cells, decreased haematocrit.
  - Respiratory system: decreased resting breathing rate, increased lung volume, increased vital capacity, increased tidal volume (in maximal exercise), increased strength of respiratory muscles, increased capillarisation around alveoli.
  - Neuromuscular system: increased myoglobin content, increased number of capillaries, increased number of mitochondria, hypertrophy of slow-twitch muscle fibres, increased stores of glycogen, increased stores of fat.
  - Energy systems: increased number of aerobic enzymes, increased breakdown of fat.
- Adaptations to anaerobic exercise:
  - Cardiovascular system: no significant adaptations.
  - Respiratory system: no significant adaptations.
  - Neuromuscular: hypertrophy of fast-twitch muscle fibres, increased content of ATP, increased content of PC, increased tolerance to lactic acid.
  - Energy systems: increased number of anaerobic enzymes.
  - Skeletal system: increased strength of bones, increased strength of tendons, increased stretch of ligaments.

Student activity 2.6

60–90 mins | P6 | P7 | M4 | D3

Taking part in long-term exercise programmes, such as four 30-minute jogging sessions per week for eight weeks, or a six-week resistance training programme, will produce stimulus to make the body adapt to the exercise so that it is able to perform the activity more readily, with less perceived effort.

Task 1

Draw a spider diagram that illustrates how each of the following systems adapts to long-term exercise:

- Cardiovascular
- Respiratory
- Skeletal
- Neuromuscular
- Energy.

Task 2

Write a report that describes, explains and analyses how the cardiovascular, respiratory, skeletal, neuromuscular and energy systems adapt to long-term exercise.

Quick quiz 4

1. Explain what cardiac hypertrophy is and how this can help an endurance athlete.
2. Explain how capillarisation around the lungs can increase the rate of gas exchange.
3. Explain how the skeletal system adapts to weight-bearing exercises.
4. Describe how the cardiovascular and respiratory system of Paula Radcliff will have adapted through endurance training.
5. Describe how the neuromuscular and skeletal system of Usain Bolt will have adapted through resistance training.

Further reading

Clegg, C. (1995) *Exercise Physiology*, Bournemouth: Feltham Press.

Crisfield, P. (1996) *Coaching Sessions: A Guide to Planning and Goal-setting*, Leeds: National Coaching Foundation.

Davis, R.J., Bull, C.R., Roscoe, J.V. and Roscoe, D.A. (2000) *Physical Education and the Study of Sport*, St Louis, Ill.: Mosby.

Dick, F. (1997) *Sports Training Principles*, London: A & C Black.

Foss, M. and Keteyian, S. (1998) *Fox's Physiological Basis for Exercise and Sport*, Maidenhead: McGraw-Hill.

Honeybourne, J., Hill, M. and Moors, H. (2000) *Advanced Physical Education and Sport for A Level*, Cheltenham: Stanley Thornes.

McArdle, W., Katch, F. and Katch, V. (2001) *Exercise Physiology: Energy, Nutrition and Human Performance*, London: WMS & Wilkins.

Useful websites

www.getbodysmart.com

Free tutorials and quizzes from an American site that looks at human anatomy and physiology, helping you to see the structure of the different body systems.

www.innerbody.com

Free and informative diagrams of the different body systems, including respiratory, cardiovascular, skeletal and muscular

www.instantanatomy.net

Free useful anatomy pictures and information, mainly from a medical viewpoint

3: Assessing Risk in Sport

3.1 Introduction

Safety is a very important factor to consider when taking part in sports or leading sporting events. If sports leaders fail to ensure that health and safety guidelines are adhered to, this could result in a charge of 'negligence' being brought against them through the civil courts. It is therefore important that learners understand the legislative factors, regulations and legal responsibilities involved while working in sporting situations.

This unit will cover ways in which a sports leader can plan and carry out a sporting activity safely under the overall supervision of a more experienced person. It includes how to carry out risk assessments, preparation of the site and participants for the activity, and maintaining the safety of participants while taking part in the activity. The unit closes with ideas on how to plan a safe sporting activity.

By the end of this unit you should:

- know the key factors that influence health and safety in sport
- be able to carry out risk assessments
- know how to maintain the safety of participants and colleagues in a sports environment
- be able to plan a safe sporting activity.

Assessment and grading criteria		
To achieve a PASS grade the evidence must show that the learner is able to:	**To achieve a MERIT grade the evidence must show that, in addition to the pass criteria, the learner is able to:**	**To achieve a DISTINCTION grade the evidence must show that, in addition to the pass and merit criteria, the learner is able to:**
P1 describe four legislative factors that influence health and safety in sport	**M1** compare and contrast the influences of legislation, legal factors and regulatory bodies on health and safety in sport	
P2 describe the legal factors and regulatory bodies that influence health and safety in sport		
P3 carry out risk assessments for two different sports activities, with tutor support	**M2** independently carry out risk assessments for two different sports activities	**D1** review the risk assessment controls and evaluate their effectiveness
P4 describe three procedures used to promote and maintain a healthy and safe sporting environment	**M3** explain three procedures used to promote and maintain a healthy and safe sporting environment	**D2** analyse three procedures used to promote and maintain a healthy and safe sporting environment.
P5 produce a plan for the safe delivery of a selected sports activity and review the plan.	**M4** explain the plan for the safe delivery of a selected sports activity and review the plan.	

3.2 Key Factors that Influence Health and Safety in Sport

P1 M1

Legislative Factors

Key terms

Legislation: a generic term for laws, which includes acts, regulations, orders and directives.

Directive: a legislative act passed by the European Union that member states must adhere to.

A number of laws and acts have been devised to try to ensure that all safety precautions are taken into account while at work and during sports participation. Any person who works should be aware of these acts and make sure they do everything possible to adhere to the legislation.

Health and Safety at Work Act 1974

The Health and Safety at Work Act became law in 1974 in response to thousands of accidents and near misses in the workplace. Its purpose is to ensure that employers take reasonable steps to ensure the health, safety and welfare of their employees while they are at work. These steps include:

- Making sure the working environment and equipment are up to the necessary standard
- Ensuring that regular and appropriate safety checks are carried out
- Ensuring the safe use, handling and storage of equipment and substances
- Providing information, training and supervision to ensure that employees can do their jobs safely
- Regular monitoring of the working environment to ensure it is hygienic and that no toxic contaminants are present.

The Health and Safety at Work Act also requires employees to take reasonable steps to ensure their own safety. They are expected to cooperate with the employer to meet legal obligations and use the equipment provided appropriately.

Both the employer and employees benefit from this Act because:

- Fewer accidents mean better health for employees
- Fewer accidents mean more regular earnings for employees
- Less sickness means money saved by the employer and the NHS.

The majority of accidents that occur in the workplace are due to the following actions and circumstances:

- Lifting and carrying
- Slips, trips and falls
- Being hit by moving objects or vehicles
- Moving machinery
- Harmful substances.

Some illness and diseases can be work-related – for example, occupational deafness, back pain and stress.

The following three factors can affect health and safety in the workplace:

1. **Occupational factors** – people may be at risk from injuries or illnesses because of the work they do.
2. **Environmental factors** – the conditions in which people work may cause problems.
3. **Human factors** – poor attitudes and behaviour can contribute to accidents.

It is the responsibility of both the employer and employees to ensure that health and safety standards are maintained.

After the Health and Safety at Work Act was passed in 1974, RIDDOR was added in 1995. RIDDOR stands for the Reporting of Injuries, Diseases and Dangerous Occurrences Regulations, which came into force on 1 April 1996. It means that all work-related accidents, diseases and dangerous occurrences should be reported to the Incident Contact Centre (ICC). These include:

- Deaths
- Major injuries
- Injuries that last for more than three days
- Injuries to members of the public where they are taken to hospital
- Work-related diseases
- Dangerous occurrences – where something happens that does not result in a reportable injury, but which could have done.

Personal Protective Equipment Regulations 2002

Personal protective equipment should be used when a hazard cannot be sufficiently controlled by other health and safety measures.

A range of PPE exists to protect various parts of the body, such as goggles for the eyes, a helmet for the head, ear plugs for the ears, and so on.

Key term

Personal protective equipment (PPE): clothes and other items worn to protect the wearer against hazards.

Control of Substances Hazardous to Health Regulations (COSHH) 2002

Hazardous substances can cause a wide range of health problems, such as dermatitis and asthma; they may also cause other problems, such as explosions or fires.

In the sports industry you may be exposed to a range of hazardous substances, such as cleaning fluids or chlorine, which is used in swimming pools. All hazardous substances should have labels that detail the nature of the hazardous substance (e.g. corrosive, irritant, poison).

You must ensure that you have been trained in how to use the equipment properly and that you wear the appropriate PPE when dealing with these substances. All hazardous substances should be kept in a locked cabinet.

> **Key term**
>
> **Hazardous substance:** any material or substance with the potential to cause illness or injury to the people who come into contact with it.

Manual Handling Operations Regulations 1992

In the sports industry you will probably find yourself having to lift, move and set up sporting equipment. Therefore it is important that you learn safe lifting techniques. Maintaining a straight back at all times is the proper way to lift items, as shown in Figure 3.1. Typical injuries from incorrect manual handling are back sprains and strains, cuts, bruises, crushing, fractures, hernias and trapped nerves.

> **Key term**
>
> **Manual handling:** using the body to lift, carry, push or pull a load.

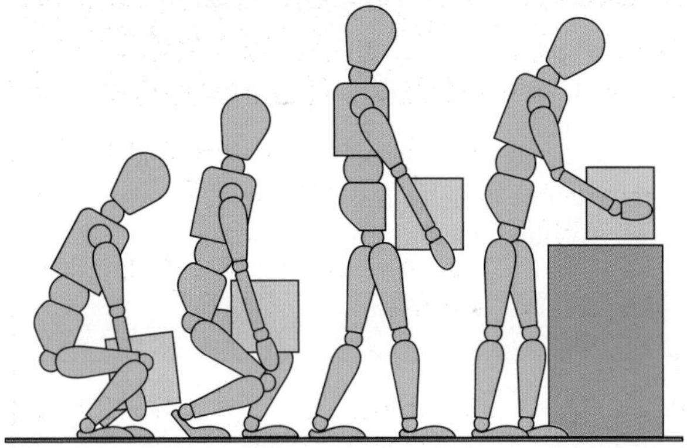

Fig 3.1 Manual handling guide

Health and Safety (First Aid) Regulations 1981

These regulations require companies and organisations to have sufficient first-aid facilities and equipment in case of illness or injury to employees. The number of qualified first-aiders will be related to the number of employees working in the organisation.

Fire Safety and Safety of Places of Sport Act 1987

This act was drawn up after the Bradford City football ground fire tragedy in 1985. It requires that all sports arenas and stadiums have sufficient means of escape in the event of a fire. Venues must also provide adequate equipment for fighting fires.

Adventure Activities Licensing Authority (AALA)

The Adventure Activities Licensing Authority was founded in 1996 and works in conjunction with the Adventure Licensing Service. Both are run by the Health and Safety Executive. Adventure Activities Licensing is responsible for inspecting activity centres and other outdoor and adventurous activity providers. If it is satisfied that a provider meets nationally accepted standards of good practice, it will issue a licence. This helps to provide the public with assurances that the activities are not exposing the participants to unnecessary danger or risks of injury.

Despite all this legislation, there are still fatalities in the workplace: in 2005–06, 220 workers were killed and 361 members of the public were fatally injured. This should remind you to remain vigilant

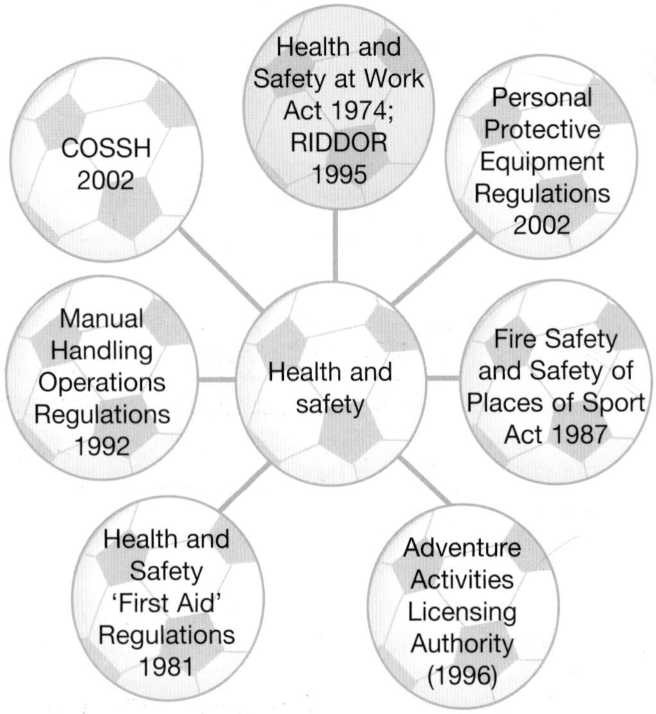

Fig 3.2 Health and Safety legislation

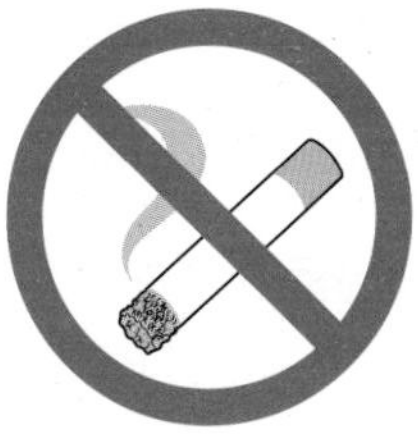

Prohibition
These signs tell you what you are not allowed to do, e.g. No smoking
Shape: Circular
Colour: White with red border and red crossbar running from top left to bottom right

Warning
These signs warn you of a danger
Shape: Triangular
Colour: Yellow with black border and letters

Mandatory
These signs tell you what you *must* do, e.g. wear ear protectors
Shape: Circular
Colour: Blue background with white symbol and letters

Warning
These signs tell you about safe areas or equipment, e.g. fire exit
Shape: Square or oblong
Colour: Green background with white symbol and letters

Fig 3.3 Safety signs

in maintaining your own and your co-workers' health and safety while at work.

Safety Signs

There are four types of safety signs (see Figure 3.3). Each type has a certain shape, colour and meaning.

Legal Factors

The court system within Britain has a structure that all legal cases have to pass through. There are a range of courts that deal with different types of charges:

- **Magistrates' court** – this is the lowest court in England and deals mainly with minor criminal matters
- **Crown court** – this deals with serious criminal charges, such as murders, with a judge and jury
- **Supreme Court** – this is the highest court in England and deals with appeals on important issues from the Court of Appeal
- **European Court of Justice** – this is the supreme law court in Europe. The decisions of this court have to be enforced by all member states.

Statutory Law

These are written laws set down by a governing authority. Any person breaking these laws is liable to be arrested by the police and prosecuted accordingly.

Civil Law

Civil law deals with the rights of private citizens and does not involve the police. An example of civil law would be when a person is suing a company or an individual for some form of negligence, or when a partner in a marriage wishes to divorce the other person.

If a company does not abide by the Health and Safety at Work Act and a person is injured as a result of this negligence, the company can be prosecuted because it has broken a statutory law. Also, the

Student activity 3.1 — 30 minutes — P1

There are a number of different types of legislation in sport today in order to help protect people from injury and ill health.

Task 1

Examine the dates on which each of the Acts came into effect. Carry out research to try to answer the following:

- What significant event occurred in 1985 which may have resulted in the Fire Safety and Safety of Places of Sport Act 1987?
- What event in 1993 may have resulted in the Adventure Activities Licensing Authority being formed?
- Why was RIDDOR added to the Health and Safety at Work Act?

Task 2

Prepare a leaflet describing four legislative factors that influence health and safety in sport.

employee who is injured can take out a civil case and sue the company for compensation.

Case Law

Case law is when a similar case has occurred previously and the accused person is prosecuted and/or sued in a similar manner to the previous case.

In Loco Parentis

In loco parentis basically means 'in place of the parent'. This means that a person or organisation has to take on the functions and responsibilities of a parent. An example of this would be a teacher supervising a student on a school trip. The teacher has overall responsibility for the child's health and safety. A person taking on a role *in loco parentis* is expected to apply the same standard of care as would a 'reasonable parent' acting within a range of reasonable responses.

Negligence

Negligence is the name given to a situation in which a person in a supervisory role basically fails to meet a 'standard' of care. The supervisor may be careless in their actions or lack of actions, such as not carrying out a full risk assessment which then results in a person taking part in the activity suffering from an injury or even death.

If a person is deemed to be negligent they may be held liable for any injuries or damages to the people involved.

Regulatory Bodies

A number of regulatory bodies have been set up to help to police employers and facilities so that they adhere to appropriate legislation. The Health and Safety Commission is in charge of health and safety regulation in the UK. The Health and Safety Executive and local authorities are responsible for enforcing these regulations. Staff from these organisations will inspect facilities and speak to staff to ensure the facility is being run appropriately. If the facility is not being run in accordance with legislation, it will be given actions to address within a set time period, or the facility may even be closed down until it is able to show that it meets health and safety guidelines.

Key learning points 1

- A range of laws is in place in order to protect the employee and employer in the workplace. These include: Health and Safety at Work Act, Personal Protective Equipment Regulations, Control of Substances Hazardous to Health Regulations, Health and Safety (First Aid) Regulations, Manual Handling Operations Regulations, Fire Safety and Safety of Places of Sport Act, Adventure Activities Licensing Authority.
- Statutory law is where a person is prosecuted, and involves the police.
- Civil law does not involve the police.
- Case law is where a case in the past is referred to.
- The Health and Safety Executive enforces regulations in the workplace.

Student activity 3.2

60 minutes P2 M1

Task 1

Design a poster with written text that describes the legal factors and regulatory bodies that influence health and safety in sport.

Task 2

Write a report that compares and contrasts the influences on health and safety in sport of the following:

- Legislation
- Legal factors
- Regulatory bodies.

Quick quiz 1

- Health and Safety at Work Act
- Magistrates' court
- *In loco parentis*
- Fire Safety and Safety of Places of Sport Act
- Civil law
- Negligence
- Health and Safety (First Aid) Act
- Crown court
- Statutory law
- Personal protective equipment

Choose a term from the list above to answer each of the following questions.

1. This means in 'place of the parent'.
2. This is where a person fails to meet a standard of care.
3. This ensures that employers take reasonable steps to ensure the health, safety and welfare of their employees while they are at work.
4. This law requires companies and organisations to have sufficient first-aid facilities and equipment.
5. This is where people who have committed serious criminal offences go to court.
6. This law deals with the rights of private citizens.
7. A shin pad is an example of this.
8. This law requires all sports arenas and stadiums to have sufficient means of escape in the event of a fire.
9. This law deals with written law set down by a governing authority.
10. This is where people who have committed minor criminal offences are tried.

3.3 Risk Assessment

P3 M3 D1

Risk assessment is a technique for preventing accidents and ill health by helping people to think about what could go wrong and devising ways to prevent problems. Risk assessment is good practice and is also a legal requirement. It often enables organisations to reduce the costs associated with accidents and ill health, and to decide on their priorities, highlight training needs and assist with quality assurance programmes. A risk assessment is usually performed by the manager or instructors working in the sports centre. It allows people to take time to consider what could go wrong while taking part in their activity. The risk assessment examines the possible hazards that may occur, the risks involved, the likelihood of them happening and how the hazards could be prevented.

Risk assessments should be logged, kept and reviewed regularly to see if they are up to date and to make sure that none of the details have changed.

Hazard

A hazard is anything with the potential to cause harm. A range of hazards can be found in any workplace. Examples include:

- Fire
- Electricity
- Harmful substances
- Damaged/wet flooring
- Unfastened shoelaces
- Jewellery worn during sports participation
- Water in a swimming pool.

Key term

Hazard: a potential source of danger.

Risk

A risk is linked to the chance of somebody being harmed by the potential hazard. Risks are often categorised into how likely they are to happen. When something is described as low-risk, it means that the likelihood of it happening is low, whereas something that is high-risk is likely to happen. Examples of risks include:

- Slipping on a wet floor and twisting your ankle
- Drowning in a swimming pool
- Tripping over your shoelaces and cutting your knee
- Catching your earring on clothing or an opponent's hand and ripping your ear.

Key term

Risk: the possibility of something bad happening.

Undertaking a Risk Assessment

Once you have highlighted the hazard, the easiest way to assess the potential problems that may arise is to use the following formula: Likelihood χ Severity.

Likelihood – is it likely to happen:

1. Unlikely.

Capsizing in a kayak	
Likelihood of it happening	Severity
2 Quite likely	1 No injury

Table 3.1 Risk assessment of capsizing in a kayak

Is the risk worth taking?	
Likelihood X Severity	Risk worth taking?
1	Yes
2	Yes, with caution
3	Yes, with extreme caution
4	Possibly, with extreme caution
5 or above	No

Table 3.2 To risk or not?

2. Quite likely.
3. Very likely.

Severity – how badly someone could be injured:

1. No injury/minor incident.
2. Injury requiring medical assistance.
3. Major injury or fatality.

For example, Table 3.1 attempts to assess the risk of capsizing in a kayak.

By multiplying the likelihood by the severity, you will be able to draw up a chart that looks at the potential problems, enabling you to make a decision about whether you want to take the risk or not (see Table 3.2).

In the example in Table 3.1, the likelihood times the severity is $2 \times 1 = 2$.

Control Measures

Hazards in the workplace should be removed whenever possible. Sometimes, however, there is no alternative but to keep a hazard. In such cases, it is important to reduce the risk – the likelihood of an accident – by introducing appropriate control measures. If some flooring is wet or damaged, for example, reducing the risk might include placing a barrier around the damage or putting up warning signs.

Other control measures could include participants wearing/using specialist protective clothing and/or equipment to help minimise the risk of injury.

The Risk Assessment Process

1. Identify the area to be assessed (e.g. resistance equipment in the gym).
2. List the hazards that you can identify (e.g. free weights incorrectly stored, wet floor).
3. Identify the risks and the people who are at risk from the hazards listed (e.g. first-time users, inexperienced users).
4. Assess the likelihood of an accident happening (e.g. if a person comes to the gym for the first time to use free weights, what is the likelihood that they may suffer from a lower back injury through an incorrect lifting technique?). Identify the likelihood, between 1 and 3, of this risk happening.
5. How severe will the outcome of the accident be, on a scale of 1 to 3?
6. Work out the level of risk.
7. Is the risk worth taking? Look at what control measures can be put in place to reduce the risk of injury (e.g. ensure all gym users are given an induction prior to using the equipment).

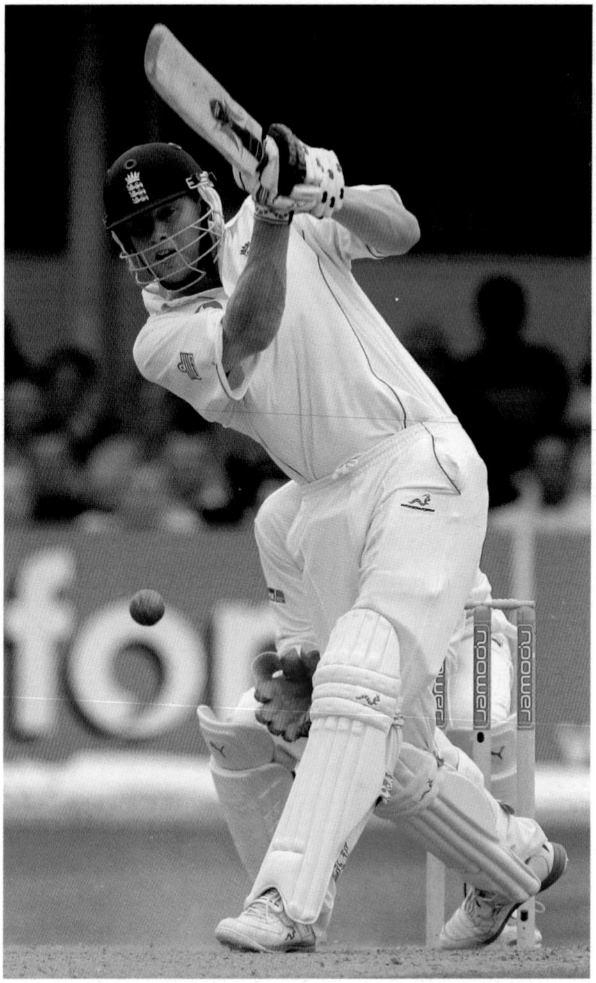

Fig 3.4 Protective clothing worn for playing cricket

Key learning points 2

- A hazard is something that has the potential to cause injury or compromise safety.
- A risk is the likelihood of something unpleasant happening.
- A risk assessment is a list of possible hazards that states the likelihood of them happening, and ways of controlling them.
- Level of risk is worked out by multiplying likelihood of risk by severity. A risk level of five or more means that either more safety precautions should be introduced or the activity should not take place.

Example of a risk assessment form

Location of risk assessment:
Risk assessor's name:
Date:

Hazard	People at risk	Likelihood	Severity	Level of risk	Control measures

Fig 3.5 Example of a risk assessment form

Student activity 3.3

60–90 mins P1 M2 D1

Task 1

Choose two of your favourite sporting activities. Make a list of:

- All the risks and hazards associated with each of your selected sports
- All the hazards associated with each of your selected sports
- All the safety equipment you need in order to reduce the risk of injury in each of your selected sports.

Task 2

Copy and complete the risk assessment form on page 59 for each of your selected sporting activities.

Task 3

Examine your risk assessments and the control measures that you have put in place and then write a report that evaluates their effectiveness.

Quick quiz 2

1. List three hazards and three risks associated with each of the following sports:
   (a) netball
   (b) rugby
   (c) high jump
   (d) shot put
   (e) hurdles
   (f) swimming
   (g) hockey
   (g) badminton.
2. List all the items of personal protective clothing and equipment that a person might wear to help protect them while participating in the following sports:
   (a) football
   (b) cricket
   (c) hockey
   (d) triathlon
   (e) windsurfing
   (f) rock climbing
   (g) mountain biking.

3.4 Maintaining the Safety of Participants and Colleagues in a Sports Environment

P4 M3 D2

The general manager and his team of managers of a sport or leisure facility are responsible for running a safe and secure environment. They will ensure that every member of staff receives training on how the facility operates, as well as two manuals that provide information on how every part of the facility should operate under normal conditions and what to do in an emergency situation – these are usually referred to as Normal Operating Procedures (NOP) and Emergency Operating Procedures (EOP).

The NOP provides instructions on how to deal with everyday situations, whereas the EOP provides instructions on how to deal with minor and major emergency situations, such as disorderly behaviour from customers or dealing with a drowning incident.

Normal Operating Procedures (NOP)

This document contains details of all the services the leisure facility provides (e.g. swimming pool dimensions, squash courts and their dimensions) and is specific to that individual facility.

The manual will indicate any potential risk factors and hazards that staff should be aware of. These may include:

- **Known hazards** (e.g. unruly behaviour by the customer, customers with prior health problems, misuse of equipment)

- **Pool hazards** (e.g. slippery poolside, diving in shallow water, blind spots in the pool)
- **Customers at risk** (e.g. weak swimmers, elderly customers, customers under the influence of alcohol or drugs).

There follow instructions on how to carry out risk assessments so that these hazards and risks can be minimised.

Methods of dealing with the public will be included in the manual, which incorporates forms of communication and rules and regulations that customers must adhere to; an example of this is the poolside rules (e.g. no running on the poolside, no pushing, no ducking).

Staff duties and responsibilities are also covered. The manual will contain details of what is expected from them (e.g. they should wear the uniform provided, lifeguards must always carry a whistle, they must never leave a pool area unattended). There are usually details of staff training requirements too (e.g. a lifeguard will usually be required to attend training sessions at least once a month so that their skills are up to date and have been practised recently).

Details of staffing requirements for a range of situations are usually included within this document (e.g. supervision of diving, the number of lifeguards required on the poolside in relation to the number of swimmers – the more swimmers there are, the more lifeguards need to be on duty).

Pool, sports hall and changing room hygiene is also an area that should be covered in this document, which gives instructions on how to carry out everyday cleaning duties. Details of first-aid supplies and how to locate a first-aider will also be in this document.

All leisure facilities will have some form of alarm system to summon help or warn people of a fire; the NOP will contain details of where these alarms are located and how to use them.

Emergency Operating Procedures (EOP)

This manual details how staff should respond to a range of emergency situations:

- Fire
- Customer suffering from a minor injury (e.g. grazed knee)
- Customer suffering from a major injury (e.g. knocked unconscious with a head injury)
- How to deal with a drowning incident
- Bomb threat
- Emission of a toxic gas
- Structural failure
- Spinal injury
- How to deal with blood, vomit and faeces.

Staff Training

Most centres will ensure their staff are up to date with their role requirements and that their qualifications are up to date, either by running in-house training or by paying for their staff to attend relevant training events elsewhere. Pool lifeguards will often be expected to attend weekly training events to ensure they are able to carry out all the different rescue techniques. In most centres, all staff will be expected to have a basic first-aid award, and will be expected to attend regular training events to ensure their first-aid skills are up to date. Staff meetings are often held on a weekly basis to update staff on any centre changes or staffing changes, and so on.

Checking Facilities

There should be regular inspections to ensure the facility is functioning as it should be. Some checks may be required on a regular basis throughout the day, and others may need to be performed at the start and end of each day. For example, examining the changing facilities to ensure they are clean and tidy, and testing the swimming pool water to assess the chlorine levels, should be carried out once every few hours; checking that all the lights are working inside and outside the building only really needs to be carried out once or twice a day.

All sports and leisure facilities have regular inspections from various authorities to ensure that the organisation is maintaining a high level of health and safety. For example, the fire department will check such things as the number and functioning of fire extinguishers and that the fire exits are easily accessible.

Equipment should be checked regularly. Although there is not a legal requirement to inspect the equipment, a centre could be prosecuted if there

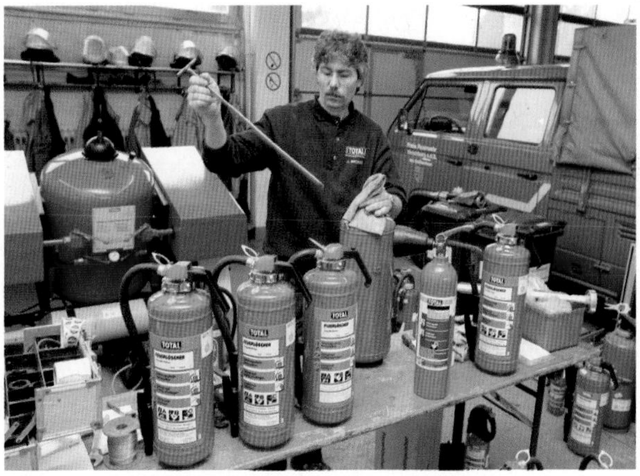

Fig 3.6 A person from the fire department checking equipment

was an accident due to faulty equipment. A typical pro forma for checking equipment should have the following headings:

- Name of equipment
- When equipment was checked
- Name of person checking equipment
- Any action taken
- Signature of the inspector
- Results of check.

Key learning points 3

- All staff have a job specification to work to, and must follow normal procedures and emergency procedures as documented in their work handbook.
- People working in a leisure or sport facility must maintain a secure and safe environment for their customers and staff.

Student activity 3.4

60–90 mins P4 M3 D2

Task 1

Go into your local sports facility or leisure centre and ask if you may have a look at its NOP and EOP. If you are able to do so, look through them and make a note of the information they contain.

Task 2

Select three different procedures used in the sports facility that you have investigated to promote and maintain a healthy and safe sporting environment. Write a report that describes, explains and analyses each procedure.

3.5 Planning a Safe Sporting Activity

P5 M4 D3

When planning a sporting activity, you will need to determine the roles and responsibilities of each member of the group.

Roles and Responsibilities

The leader of the activity is responsible for the planning and preparation and the smooth running of the event. Prior to the activity, the leader should:

- Determine who will be taking part in the activity
- Undertake a risk assessment of the proposed activity
- Determine the staffing requirements of the activity – this should include an appropriate number of qualified first-aiders
- Ensure that you or your centre has adequate insurance to run the activity
- Plan transport arrangements, if required
- Visit the site or facility where you plan to hold the activity
- Plan contingency and emergency arrangements
- Inform parents of any children taking part in the activity and obtain parental and medical consent.

The Site, Equipment and First-aid Provision

The site chosen must be suitable for the activity. If it is an indoor event, you must ensure that the facility is an appropriate size, that it has suitable lighting, suitable changing facilities, first-aid provision, all the equipment you require, and so on. Basically, it has to suit the needs of the chosen activity and the needs of the participants, and still adhere to health and safety guidelines. If the activity is to be held outside, you should always take into account environmental factors that may adversely affect your activity. For example, a lot of rain could waterlog a sports field, which could then become dangerous to play on. Always have a contingency plan that allows you to run an activity but does not put the participants' health at risk. For example, a football game that was due to be played outside could be changed to a five-a-side match inside.

It is important that all equipment is checked prior to being used to ensure that it is complete, in working order and not faulty or damaged.

Adequate arrangements must be made for first aid, including responsible people, equipment and facilities.

You should always carry a basic first-aid kit with you, or ensure you have access to one when you are running a sports activity. A basic first-aid kit should contain:

- Ten plasters of various sizes

- Two large sterile dressings for the management of severe bleeding
- One medium sterile dressing for the care of larger wounds
- Four triangular bandages to support suspected broken bones, dislocations or sprains
- One eye pad in case of a cut to the eye
- Four safety pins to secure dressings
- Disposable gloves.

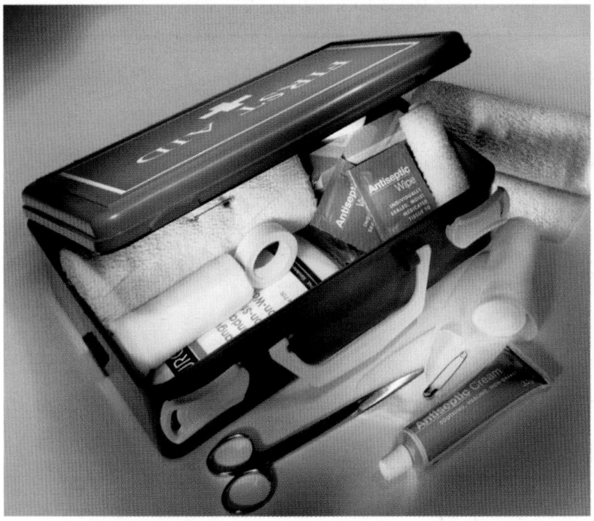

Fig 3.7 A first-aid kit

Suitability of Participants to the Activity

One of the main factors to help determine the suitability of a participant is to consider their age. If the participants are people of a different age to yourself, you should always speak to a person who has experience of dealing with this age group. You can then discuss your idea for your activity and determine whether it is suitable. From this you will be able to gauge what sort of equipment you should use, any adaptations required to make the activity more suitable and the staffing ratio required.

For example, if you wanted to run a cricket activity with (a) primary-school-aged children or (b) a group of 18-year-olds, you would have very different plans.

For the primary-school-aged children, you would use soft balls because hard balls would be more likely to cause injuries, as the children are less experienced in throwing and catching compared with most adults. You would probably adapt the game so that more people are active more of the time (e.g. you may have four teams of eight children playing quick cricket). You would need more staff to supervise the children to ensure their health and safety.

For a group of 18-year-olds you would use the usual cricket equipment, the game would be played to the usual cricket rules, and the only staffing required would be to umpire the event and ensure there is appropriate first-aid provision.

Health and Safety Review

After an event has taken place, you should always review your health and safety planning and procedures to see whether they were effective or if they could be improved. Examine if there were any injuries or near misses, how they occurred and if you could have done anything to reduce the likelihood of each incident happening. Determine if the participants were a suitable group for the activity: Were they the right age, of the right ability, and so on? Did the staff receive a suitable briefing so that they were able to carry out their roles and responsibilities effectively? Was the equipment suitable? Could you have used anything else to improve the health and safety of the participants during the activity?

This information will help you to improve your awareness of health and safety, and to ensure that you are doing everything possible to reduce risks and maintain the health and safety of yourself and others.

Key learning points 4

- In order to pay full attention to health and safety, a sporting activity should be planned effectively, with attention given to risk assessments, equipment, the site, the participants, first-aid provision, contingency plans, and the roles and responsibilities of each team member.

Student activity 3.5

60 minutes P5 M4

Task 1

Select a sports activity of your choice. Produce and write a report to explain a plan for this sports activity that takes into account a range of different health and safety procedures.

Task 2

Write a report that reviews the plan you have produced, to determine how effective it is in managing the associated risks involved in the selected sports activity and the suitability of the participants, site and equipment used.

Useful websites

www.safesport.co.uk

Advice and safety tips on a wide range of sports & athletic abilities

http://www.uka.org.uk/governance/health-safety/

Advice on carrying out a risk assessment for sports; includes a sample template for an online incident report form

4: Fitness Training & Programming

4.1 Introduction

Developing the correct training programme is vital to the success of the individual athlete and the team. Top-class athletes build their life around the requirements of their fitness training and have a dedicated coach for this purpose. Fitness will be important to any individual who is involved in physical activity to give them the best chances to succeed.

By the end of this unit you should:

- know different methods of fitness training
- be able to plan a fitness training session
- be able to review a fitness training programme.

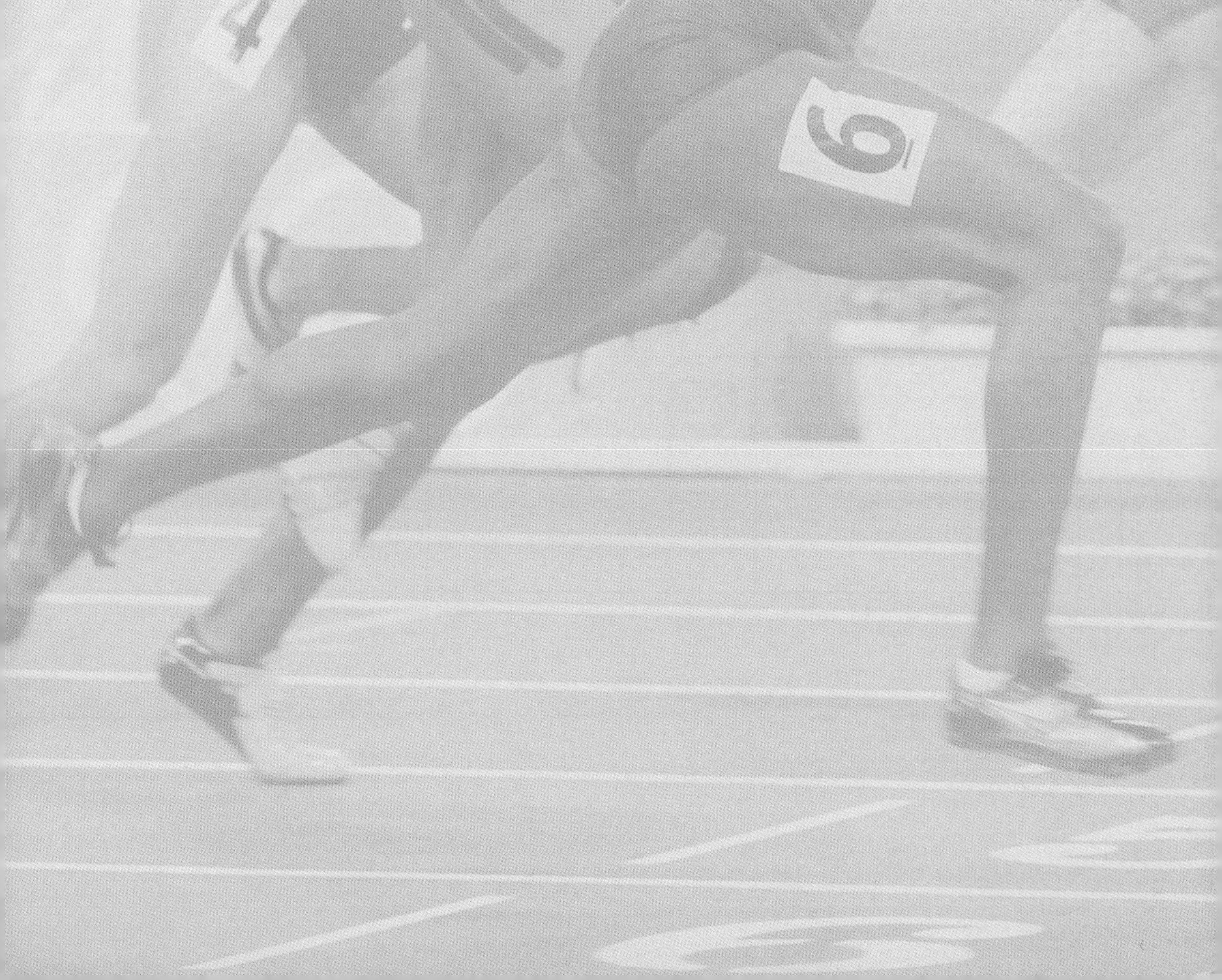

Assessment and grading criteria		
To achieve a PASS grade the evidence must show that the learner is able to:	**To achieve a MERIT grade the evidence must show that, in addition to the pass criteria, the learner is able to:**	**To achieve a DISTINCTION grade the evidence must show that, in addition to the pass and merit criteria, the learner is able to:**
P1 describe one method of fitness training for six different components of physical fitness	**M1** explain one method of fitness training for six different components of physical fitness	
P2 produce training session plans covering cardiovascular training, resistance training, flexibility training and speed training	**M2** produce detailed session plans covering cardiovascular training, resistance training, flexibility training and speed training	**D1** justify the training session plans covering cardiovascular training, resistance training, flexibility training and speed training
P3 produce a six-week fitness training programme for a selected individual that incorporates the principles of training and periodisation		
P4 monitor performance against goals during the six-week training programme		
P5 give feedback to an individual following completion of a six-week fitness training programme, describing strengths and areas for improvement.	**M3** give feedback to an individual following completion of a six-week fitness training programme, explaining strengths and areas for improvement.	**D2** give feedback to an individual following completion of a six-week fitness training programme, evaluating progress and providing recommendations for future activities.

4.2 Different Methods of Fitness Training

P1 M1

Components of Fitness

Fitness can mean different things to different people and has been defined in different ways. When we examine fitness we need to ask 'What does this person have to be fit for?' or 'What functions does this person have to perform?' From this starting point we can build up a picture of their fitness requirements and then look at what can be done to develop their fitness.

Fitness is defined by the American College of Sports Medicine (ACSM) (1990) as:

> 'a set of attributes that people have or achieve that relate to their ability to perform physical activity.'

Fitness is clearly related to performance and developing the attributes to achieve this performance.

Physical Fitness

Physical fitness can be seen to be made up of the following factors.

Aerobic endurance is also called cardiovascular fitness or stamina. It is the individual's ability to take on, transport and utilise oxygen. It is a measure of how well the lungs can take in oxygen, how well the heart and blood can transport oxygen, and then how well the muscles can use oxygen. When working aerobically we tend to perform repetitive activities using large muscle groups in a rhythmical manner for long periods of time.

Muscular endurance is how well the muscles can produce repeated contractions at less than maximal (submaximal) intensities. When training for muscular endurance we usually do sets of 15 to 20 repetitions. Most movements we produce in sport and everyday activities will be at submaximal intensities and all people will benefit from muscular endurance training.

Flexibility is the range of motion that a joint or group of joints can move through. Flexibility is often not given the amount of attention it should have in a training programme because people do not always see its importance. However, improving flexibility can improve performance because a greater range of motion will result in greater power development and will help to prevent injury and pain caused through restrictions in movement.

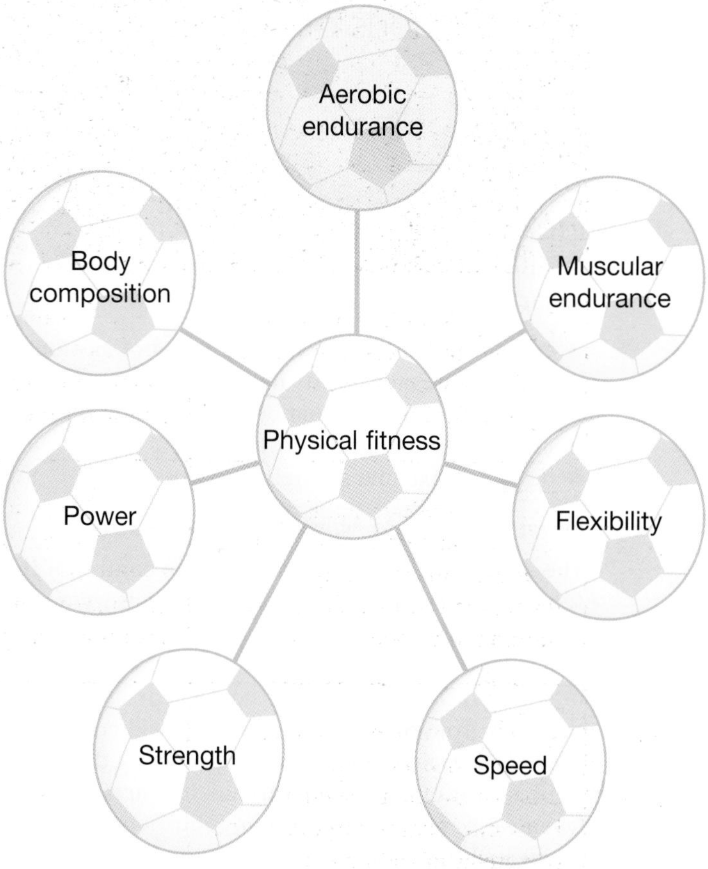

Fig 4.1 Physical fitness

Speed is the rate at which the body or individual limbs can move.

Strength is the maximum force a muscle or group of muscles can produce in a single contraction. Heavy weight lifting or moving a heavy object will require strength. For example, if you have to push-start a car the success or failure of this effort will be an expression of your muscular strength. To train for strength we usually do sets of 1 to 5 repetitions.

Power is the production of strength at speed and can be seen when we throw an object or perform a sprint start. To move a heavy load quickly we need to use our power. Activities such as jumping to head a ball or a long jump will require us to express our power.

4.3 Methods of Physical Fitness Training

P1 M1

Flexibility Training

Flexibility is the 'range of motion available at a joint' and is needed in sports to:

- enable the athlete to have the range of motion to perform the movements needed
- prevent the athlete from becoming injured
- maintain and improve posture
- develop maximum strength and power.

What Happens to Muscles When we Stretch?

The stretching of muscles is under the control of the sensory nerves. There are two types of sensory nerves which are involved in allowing muscles to stretch and relax. They are muscle spindles and Golgi tendon organs (GTOs). The sensory nerves work to protect the body from becoming injured and will contract if they think a muscle is at risk of becoming damaged. This is one of our basic survival instincts because when we were hunter-gatherers injury would render us incapable of finding food and our families would starve.

The muscle spindles are sensory receptors which become activated as the muscle lengthens (due to its potential danger). When the muscle has reached a certain length they tell the nervous system to contract the muscle and prevent it being stretched any further. This protects the muscle against damage. If you perform the patella knee tap test this activates the muscle spindles. When this test is conducted, the knee extends due to the contraction of the quadriceps muscle activated by the muscle spindle. This is also called 'the myotatic stretch reflex'.

When we stretch a muscle we try to avoid this by stretching in a slow and controlled manner. The muscle spindles contract the muscle, which makes it feel uncomfortable or slightly painful. This is called the 'point of bind' where the muscle has contracted to avoid any damage.

When the point of bind is reached the stretch should be held for around ten seconds. This is because after ten seconds the muscle will relax and the pain will disappear. This relaxation is brought on by the action of the GTOs. GTOs are found in tendons and they sense how much tension there is in the muscle. Once the GTOs sense that the muscle is not in danger of damage they will override the muscle spindles and cause the muscle to relax. This is the effect that you want a stretch to have; it is called 'the inverse stretch reflex'. Once the muscle has relaxed you can either stop the stretch there or stretch the muscle a bit more until the point of bind is reached again and the process starts again.

There are various methods of stretching muscles.

Static Stretching

This is when a muscle is stretched in a steady, controlled manner and then held in a static or still position. It is taken to the point where the muscle contracts and a slight pain is felt. This is called 'the point of bind'. At this point the stretch is held until the muscle relaxes and the discomfort disappears.

A static stretch can be a maintenance stretch or a developmental stretch. A maintenance stretch is held until the discomfort disappears and then the stretch is stopped. A developmental stretch is different because when the muscle relaxes and the discomfort disappears the stretch is applied further to a second point. It is taken to a point when the discomfort is felt again, it is held until the muscle relaxes and then applied again. It lasts for around 30 seconds while a maintenance stretch will last for around 10 seconds.

Proprioceptive Neuromuscular Facilitation

This type of stretching, known as PNF, is an advanced type of stretching in order to develop the length of the muscle. It needs two people to be involved: one person to do the stretching and one to be stretched.

It is carried out in the following way.

- The muscle is stretched to the point of bind by the trainer.
- At this point the trainer asks the athlete to contract the muscle and push against them at about 40 to 50 per cent effort.
- This contraction is held for 10 seconds.
- When the muscle is relaxed the trainer stretches the muscle further.
- Again a contraction is applied and then the muscle is re-stretched.
- This is done three times.

This is a more effective way of developing the length of the muscle as the contraction will actually cause the muscle to relax more quickly and more deeply.

Ballistic Stretching

This means a 'bouncing' stretch as the muscle is forced beyond its point of stretch by a bouncing movement. Ballistic stretches are performed in a rapid, repetitive bouncing movement. It is a high-risk method of stretching due to the risk of muscular damage but it may be used in specific sports such as gymnastics. It must never be used on people training for health and fitness reasons rather than sports.

Resistance Training

Resistance training means using any form of resistance to place an increased load on a muscle or muscle group. Resistance training can be done to develop muscular endurance, strength or power depending upon the number of repetitions chosen, resistance chosen and speed the movements are performed at. Muscular endurance training involves a high number of repetitions (12–20) performed with relatively low weights, while strength training involves low repetitions (1–5) with relatively heavy weights and power training is performed by moving weights at speed so involve low repetitions (1–5) with relatively heavy weights.

Resistance can be applied through any of the following methods:

- free weights
- resistance machines
- cable machines
- gravity
- medicine balls
- air
- water
- resistance bands
- manually.

The following are popular methods of resistance training:

- resistance machines
- free weights
- cables
- plyometrics
- circuit training.

A range of resistance machines have been developed to train muscle groups in isolation. They were originally developed for body builders but their ease of use and safety factors make them a feature of every gym in the country. These machines target individual muscles and replicate the joint actions these muscles produce.

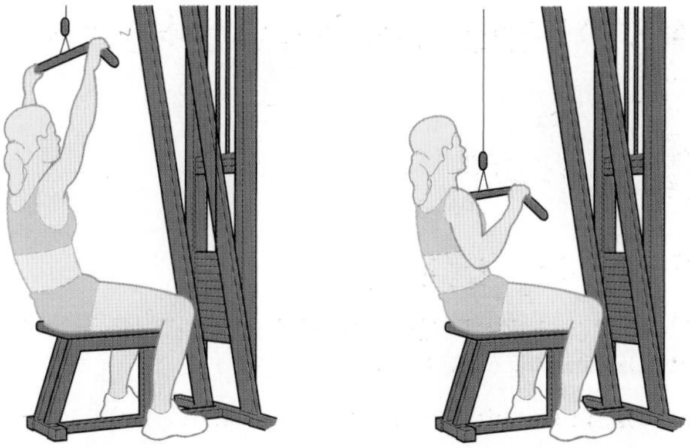

Fig 4.2 Resistance training with a machine

Free weights involve barbells and dumbbells and are seen to have advantages over resistance machines. Mainly, they allow a person to work in their own range of movement rather than the way a machine wants them to work. Also, when a person does free weights they have to use many more muscles to stabilise the body before the force is applied. This is particularly so if the person performs the exercise standing up. They also have more 'functional crossover' in that they can replicate movements that will be used in sports and daily life. This is seen as a huge advantage.

Cable machines are becoming increasingly popular because, again, they involve the use of many more muscles than resistance machines, and therefore burn up more calories. Once again, they can produce

Objective	Muscular strength	Muscle hypertrophy	Muscular endurance	Power
Repetitions or duration	1–5	6–12	12–20	1–2 for single-effort events 3–5 for multiple-effort events
Recovery period	3–5 mins	1–2 mins	30–60 secs	2–5 mins
Sets per exercise	2–6	3–6	2–3	3–5
Frequency per week	1–2 on each muscle group	1–2 on each muscle group	2–3 on each muscle group	1–2 sessions

Table 4.1 Shows the repetition ranges for targeting components of fitness.
(Adapted from Baechle and Earle, 2000)

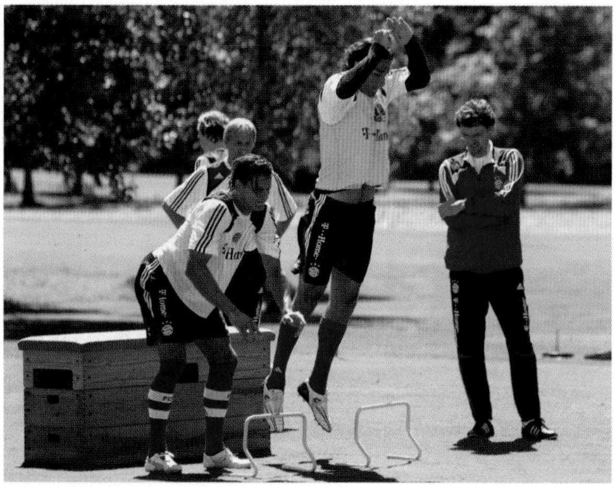

Fig 4.3 Depth jumping is one example of plyometric activity

movements that are not possible on resistance machines. For example, a golfer will need to perform rotation-type movements and can do these on cable machines.

Plyometrics

Plyometric training develops power, which is producing strength at speed. It usually involves moving your body weight very quickly through jumping or bounding. Any sport that involves jumping in the air or moving the body forwards at pace will need power training.

Examples of plyometric training include:

- jumping on to boxes and over hurdles
- depth jumping
- vertical jumps and standing long jump
- medicine ball throws
- hopping
- bounding
- squat and jump
- press-up and clap.

It is a very strenuous type of training and an athlete must have well-developed strength before performing plyometrics. Before you take a plyometric session you must make sure the athlete is well warmed up and that you have checked the equipment and the surfaces thoroughly. Ideally, you should use a sprung floor or a soft surface.

Circuit Training

A circuit is a series of exercises arranged in a specific order and performed one after the other. There are normally eight to twelve stations set out and organised so that each muscle group is worked in rotation. Each exercise is performed for a certain number of repetitions or a set time period. Circuits are used predominantly to develop muscular endurance or aerobic fitness – this depends upon the resistances used, the speed of the movements and the length of time on each station. For muscular endurance the participant works flat out on each station for about 30 seconds, while to develop aerobic endurance the time period on each station is increased to 45 seconds with a slower speed of movement. They can be made specific to various sports by including exercises for the muscles used in that sport and some of the skills specific to that sport.

When planning a circuit you need to ask several questions:

- What is the objective of the session?
- How many participants will I have?
- What is their level of fitness?
- How much space have I got?
- What equipment is available?

A basic circuit session should contain exercise to improve aerobic fitness or raise the pulse rate, exercises to work the upper body, lower body and the core. When designing the circuit layout be careful not to place all the exercises for the same muscle group beside each other as this will cause undue fatigue. The circuit should follow the normal structure of a routine:

- warm-up
- main session
- cool-down
- flexibility.

The warm-up will include a pulse raiser, mobility and dynamic stretches. For example:

- walk
- walk with bicep curls and shoulder presses
- slow jog with shoulder circles
- jog
- dynamic stretches such as squat and press, step back and chest stretch
- jog with knee raises and heel flicks
- run
- jumps and hops
- sprint.

The main session should include eight to twelve exercises from Table 4.2.

Aerobic fitness or pulse raisers	Shuttle runs Skipping Box step-ups Box jumps Jumping jacks Star jumps Spotty dogs Grapevines
Upper body	Press-ups Bench press with dumbbells Cable seated rows Bent-over row Shoulder press Bicep curls Tricep curls Lateral raises Dumbbell pullovers Medicine ball chest passes Medicine ball chest pass & press-up Medicine ball overhead throws
Lower body	Squats Lunges Split squats Side lunges Squat thrusts Hurdle jumps Ladder work Step-ups with dumbbells
Core exercises	Swiss ball curls Swiss ball back extension Plank Bridge Superman Rotations with medicine ball Medicine ball rotate and throw

Table 4.2

The cool-down should progressively lower the pulse, but it can be combined with some stretching as well. It could follow this example:

- run (1 minute)
- jog (1 minute)
- brisk walk (1 minute)
- stretch trapezius, pectoralis major, latissimus dorsi, triceps, deltoids
- standing stretches of adductors, calves and quads
- kneeling stretches of hip flexors and lower back
- lying stretches of hamstrings and gluteus medius and minimus.

Aerobic Endurance Training

Continuous training is also called 'steady-state' training and involves an individual maintaining a steady pace for a long period of time. To be effective it needs to be done for a period of over 20 minutes. It is useful for developing a strong base of aerobic fitness, but it will not develop speed or strength.

While continuous training has a role to play it can be limited in its benefits, particularly if the athlete does the same session each time they train. While initially it will have given them fitness gains there will be limited benefits after about four weeks once the body has adapted to the work. It may also produce boredom and a loss of motivation to train.

Interval training is described as having the following features: 'a structured period of work followed by a structured period of rest'. In other words, an athlete runs quickly for a period of time and then rests at a much lower intensity before speeding up again. This type of training has the benefit of improving speed as well as aerobic fitness. Interval training also allows the athlete to train at higher intensities than they are used to, and thus steadily increase their fitness level and the intensity they can work at. The theory is that you will be able to run faster in competition only if you train faster – and interval training allows this to occur. Intervals can be used to improve performance for athletes and fitness levels for people involved in exercise.

Interval training can be stressful to the systems of the body and it is important to ensure that an individual has a good aerobic base before raising the intensity of the training.

Once an athlete has reached the limit of their aerobic system they will start to gain extra energy from their anaerobic system (lactic acid system); this is demonstrated by an increased accumulation of lactic acid in the blood. The point where blood lactic acid levels start to rise is called the lactate threshold. Interval training can be designed to push an athlete beyond their lactate threshold and then reduce the exercise intensity below the lactate threshold. This has the effect of enabling the athlete to become better at tolerating the effects of lactic acid and also increasing the intensity they work at before lactic acid is produced. Well-designed interval training sessions can produce this desirable effect.

The intensity of interval training is higher than continuous work and thus there will be more energy production to sustain this high-intensity work. More energy production equals more calories burnt during training, which could lead to a faster loss of body fat (if the nutritional strategy is appropriate). As the intensity is higher more waste products are built up, resulting in a greater oxygen debt and a longer period of recovery. This longer period of recovery results in more oxygen being used post-exercise and more energy used to recover. Therefore, more energy is used during exercise and also after exercise, multiplying the potential effects of fat loss.

The main benefits of interval training are:

- improved speed
- improved strength
- improved aerobic endurance
- improved ability to tolerate the effects of lactic acid
- increased fat burning potential
- increased calorie output
- improved performance.

Interval training can be used to develop aerobic fitness as well as anaerobic fitness. When designing interval training sessions you need to consider how long the periods of work are in relation to the periods of rest. The following are recommended guidelines for training with each of the three energy systems.

- Aerobic interval: 1 or half a unit of rest for every unit of work.
- Lactic acid intervals: 2 to 3 units of rest for 1 unit of work.
- ATP/CP intervals: 6 units of rest for 1 unit of work.

As the intensity increases, more rest is required to guarantee the quality of each interval. If you were training for aerobic fitness you may do four minutes' work then have two minutes' rest (1:1/2). If you were training for lactic acid intervals you would have one minute's work and two or three minutes' rest.

Sample Aerobic Interval Session

First estimate the maximum heart rate as 220 minus age and then you can work out the percentage of maximum heart rate.

For a 20 year old:
Maximum heart rate = 220 − 20 = 200 bpm
70% of max HR = 200 × 0.7 = 140 bpm
80% of max HR = 200 × 0.8 = 160 bpm
90% of max HR = 200 × 0.9 = 180 bpm

You will need to find out what workload (speed) produces each heart rate when you are running.

Basic interval
Work = 4 minutes   Rest = 2 minutes
4 sets of 4 minutes at 70% effort with 2 minutes' rest in between

Pyramid interval
Work = 3 minutes   Rest = 1.5 minutes

Warm-up
3 mins @ 80% of max HR

Rest
3 mins @ 85% of max HR

Rest
3 mins @ 90% of max HR

Rest
3 mins @ 85% of max HR

Rest
3 mins @ 80% of max HR

Cool-down

Treadmill hills pyramid
Find the speed that produces 70% of max HR and stay at this speed throughout the interval programme; then vary the gradient on the treadmill.

Work = 2 mins   Rest = 1 min

Warm-up
2 mins @ 2% gradient

Rest
2 mins @ 4% gradient

Rest
2 mins @ 6% gradient

Rest
2 mins @ 4% gradient

Rest
2 mins @ 2% gradient

Cool-down

Alternately the gradients could be set at 3%, 6%, 9%, 6% and 3%.

Sample Anaerobic Session

Lactic Acid System

6 sets of 45 seconds (or 300 m) at 90–95% effort with 90 seconds' rest
4 sets of 75 seconds (or 500 m) at 80–85% effort with 150 seconds' rest

ATP/PC System

10 sets of 50 metres at 100% effort with 1 minute rest

Fartlek is a Swedish term; it literally means 'speed play' and it involves an athlete going out and running at a range of different speeds for a period of 20 to 30 minutes. This type of training is excellent for replicating the demands of a sport such as football, rugby or hockey where different types of running are required at different times. It can be used to develop aerobic or anaerobic fitness depending on the intensity of the running. It can also be used in cycling or rowing training. Fartlek running involves finding a base speed at around 60 to 70 per cent of maximum intensity and then fast bursts of work at 75, 80, 85 and 90 per cent mixed up into longer or shorter time periods. It can be used to challenge the different energy systems and demands of sports as well as reducing the boredom of training for long periods of time.

Core Stability

If we were to take our arms and legs off our body we would be left with the body's core, which can be said to be the working foundation of the body and is responsible for providing the base to develop power. If we have a strong core we will be able to generate more force and power through the arms and legs; this is important when we kick a football or hit a tennis ball.

The body is made up of layers of muscles and the abdominal area is no different as it has deep, middle and outer layers which work together to provide stability.

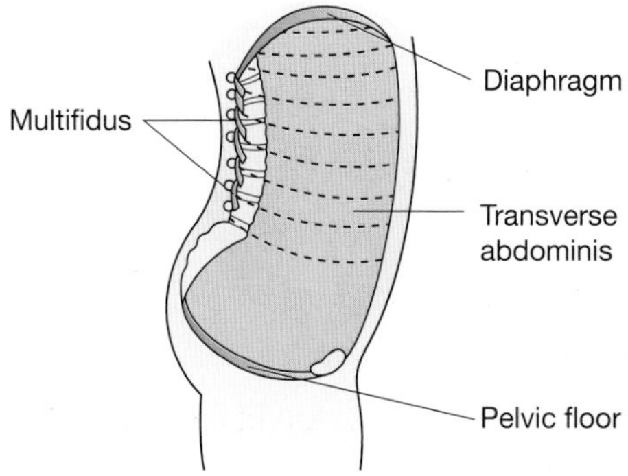

Fig 4.4 Outer layer of core muscles

The outer layer of muscles are the best known abdominal muscles with the rectus abdominis at the front, the erector spinae at the back and the internal and external obliques at the sides.

The middle layer is deeper muscle, which forms a cylinder or unit around the vertebrae. At the top we have the diaphragm and at the bottom the pelvic floor muscles, while across the back we have the multifidus, and around the front and sides we have the transverse abdominis (TVA). The TVA is the key muscle here and is described as being 'the natural weight belt' because a weight belt replicates its shape and function.

The role of the inner muscles is to stabilise the vertebrae, ribs and pelvis to provide the stable working base or foundation. These muscles contract a fraction of a second before the arms or legs are moved when the body is functioning correctly. If this does not happen the chances of damaging the spine are increased.

The deep layer is tiny muscles which sense the position of the vertebrae and control their movement to keep them in the strongest position and prevent injury.

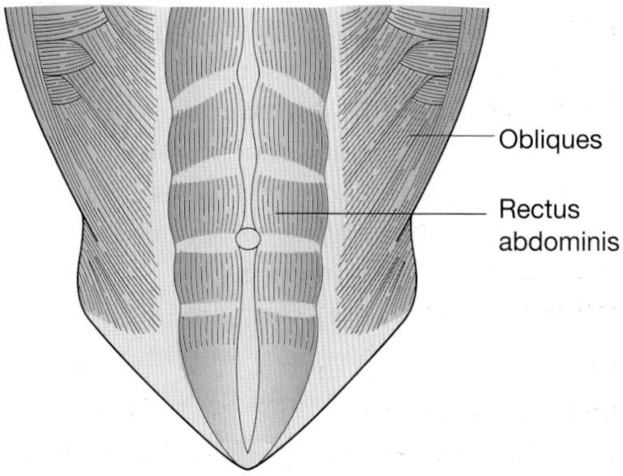

Fig 4.5 Inner layer of core muscles

Activating the core muscles can be done in two ways. First, by hollowing or pulling in the abdominals or by bracing, which means contracting the muscles without them moving out or in. Different trainers will recommend different techniques depending upon their own experiences and training.

Abdominal Training

The concepts of abdominal training are changing rapidly. The traditional method has been to do hundreds of sit-ups in pursuit of a perfect six-pack and then, in the late 1990s, abdominal cradles were introduced into gyms to aid people further. The 2000s have seen the introduction of Swiss balls and functional abdominal exercises into training programmes. There is still some confusion over what is the best way to train the abdominals. We need to look at a couple of misconceptions first before looking at what is the best way to train.

'Sit-ups will help me lose fat in the abdominal area'

No, you cannot spot-reduce fat because the muscle below the abdominal fat is separate from the fat itself and you can never be sure from where the losses in fat due to exercise will come. The way to lose abdominal fat is to increase activity level and have a correct nutritional strategy.

'Sit-ups will give me the six-pack I want'

Not necessarily, because overdoing abdominal work can cause a shortening of the abdominal muscles and pull your posture forwards, making the abdominal area shorter, squeezing the fat together and making you look fatter. In fact, if you perform back extensions it will make your posture more upright and help to keep the abdominals contracted and make them look more toned.

'Sit-ups are the best abdominal exercise'

This is debatable because sit-ups produce concentric and eccentric muscular contractions. The abdominals will contract isometrically when we train and move around in daily life. Therefore, surely we should replicate this isometric contraction when we train as it will have the best 'functional crossover' to daily life.

When we train the core muscles we need to target the deeper muscles; this is done by producing isometric or static contractions.

Any exercise where you are standing up or supporting your body weight will be a core exercise. For example, a press-up is an excellent core exercise because the core muscles work to keep the back straight and the back will start to sag when these muscles become fatigued. All standing free weight and cable exercises require the core to stabilise the vertebrae while they are being performed. However, there are some specific core exercises that can be performed (see Figure 4.6).

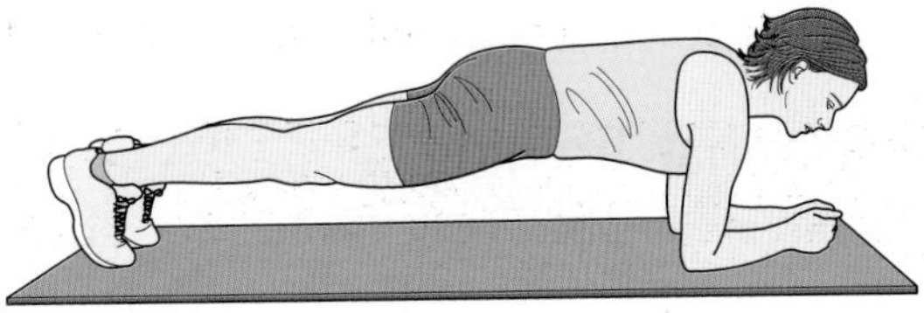

Fig 4.6a Plank

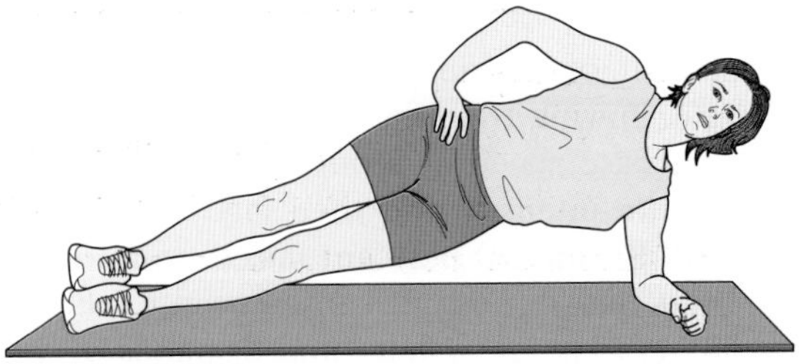

Fig 4.6b Side plank

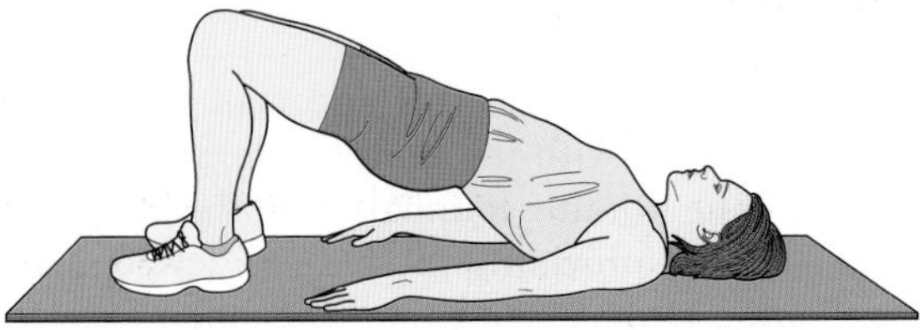

Fig 4.6c Bridge

The use of a Swiss ball to perform exercises requires an extra load on the core muscles and works them harder, as will using cables to exercise.

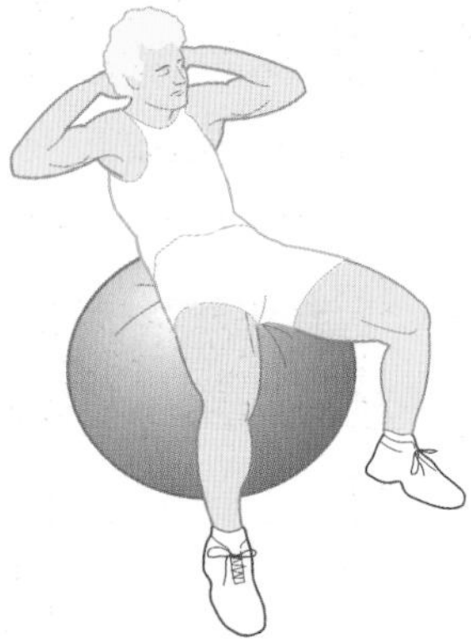

Fig 4.7 Swiss ball abdominal crunches

Q Quick quiz 1

Match the following: (a) the definition to the component of fitness and (b) the training method to the correct component of fitness that it works on.

Component of fitness	Definitions	Training methods
Aerobic endurance		
Muscular endurance		
Flexibility		
Speed		
Strength		
Power		

(a) Choices of definition
- The range of motion a joint or group of joints can move through
- The ability to take on, transport and utilise oxygen
- The rate that individual limbs can move
- The production of strength at speed
- The maximum force a muscle or group of muscles can produce in a single contraction
- The ability of muscles to produce repeated contractions

(b) Training methods
- plyometrics
- PNF stretching
- Resistance training (high weights, low repetitions)
- Resistance training (Low weights, high repetitions)
- Steady state running
- Interval training.

Student activity 4.1

40 minutes P2 M1

Methods of fitness training

Complete the table below to describe and explain different methods of fitness training for six different components of fitness.

Component of fitness	Describe one method of fitness training for this component	Explain one method of fitness training for this component
Aerobic endurance		
Muscular endurance	E.g. Resistance training, which would be 8–10 exercises with a low weight but high repetitions.	E.g. Resistance training on free weights, resistance machines or cables using a low weight (about 60–70 of maximum) and high repetitions (12–20). Working all muscle groups and doing 2–3 sets per exercise.
Flexibility		
Speed		
Strength		
Power		

4.4 Planning a Fitness Training Session

P2 M2 D1

Principles of Training

To develop a safe and effective training programme you will need to consider the principles of training. These principles are a set of guidelines to help you understand the requirements of programme design. The principles of training are:

- Frequency
- Intensity
- Time
- Type
- Overload
- Reversibility
- Specificity.

Frequency means how often the athlete will train per week, month or year. It is recommended that a beginner trains three times a week while a competitive athlete may train ten or twelve times a week.

Intensity is how hard the athlete works for each repetition. It is usually expressed as a percentage of maximum intensity. Intensity can be increased by adding more weight to be lifted, or increasing speed or gradient on the treadmill.

Time indicates how long they train for in each session. The recommended length of a training session is around 45 minutes before fatiguing waste products build up and affect training technique.

Type shows the type of training they will perform and needs to be individual to each person. A training effect can be achieved by varying the exercises an individual does – moving them from a treadmill to a rower, or a seated chest press to a free weight bench press.

Overload shows that to make an improvement a muscle or system must work slightly harder than it is used to. The weight that produces overload depends upon what the individual is currently used to at that moment. This may be as simple as getting a sedentary person walking for ten minutes or getting an athlete to squat more weight than they have previously. Overload can be achieved by changing the intensity, duration, time or type of an exercise. Reversibility says that if a fitness gain is not used regularly the body will reverse it and go back to its previous fitness level. Any adaptation which occurs is not permanent. The rule is commonly known as 'use it or lose it'.

Specificity states that any fitness gain will be specific to the muscles or system to which the overload is applied. Put simply, this says that different types of training will produce different results. To make a programme specific you need to look at the needs of the athletes in that sport and then train them accordingly. For example, a footballer would need to run at different speeds and have lots of changes of direction. A golfer would need to do rotational work but sprinting speed would not be so important. A runner would need to do running predominantly, and they may get some aerobic gain from swimming or cycling but it would not achieve the best result.

There are other principles too.

Progressive Overload

To ensure an athlete continues to gain fitness they need to keep overloading their muscles and systems. This continued increase in intensity (how hard they work) is called progressive overload. If you keep training at the same intensity and duration the body will reach a plateau where no further fitness gains are made. Therefore, it is important to keep manipulating all the training variables to keep gaining adaptations.

Who Will You Train?

You need to be prepared to train a range of individuals including elite performers, trained or well conditioned individuals and untrained or de-conditioned individuals. You may also train individuals who are training for a specific sport or have special requirements or medical conditions. You will have been able to identify the strengths and weaknesses of each individual by carrying out the health screening questionnaire, performing the static health tests and the dynamic fitness on the individual and then analysing their strengths and areas that need improvement.

Planning the Programme

Once you have identified the training needs of the individual through the screening process then you can design their training programme. Each programme will have a different content dependent upon the goals of the individual; however, the structure of the training programmes will be fairly similar. It should look like Table 4.3.

Type of training	Description of amount	Guidance
CV training – warm up	3–5 minutes	This involves a gradual increase of intensity to raise the heart rate steadily
Flexibility	2–3 dynamic stretches	These stretches involve moving the joints and muscles through the full range of movement in a controlled manner to replicate movements coming up in the main session
Resistance 1	4–5 exercises to cover the main muscle groups (pecs, lats, glutes, quads and hamstrings)	Sets and repetitions are dependent upon the training goals of the individual. Exercises could include free weights, resistance machines or cable exercises
CV training	Between 5 and 20 minutes, dependent upon the goals of the individual	Could involve steady state work or intervals. It may be done for speed or aerobic endurance and involve running, rowing or cycling
Resistance 2	4–5 exercises to cover a selection of the minor muscle groups (biceps, triceps, deltoids, claves)	Sets and repetitions are dependent upon the training goals of the individual. Exercises could include free weights, resistance machines or cable exercises
CV training	Between 5 and 20 minutes dependent upon the goals of the individual	Could involve steady state work or intervals. It may be done for speed or aerobic endurance and involve running, rowing or cycling
Core training	2–3 exercises to cover the abdominals, back muscles (erector spinae) and obliques	This could include dynamic exercises, such as sit ups, crunches or back extensions or static exercises, such as the plank or a bridge
CV training – cool down	3–5 minutes	This involves a gradual decrease of intensity to lower the heart rate steadily
Flexibility	8–10 stretches on all the muscles worked in the session	This would include developmental stretches on those muscles which are tight (e.g. pecs, hamstrings) and static stretches on all the other muscles worked

Table 4.3 The structure of a typical training programme

A typical training session for an untrained beginner may look like Table 4.4.

Type of training	Name of exercise	Amount
CV training – warm up	Treadmill	5 minutes
Flexibility	Dynamic stretches: chest, back, legs	×10 on each exercise
Resistance 1	Squats Bench press Seated row Leg extension Leg flexion	2 × 15 on each exercise with 20–30 seconds rest between sets and exercises
CV training	Rower	5–10 minutes
Resistance 2	Shoulder press Bicep curls Tricep press Calf raises	2 × 15 on each exercise with 20–30 seconds rest between sets and exercises
CV training	Static bike	3–5 minutes
Core training	Sit ups on stability ball Back extensions on stability ball	2 × 10 repetitions on each exercise
CV training – cool down	Treadmill	3–5 minutes
Flexibility	Quads Hamstrings (developmental) Pecs (developmental) Lats Glutes Biceps Triceps Deltoids Calves	All stretches to be held for 10 seconds, except the developmental stretches, which will be held for 30 seconds.

Table 4.4 A typical training session for an untrained beginner

Quick quiz 2

Match the components of fitness to their correct definition:

Component of fitness	Definition
Frequency	
Intensity	
Time	
Type	
Overload	
Reversibility	
Specificity	

Choice of definitions:

- if a fitness gain is not used it will be lost
- how often the athlete will train per week, month or year
- the individual's choice of training
- any training gain will only be of benefit to the muscles/energy system to which it is applied
- how hard the individual works
- working a muscle or system slightly harder than it is used to
- how long each session will last

4.5 Planning a Fitness Training Programme

P3

Collecting Information

As an effective fitness coach it is important to be able to write an appropriate fitness training programme. There is a process that you need to go through to write an effective training session for a client.

Stage 1 – Gathering information: the first step is to gain relevant information about the person so that you can plan a personal training programme. The key is to build up a picture of the individual and what their life is like. Then you can look at what exercises you will plan for them. This is done through a questionnaire, which the client will fill out on your first meeting. (See Unit 8 Fitness Testing for Sport & Exercise, for a sample questionnaire.)

What a person does or does not do in their life will have an effect on their health and fitness levels as well as their chances of being able to keep the training programme going. The following factors need to be taken into consideration.

- Occupation – hours worked and whether work is manual or office-based.
- Activity levels – amount of movement they do on a daily basis.
- Leisure time activities – whether these are active or inactive.
- Diet – what, how much and when they eat.
- Stress levels – either through work or their home life and how they deal with it.
- Alcohol intake – how much they consume and how often.
- Smoking – whether they are a smoker or ex-smoker and the amount they smoke.
- Time available – the client needs to fit the training into their schedule and the fitness trainer needs to be realistic when planning the programme.
- Current and previous training history – this will give an idea of the current fitness level of the client and also their skill level.

Stage 2 – Establishing objectives: to ensure the success of the fitness programme it needs to be specific to the outcome a person wants. Once we have found this out we can establish goals. Their objective could be any of the following:

- cardiovascular fitness

- flexibility
- muscular strength
- muscular size
- muscle tone
- power.

Once the objectives have been established it is time to set goals to achieve these objectives.

Stage 3 – Goal setting: when setting goals it is important to ensure they follow the SMART principle – that they are specific, measurable, achievable, realistic and time-constrained. These goals should be set for the year or season, then for three months, one month and down to one week or one day. (For a full guide on how to set goals effectively see pages 268–270.)

This goal-setting information should be kept in the training diary along with records of each training session.

Periodisation

Periodisation means a progressive change in the type of training that is being performed to gain maximum fitness benefits. It needs to be carefully planned and would show progression from one type of training to another. For example, a sprinter will focus on developing their strength base and muscular endurance in the autumn before working on improving power and speed as they get closer to the competitive season. All training for sports performance needs to be periodised. For people training in the gym, they can periodise their training by changing the volume and intensity of their training so that they train different energy systems and for different components of fitness.

For example, consider a competitive sports performer who has six weeks to prepare for the new season. They may realise that they need to train for aerobic endurance, anaerobic endurance and speed, as well as muscular endurance and power. They will periodise their cardiovascular training and their resistance training by manipulating the volume and intensity of their training. An example is provided in Table 4.5.

Macrocycle, mesocycle and microcycle are terminology specific to periodisation. The macrocycle is the largest unit of the training cycle and would cover the overall objective of the training. It will last for the length of a season or a training year. It is broken down into smaller units or mesocycles. A mesocycle is an individual phase of training and would cover a period of around a month depending upon the objective of the phase of training. A microcycle would represent each individual training session and its content. The plan would be periodised by looking at the big picture, or the macrocycle, then broken down into mesocycles, each contributing to the big picture and then the small detail of each session would be to consider how to achieve the aim of each mesocycle.

A Training Diary

A training diary is used to record all the training sessions completed, to enable the individual to monitor their progress. It should include the following details:

- date of each session
- detail of what was done in each session
- a record of the performances in training
- notes on how the athlete felt
- reasons as to why the athlete felt that way
- competition results
- fitness testing results
- performance reviews with their coach.

This can then be used to demonstrate progress, keep the athlete motivated and then to understand any improvements which have been made (or not).

Number of sets × number of repetitions	Week 1	Week 2	Week 3	Week 4	Week 5	Week 6
2 × 20	2 × 20					
2–3 × 15		2–3 × 15				
3 × 12			3 × 12			
3 × 10				3 × 10		
4 × 8					4 × 8	
5 × 5						5 × 5

Table 4.5 Example of a periodised six-week training plan for resistance training

Student activity 4.2

90 minutes P2 P3 P4 M2 D1

Developing a six-week training programme

Read the following case study and then answer the questions that follow:

CASE STUDY

Harry is a 21-year-old who wants to start playing tennis again after having stopped playing when he left school 3 years ago. Since then he has been working in a sedentary job, which involves him sitting in front of a computer every day, and his favourite leisure activities are playing computer games and going to the cinema to watch horror films. He knows his diet is poor as he eats a lot of fried chicken and he is starting to put on a bit of weight around the middle. At his consultation he says he wants to get fit enough to start playing tennis again, and he is particularly worried that he gets breathless very easily.

At the consultation Harry and his trainer decide upon the following goals:

- Improve his aerobic fitness to help him keep going during his matches.
- Improve his speed so he can move around court quickly.
- Improve his muscular strength and endurance to his improve his hitting.
- Develop his flexibility so he can stretch for the ball.
- Develop his core strength so he can produce the strength and power he needs.

(a) Using the layout presented easlier in this unit, produce a training session for Harry covering cardiovascular training, resistance training, flexibility and speed training.

P1

To gain a merit the programme needs to be produced with detail, and to gain a distinction you need to justify your training programme by explaining why you have chosen the exercises that you did for Harry.

M1 D1

(b) Harry has got 6 weeks until he has his first tennis match. Using the template below, show how his training will develop over this six-week period. You need to consider the principles of training and how frequency, intensity, time and type will change over the six weeks to ensure progressive overload on the muscles and energy systems.

(c) How will you monitor Harry's performance over the six weeks of the training programme?

P4

This is an example for you to use as a practice before you prepare a six-week training programme for a selected individual, and then monitor their progress over the six weeks.

Component of fitness	Week 1	Week 2	Week 3	Week 4	Week 5	Week 6	Comments
Cardiovascular training							
Resistance training – Muscular endurance							
Resistance training – Strength							
Speed							
Flexibility							

4.6 Reviewing a Fitness Training Programme

P4 P5 M3 D2

The programme is planned out in detail and implemented with great energy and enthusiasm; likewise it must be evaluated in an organised manner. The athlete must keep a training diary for every session, whether it covered physical training, technical development or mental skills. Only then can it be accurately and systematically evaluated.

The athlete can evaluate the success and effectiveness of their training in the following ways:

- repeating their fitness tests
- evaluating performances
- reviewing their training diary
- measuring whether their goals have been achieved.

Based on all this information, the next stage of the training programme can be developed.

The diary can also be used to evaluate the reasons why the athlete did or did not achieve their goals, and any modifications or interventions can then be planned.

Further reading

Ansell, M., (2008) *Personal Training*, Exeter: Learning Matters.

Baechle, T. and Earle, R., (2008) *Essentials of Strength Training and Conditioning*, Human Kinetics.

Coulson, M., (2007) *The Fitness Instructor's Handbook*, London: A&C Black.

Dalgleish, J. and Dollery, S. (2001) *The Health and Fitness Handbook*, Harlow: Longman.

References

Baechle, T. and Earle, R. (2008) *Essentials of Strength Training and Conditioning*, Human Kinetics.

Elphinston, J. and Pook, P. (2009) *The Core Workout: a Definitive Guide to Swiss Ball Training for Athletes, Coaches and Fitness Professionals*, Core Workout.

Useful websites

www.topendsports.com/testing/tests.htm

Over 100 fitness tests to try, all divided into different fitness categories.

www.netfit.co.uk/previous.htm

Extensive range of exercise and training techniques, some sports specific, others more general

Student activity 4.3 — 45 minutes — P5 M3 D2

Reviewing the training programme

Once the selected individual has completed the six-week training programme, you need to review their progress and then prepare to give them feedback. You can use the following information to base your review on:

- Information in the training diary on their progress over the six weeks.
- Progress towards their goal.
- Feedback from other people involved in the training.

To achieve a pass you need to give feedback and then describe their areas of strength and those that they need to improve on; to move to a merit you need to explain their areas of strength and those requiring improvement and to achieve a distinction you need to evaluate their progress by looking at the factors that have contributed to their progress or worked against it and then offer recommendations for future training activities.

5: Sports coaching

5.1 Introduction

Sports coaches are vital to the success of a number of programmes across a range of sports. They are at the heart of participation and performer development. Whether the coach of an after-school club or a top international coach with support staff, coaches are at the very centre of the development of sport.

This unit will assist those starting on the coaching ladder to learn the rules and responsibilities, the qualities and characteristics of sports coaches. It will provide an understanding of the role of the coach in promoting a positive coaching experience.

By the end of this unit you should:

- know the roles, responsibilities and skills of sports coaches
- know the techniques used by coaches to improve the performance of athletes
- be able to plan a sports coaching session
- be able to deliver and review a sports coaching session.

Assessment and grading criteria		
To achieve a PASS grade the evidence must show that the learner is able to:	**To achieve a MERIT grade the evidence must show that, in addition to the pass criteria, the learner is able to:**	**To achieve a DISTINCTION grade the evidence must show that, in addition to the pass and merit criteria, the learner is able to:**
P1 describe four roles and four responsibilities of sports coaches, using examples of coaches from different sports	**M1** explain four roles and four responsibilities of sports coaches, using examples of coaches from different sports	**D1** compare and contrast the roles, responsibilities and skills of successful coaches from different sports
P2 describe three skills common to successful sports coaches, using examples of coaches from different sports	**M2** explain three skills common to successful sports coaches, using examples of coaches from different sports	
P3 describe three different techniques that are used by coaches to improve the performance of athletes	**M3** explain three different techniques that are used by coaches to improve the performance of athletes	**D2** evaluate three different techniques that are used by coaches to improve the performance of athletes
P4 plan a sports coaching session		
P5 deliver a sports coaching session, with tutor support	**M4** independently deliver a sports coaching session	
P6 carry out a review of the planning and delivery of a sports coaching session, identifying strengths and areas for improvement.	**M5** evaluate the planning and delivery of a sports coaching session, suggesting how improvements could be reached in the identified areas.	**D3** justify suggestions made in relation to the development plan.

5.2 The Roles, Responsibilities and Skills of Sports Coaches

P1 P2 M1 M2 D1

Effective coaches tend to find new ways of improving existing practices or theories. Some adapt the way in which they practise, others deal with how to play specific strategies in differing situations. Other coaches integrate new developments or technologies to improve performance. Consider the trampoline coach who adapts a harness that supports a performer for use while learning somersaults, allowing them the freedom to twist at the same time and add to the range of skills and techniques achievable. Performers who work with innovative coaches speak about how they are never bored and always trying something new.

Trainer, educator and instructor

The difference between a teacher, educator and instructor is hard to discern. Teaching implies a transfer of learning through demonstration, modelling or instruction. Coaches can also teach emotional and social skills. Young performers in particular can be encouraged to increase their social awareness, learn to cope with losing and winning, and develop self-confidence. Good coaches will be aware that people learn in different ways. They then adapt and use a range of techniques to ensure that learning takes place.

In some cultures trainers and coaches are taken to mean the same thing. Since all sport requires some kind of physical exertion, it is important that these physical demands are recognised and that allowance for these demands is incorporated into coaching programmes.

A sound knowledge of anatomy, physiology and fitness theory is essential for coaches. In the role of trainer, you might expect to design and implement training programmes for your performers.

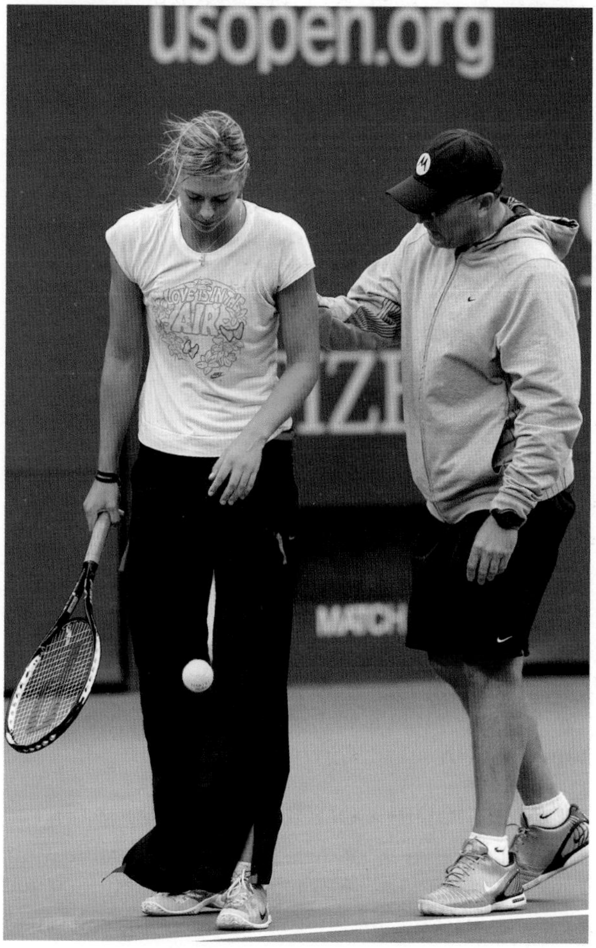

Fig 5.1 A tennis coach and player

Motivator

Motivation can come merely by providing a stable environment in which to learn, in a positive and safe atmosphere. Performers who constantly find negativity are certain at some point to become despondent and suffer a reduction in self-confidence and improvement.

Evidence suggests that performers who receive praise and positive feedback are likely to get more from their performances. When providing feedback to performers you would employ the following technique: KISS, KICK, KISS.

This technique would be applied in providing feedback such as in skill learning. When communicating with performers, the emphasis with this technique would be to start your feedback with a positive comment. There is nearly always something that is positive in any performance. Second, a corrective comment can be presented in as positive a manner as possible. Finally, leave the interaction with a positive comment and possibly an action plan. Consider a tennis player struggling to make a particular shot:

KISS – 'Good positioning prior to the shot and you watched the ball well.'
KICK – 'You should consider how you back-lift the racket; you could prepare your grip earlier.'
KISS – 'If you practise these changes you will almost certainly improve.'

Role model

In almost every coaching situation players will look mostly, if not entirely, to the coach as their source of inspiration and knowledge, never more so than when working with children. Children often imitate the behaviour and manner of their coach. For this reason it is vital that coaching is safe and responsible, and that behaviour is considered good practice.

The coach can influence player development in a number of ways.

- Social – sport offers a code of acceptable social behaviour, teamwork, citizenship, cooperation and fair play.
- Personal – players can be encouraged to learn life skills, promote their self-esteem, manage personal matters like careers or socialising, and develop a value system including good manners, politeness and self-discipline.
- Psychological – coaches can create environments that help performers control emotions and develop their own identities. Confidence, mental toughness, visualisation and a positive outlook on life can be developed or improved.
- Health – in taking care to design coaching or training sessions to include sufficient physical exercise, good health and healthy habits can be established and maintained.

The responsibilities of a coach

Many expectations are put upon a coach. Some of these responsibilities are clear-cut, others less so. Coaching and playing sport should always be enjoyable, and to that end coaches should not be overburdened by expectation. Common sense and a good knowledge of safety and ethics will provide the basis of a responsible coach.

As coaching is now considered a profession, so coaches will increasingly be measured and assessed, whether paid or voluntary, and increasingly expected to work to a code of practice.

A coaching code of practice

So that performers achieve their potential, coaches should:

- remain within the bounds of adopted codes of practice
- maintain safe and secure coaching environments
- make best use of all facilities and resources
- establish good working relationships with all involved
- control the behaviour of participants where possible.

Many sports governing bodies and sports coach UK have established a code of conduct for sports coaches, which includes the following sections.

- Rights – coaches must respect and champion the right of every individual to participate in sport. Coaches should ensure that everyone has an equal opportunity to participate, regardless of age, gender, race, ability, faith or sexual orientation. For example, you would organise sessions in a place that has childcare arrangements, and you would be sensitive to religious festivals of all denominations and make allowances for the absences of performers on notable religious dates. Coaches also have a responsibility to ensure that no discriminating behaviour occurs during their working sessions. Every member of the coaching group should have the right to feel part of the group, free from prejudice.
- Relationships – coaches need to establish relationships with performers that are based on openness, trust and mutual respect. This is not just about effective communication. Good coaches understand how their performers think and what is best for them. Performers will also learn better in an atmosphere of trust and respect for their coach. Involving performers in the decision-making process is an excellent way of establishing an effective relationship with a performer. When deciding what is best for a performer or group of performers, an example could be a situation where the coach presents the performers with information about their performance, such as a particular phase of play in a tennis competition. Having supplied that information and perhaps offering their opinion, the coach could present the performer with a range of options that relates to the best course of action – how to improve on the last period of play. The performer who has an input into the decision in this process will come to appreciate the knowledge and analytical skills of the coach and over time their relationship will develop based on trust and respect.

Coaches should also anticipate and deal with potential relationship problems such as:

- dealing with parents
- dropping players from squads
- assuming control as a carer.

Personal standards

Coaches should demonstrate model behaviour at all times. Their influence should always be positive and would usually mean working to a code.

Professional conduct

It is not enough to achieve a coaching qualification. Coaches should have a commitment to continual and ongoing learning or professional development. This could include:

- attaining higher-grade qualifications
- attending workshops and seminars
- being aware of changes to their sport.

Skills of sports coaches

The essential skills required of a sports coach are illustrated in Figure 5.2.

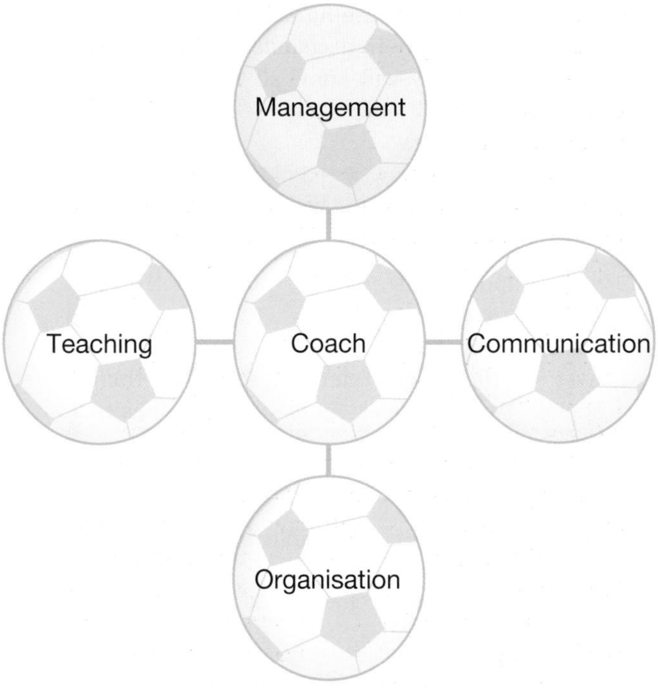

Fig 5.2 Skills of sports coaches

Management

The key ways to demonstrate good leadership in coaching are:

- checking that participants are well prepared and organised
- checking that participants and appropriate others are well deployed
- safe management and coordination of equipment and facilities
- safe and well-delivered sessions
- maintaining support and guidance to participants
- establishing and maintaining effective communication with appropriate others within the coaching environment.

It is important that coaches motivate participants by ensuring that they remain interested and challenged. Coaches will get the best from their sport if they are self-motivated and working in an atmosphere that allows them to:

- enjoy their coaching sessions
- share their experiences with others and socialise with peers and friends
- compete in a safe and non-threatening environment
- achieve negotiated goals
- remain fit and healthy
- achieve success or reward
- please others and receive praise
- create a positive self-image.

Organisation

Planning and organisation are critical to the success of coaching. When planning a session there is much to consider, but the main points are to:

- have identified a set of goals for the session
- have an awareness of the resources available
- have enough information about the participants
- have developed a plan that allows participants to achieve.

During a session coaches need to be constantly making judgements about the following:

- Is the practice working?
- What could be adapted and how?
- Are the facilities being used to full advantage?

Many coaches now keep records, usually in the form of logbooks. Many coaching qualifications require candidates to complete logbooks as part of the formal assessment process. Few coaches have the privilege of just turning up, coaching and going home. Often coaches are also involved in booking facilities, arranging equipment or contacting participants,

Role	Responsibilities
Coach	Team selection
Assistant coach	Warm-up, cool-down & general preparation
Player 1	Calling players to arrange meeting place for away fixtures
Player 2	Washing & looking after kit
Player 3	Contacting officials prior to games
Player 4	Maintaining website & making travel arrangements
Player 5	All communication with league
Player 6	Introducing new players & schools liaison
Player 7	Seeking sponsorship

Table 5.1 Responsibilities and roles within a senior women's volleyball team

which involves a great deal of organisation. Some coaches delegate these responsibilities as in the example for a senior women's volleyball team shown in Table 5.1.

In some clubs such as this, some or all of these responsibilities and others are undertaken by appropriate others, usually with the coach in control of exactly who is capable and most responsible for the task.

Communication

Perhaps the single most valuable skill is the ability to convey your thoughts and ideas in such a way as to be easily understood. It is not enough to just present your opinions: you must be able to send effective messages – these are mostly non-verbal signals. Consider the body language of a coach in a variety of scenarios. The main feedback a performer receives in almost every sport is non-verbal body language from their coaches.

Talking too much can lead to confusion. The pace, tone and volume of the spoken word will all have a marked effect on participants. The coach who spends most of their time shouting abuse will quickly lose the respect of their participants and will be less likely to be successful.

You must also be able to receive incoming messages. This particular skill is concerned with understanding and interpreting the signs and signals of other players, officials, etc. You must also listen to opinions from players regarding tactical decisions, drills in practice or perhaps even concerning opponents.

You must also be able to check message reception. Good coaches will question their players and check their understanding. If an instruction is not understood, this is the fault of either the performer lacking concentration or the coach in the quality of the message. One way of ensuring understanding is to ask players to explain a concept in their own words.

Teaching

One of the key processes of teaching is an understanding of how people learn. Drills and practices need to be designed in a way that allows participants to progress at an appropriate pace. As a rule of good practice, the following model is useful when teaching skills:

- introduce and explain the technique
- demonstrate the technique
- practise (allow performers to experience the technique)
- observe and analyse the participants
- identify and correct errors.

It is vital that learning is achieved in simple, short and logical steps. The most valuable knowledge that a coach can gain is through learned experience, judging for themselves and from their performers what is effective and what is not.

Coaching is a continuous process which lends itself to self-reflection and evaluation. Since the knowledge and skills required to be a successful coach are constantly changing and developing with the sport, it is unlikely that coaches will ever reach the point where they will know all that there is to know!

Key learning points 1

- The roles of a sports coach are many and varied, and include teacher, trainer, motivator and instructor.
- Coaches can have a direct influence on the lives of their performers in terms of their social, psychological, personal and health development.
- Most coaches in the UK work to a code of conduct or practice that is established to set the parameters of acceptable behaviour and effective coaching.
- The essential skills toolkit of a successful sports coach includes:
  - management
  - communication
  - teaching
  - organisation.

Q Quick quiz 1

Fill in the blanks in the following paragraph.

Coaches will perform many different roles as they work with their performers. They will act as a _________ as they demonstrate and model skills. They will need to have a good knowledge base, including ________ and ________ . Coaches will need to pick out the good points so that performers remain motivated and also act as a _____ _____ so they influence performers in a positive way.

Student activity 5.1

60 minutes | P1 | P2 | M1 | M2 | D1

Roles and responsibilities of a sports coach

Part 1

Investigate the roles, responsibilities and skills of the sports coach by filling in the following table.

Role/Responsibility	Describe each of the roles/responsibilities, using examples of coaches from different sports	Describe each of the roles/responsibilities, using examples of coaches from different sports	Compare and contrast the roles, responsibilities and skills of successful coaches from different sports
Role 1: Trainer			
Role 2: Educator			
Role 3: Role model			
Role 4: Motivator			
Responsibility 1: Working within a code of practice			
Responsibility 2: Maintain a safe and secure environment			
Responsibility 3: Equal opportunities			
Responsibility 4: Professional conduct			

Part 2

Take three coaches of your choice:

(a) Describe how they use the skills of communication, organisation and analysis to improve the performance of athletes:

Coach	Communication	Organisation	Analysis
Coach 1:			
Coach 2:			
Coach 3:			

(b) To achieve a merit you need to explain these three techniques.

(c) To achieve a distinction you need to evaluate the effectiveness of each of the three techniques.

5.3 Techniques used by Coaches to Improve Performance

P3 M3 D2

Coaches in all sports have a number of techniques at their disposal that they can use to improve the performance of their athletes.

Coaching diaries/logbooks

Diaries come in different sizes, paper or electronic. They can be used to record personal thoughts, make appointments or log training sessions. Diaries can be useful in aiding self-reflection, planning and evaluation of coaching sessions.

Guidelines for getting the most from your diary are as follows:

- Complete the diary soon after the coaching session.
- Write down what happened in order.
- Focus on what went well first.
- Describe what needs improvement.
- Action plan to develop what needs to be improved.

The benefits of diaries are that they can show progress over a period of time and are usually honest and describe how you felt about a situation at that time.

Performance profiles

If a trampolinist is not performing a somersault correctly or is not coping with the physical demands of the sport, the coach or trainer can design a suitable exercise or coaching programme. But what if the trampolinist has trouble with their nerves before the start of the competition, or they have some kind of mental block that stops them from executing a skill?

Although not always obvious, the following psychological factors can affect sporting performance:

- confidence: belief in yourself and your abilities
- concentration: the ability to attend to relevant cues, not being distracted
- control: the extent to which you feel able to influence events
- commitment: the level to which you apply yourself
- re-focusing after errors: the ability to adjust to negative outcomes in a positive way
- enjoyment: the amount of fun that you can have.

To use a performance profile you would talk with the performer and ask them to tell you how they feel about their sport. Do they ever feel anxious, and if so, when? Do they understand the terms above and if so, how do they rate them?

In Table 5.2, a performer has been asked to rate out of ten the importance of each of the factors and then rate their own proficiency in that factor.

It seems that the performer's main emphasis for any intervention should be focused on the areas that they identify as a weakness, in this case re-focusing after errors and concentration.

Key term

Intervention: an interruption that brings about change (in sporting performance).

In the same way, coaches can adapt this approach and apply it to their own coaching (as in the example below).

Observation and analysis

It is possible to be observed and analysed by your team or club mates, your coach and yourself, particularly if you have access to a video of your performance.

Interviews

It is possible to get a great deal of information from an interview. You could ask a performer about what

Performance factors	Importance to performer	Self-assessment
Confidence	9	9
Commitment	10	10
Concentration	9	6
Control	9	8
Re-focusing after error	10	6
Enjoyment	7	9

Table 5.2 Factors and proficiency

Strengths A good relaxed swing Excellent body positioning in relation to the ball A low-risk safety-first approach	**Weaknesses** Not accurate with driving clubs Putting is inconsistent Poor technique in short iron game (head up too early)
Opportunities Short game practice has improved in recent weeks Has learned how to mentally rehearse Opponent has no knowledge of the course	**Threats** Can be prone to getting annoyed easily and letting it spoil their game Environment – windy day Opponent is a better player

Table 5.3 SWOT analysis of a golfer

they consider to be their strengths and weaknesses, or you could ask them about what tactics they might use against a particular opponent.

SWOT analysis

This is a subjective analysis of a performance or a performer's ability. Table 5.3 shows an example of a SWOT analysis carried out on a golfer.

Simulation or conditioned practice

This is about artificially creating a competition-like situation in a practice session, or a particular condition that may be likely to happen in a competitive situation. A basketball coach might consider the merits of initially removing defenders, or outnumbering them in a practice situation that is aimed at improving a particular attacking focus. Defenders

Coaching factors	Importance to coach	Self-assessment
Planning & preparation	9	9
Needs of participants considered	10	10
Technical progression & sequencing	9	6
Health & safety observed	9	8
Goals defined at start of session	10	6
Technically accurate instructions/demonstrations	7	9
Appropriate content & structure		
Variety of drills		
Monitored progress		
Skills related to game situation		
Errors identified & corrected		
Control & behaviour of group		
Time management		
De-brief & feedback to participants		
Checked player understanding		
Stopped & brought group together		
Evaluated against objectives set		
Made provisions for future planning		

Table 5.4 Assessment of factors for coaching

can be added when the techniques are well practised. Or, conversely, extra defenders could be added so that the attacking technique could be practised under greater pressure. Similarly, defenders in these practices could be asked to take one of three roles according to the conditions required by the coach:

- passive, offering little resistance other than presence
- active, playing under normal conditions, tempo, intensity
- pressure, playing with extra intensity.

Conditioned games are used when a coach wants to create a situation that is likely to happen in a game, such as practising defending free kicks in football. Or simply adding a condition that emphasises a teaching point, such as choosing a target area on a tennis court with a chalk circle or hoop where the player is expected to return the balls in a practice drill.

Video analysis

Video gives the person who watches it an objective record of a performance. The greatest benefit of video is the playback feature, including slow motion, which can be used to demonstrate skill execution, tactical efficiency or a more general generic performance evaluation.

Here are some guidelines on the use of video analysis in sport:

- Do not try to film your performers and coach them at the same time. Ask someone reliable to do the filming and brief them on what you want – follow the player or the ball, try to capture tactics or specific techniques, etc.
- Try to pick up all of the sound as it can provide useful feedback.
- Start the recording before the action and end it well after, judging players' body language before and after performance.
- Label and date the film immediately, to keep a record.

Notation

Notation is a way of collecting data and can be done by hand or with a computer. Hand notation is a system of recording detailed analysis of a sport and literally noting the data on a sheet of paper using a predefined set of symbols. Systems like this exist for many sports, such as tennis, archery and football.

The advantage of these systems is that they are inexpensive and, if completed by a skilful recorder, will produce quick information in real time, so that the coach or performer can have instant access to detailed information. The main disadvantages of this system are that it is open to human error, can be difficult to interpret and can be difficult in certain conditions such as bad weather.

On the next page there is an example of a match analysis sheet for a team sport. This could be filled in by the performer, a peer or a neutral observer, scoring 1 to 10 for both achieved and target scores.

Key learning points 2

- Coaches can make good use of reflective diaries in order to improve their coaching performance.
- Performance profiles can be used for performers and coaches alike.
- Coaches are expected to make interventions to improve performance, having identified areas for development.
- Coaches can condition games to facilitate the teaching of a specific skill or tactic.

Q Quick quiz 2

Which coaching techniques are the following sentences a description of?

(a) Watching the individual performing skills.

(b) Identifying strengths and weaknesses.

(c) Recording data about performance by hand or using a computer package.

(d) Getting a performer to rate different aspects of their performance out of 10.

(e) Creating similar conditions to those of competition.

Possible answers:

SWOT analysis, performance profiling, observation, simulation, notational analysis.

Student activity 5.2 — 45 minutes — P3 M3 D2

Techniques used by a sports coach

Fill out the following table to show your understanding of different techniques used by coaches.

Coaching technique	Describe the techniques used by coaches to improve the performance of athletes	Explain the techniques used by coaches to improve the performance of athletes	Evaluate the techniques used by coaches to improve the performance of athletes
Observation analysis			
Performance profiling			
Coaching diaries			

5.4 Plan a Coaching Session

P4

Planning can be separated into the following stages:

- collecting and reviewing relevant information
- identifying participant needs
- goal setting
- identifying appropriate resources
- identifying appropriate activities to enable goals to be achieved
- planning coaching sessions and/or programmes.

Before you coach any session you need to answer the following questions:

- What is the starting point, what are their skill levels, who are they?
- Where do they want to be and what do they want from you?
- How will you achieve this?
- What will you need to do this – facilities, equipment, etc.?
- How will you/they know if they have improved?

To plan an effective coaching session or programme of sessions, the coach needs to establish:

- the number of participants, as this will affect the kinds of practices that the coach can employ
- the age of participants, as this will affect the kinds of practices that the coach can use, and even how they might approach coaching that group
- the level of experience and ability of the participants
- whether the participants have any special requirements relating to diet, health, culture or language.

An example of a session planner is reproduced in Table 5.5.

Setting SMART goals

It is a good idea to use the SMART principle when planning your sessions or season.

Key terms

Specific: this means that the session meets what you want it to meet, and is specific to the sport. For example, you could focus a cricket batting session on dealing with short-pitched, fast deliveries, thus being explicit and specific.

Measurable: this is the way in which you measure your results. If you have identified that you want to improve a basketball player's jump shooting, then you might measure this by counting how many shots are successful in a training or game situation and then measure again after the training programme.

Achievable: what you set out to improve must be possible. It would not be fair to ask a beginner in trampolining to complete a complicated routine with multiple somersaults.

Realistic: it must be possible and realistic to achieve what you intend to achieve.

Time-constrained: there should be a reasonable amount of time to achieve the learning goal. Some goals will be short term in nature and established to be achieved in the next session, others more long term and established for the entire season.

Session planner	
Date	Venue
Time	Duration
Group	No. of participants
Equipment required	Aims of session
Safety checks required	
TIME	CONTENT
	Warm-up
	Fitness work
	Main technical skills work
	Game play/tactical work
	Cool-down
Injuries/issues arising	
Evaluation of session	

Table 5.5 Example of a session planner

Health and safety

The health and safety of all involved in sport should be the most important of the coach's considerations. In most cases it is necessary to ensure that facilities and equipment are safe and well maintained, and that performers are adequately aware of key health and safety issues, particularly relating to their own safety and the safety of others.

Coaches should consider the following as a checklist, though it is by no means exhaustive.

- The context in which the sport will take place – the facilities and equipment. Does the provider have a normal operating procedure and emergency action plan? This should cover number of players allowed, coach:learner ratio, conduct and supervision, hazardous behaviours, fire and evacuation procedures.
- The nature of the sport, for playing and training:
  - what to do when rules are not observed
  - what to do with injured players
  - not teaching activities beyond the capabilities of the performers
  - in competitive situations, matching performers where appropriate by size, maturity or age.
- The players:
  - are you aware of any special individual medical needs, and the types of injuries common to the sport?
  - safety education – informing players of inherent risks and establishing a code of behaviour
  - teammates and opponents to be aware of their responsibilities to each other
  - players should be discouraged from participating with an existing injury.
- The coach:
  - safe practices
  - safe numbers for the area
  - arranging appropriate insurance
  - dealing with and reporting accidents
  - being aware of emergency actions.

Risk assessments

Risk assessments are not just forms to fill out. A risk assessment is a skill that helps prevent accidents or serious events. You need to consider what could go wrong and how likely it is.

Risk assessments should be kept and logged, and stored in a safe place. Examples of risk assessments for sporting activities are wide ranging and will depend upon who they are prepared for, the nature of the sport and the competence of the person making the assessment.

Contingency planning

Nothing ever goes completely to plan and for that reason it is good practice to plan for the unexpected so that everyone remains safe and continues to learn. Consider the following as examples of what can happen and what you could plan for.

- Weather threatens your outside session.
- You fall ill and are no longer able to continue as coach.
- There are not enough participants for the session.
- The facility is double-booked when you arrive for the session.
- The group is not responding to your style of coaching or the practices that you have chosen.

The components of a session

While the demands of the structure of sessions for different sports are quite different, the general rules for the layout of sessions are common to all sports.

Key terms

Warm up: to physically and mentally prepare and focus the performers.

Skill learning phase: the objectives of the session are established and employed through a series of drills or practices, perhaps with a competition, followed by an evaluation.

Cool-down: the final and often ignored phase that is concerned with restoring normality to body functions and that has a role to play in injury prevention and emotional control.

Key learning points 3

- Planning is the first stage of coaching and requires the gathering of information relating to performers, facilities and resources.
- Effective coaches use session planners to show what they have planned for a session and to maintain a record.
- Health and safety is the most important consideration in the planning and delivery of coaching sessions.
- Contingency plans are back-up plans that can be used in the event of an unforeseen circumstance that threatens the safety or quality of the coaching session.

Student activity 5.3 — 45 minutes — P4

Planning a coaching session

Using the session planner provided, plan a sports coaching session for a group or individual of your choice.

5.5 Delivering a Coaching Session

P5 P6 M4 M5 D3

This is concerned with the actual 'doing' part of coaching, and will help with the principles of coaching sessions.

Like the planning of a session, delivering a session follows a logical path.

- Ensure the session plan fits all.
- Identify any risks to the delivery of the session.
- Introduce and start planned activities.
- Manage the behaviour of all involved.
- Monitor and adapt the session as it progresses.
- Summarise and conclude the coaching session.

Once the session is under way, the coach should work to maintain what is going well, and the role of the coach changes to become more of a manager/supervisor.

Skills should be introduced, followed by an explanation which could help performers understand their relevance and when they could be used in a competitive situation.

A competent demonstration should follow, which

could be from the coach or with the aid of a video model. This must be a technically correct example and should be thorough, without too much explanation. There should be a balance between verbal instruction and visual demonstration. There will also need to be a balance between activity, instruction and discussion depending on the age, experience and maturity of performers. It is essential for the coach to note the differing rates of learning of individuals.

Performers will then need time to practise the skill or technique. Coaches can use questions to check understanding. The role of the coach changes again to become one of observer/analyst, and it is here that the coach will be looking to assist learners and correct any faults.

To improve performance the coach must have highly developed awareness relating to how to identify errors, compare to a perfect model example and, most importantly, knowledge of how to bridge the gap using feedback, observation and application of a range of suitable techniques.

There is no substitute for practice at this stage. A session that is continually interrupted by a coach for whatever reason is less likely to be successful. It is also important that a coach does not attempt too much in one session.

Most coaches enjoy this part of the coaching process the most, but it is too easy to forget what the aims of the session are and how to keep track of achievement.

Reviewing a session

It is important to consider that coaching does not finish at the end of a session when everyone has cooled down or even gone home. Coaching is a continuous process, and the best coaches reflect on what happened and, more importantly, how to improve. A well-considered evaluation should aid the improvement of subsequent sessions.

The process is as follows:

- Collect, analyse and review – information about the session from feedback, self-reflection and from others.
- Session effectiveness – identify the effectiveness of the session in achieving objectives.
- Review key aspects – drills or practices.
- Identify development needs and take steps to action them.

When evaluating a session a coach should consider the following:

- Performance against pre-set goals: effective coaches will be familiar with the goals for the season, both long and short term. There should be an opportunity to decide to what extent, if at all, the session objectives were met and to what extent this matched the other goals.
- Participants' progress: the review will enable coaches to monitor the performer's progress over a period of time, and help plan for future sessions. Typical review questions could be:
  - How well did the performers learn the skills or techniques introduced to them?
  - What performance developments were evident for each participant?
  - Are the performers ready to progress to the next session?
- Coaching ability: this is the part where the coach can review their own performance:
  - What went well?
  - What went less well?
  - How did the performers respond?
  - Were the performers bored or restless?
  - Did the coach behave acceptably?
- Future targets: this is all about planning for future goals and objectives based on achievements and progress made by participants.

Tools for the review process

There are a number of tools that coaches can use.

- Videos – an excellent way of improving your coaching effectiveness. Videos can be used to judge coaching actions, interaction with your performers, facial expressions and gestures, as well as what you say.
- Critical analysis and self-reflection – self-reflection allows you to explore your perceptions, decisions and subsequent actions to work out ways in which performers can improve technical, tactical or physical ability.
- A mentor – a mentor coach can help provide you with a role-model figure who can offer you practical solutions, work as a sounding board and generally provide you with a range of support.
- Coaching diaries – these can act as a permanent source of information to record your thoughts and feelings, and serve as a true account of what happened and when. Diaries or logs can certainly help with self-reflection and form the basis of action plans for improvement.

Formative and summative reviews

A formative review occurs during the process of coaching and changes can be made immediately. A summative review is done at the end of the coaching session as you reflect on the process overall.

Student activity 5.4 — 45 minutes — P5 P6 M4 M5 D3

Delivering a sports session

Part 1

Once you have planned your session, arrange with your tutor when you are going to deliver your session.

Part 2

When you have delivered your coaching, you need to carry out a review of the planning and delivery of the session in the following manner:

1. Gain as much feedback/information as you can about the planning and delivery of your session by asking open questions to:
   - the participants in your session
   - your tutor
   - other people who were observing your session.

   You want to find out what was good and what was not so good about your session.

   Then think deeply about your session and the parts that you thought were good and not so good.
2. What will you ask them about? The more specific you can be in your questioning, the better information you will receive and the more you will learn.

   First, ask them:
   - whether the aims and objectives of the session were met
   - what parts went particularly well
   - what parts went particularly badly.

   Then, ask them about the skills you used to coach during the session:
   - communication
   - organisation
   - observation
   - decision-making
   - time management.
3. Once you have gained the information to achieve a pass you need to identify the strengths and weaknesses of your session.

To achieve a merit you need to dig a bit deeper and think about what it was about each of these factors that made it a strength or a weakness. For example, if you felt your communication was good, what was it about your communication that was good? Did you use the right tone of voice, did you explain things well, did you use language that was appropriate? When you have evaluated all your strengths and weaknesses, you can then make suggestions about how you could improve your performance for the next session.

To achieve a distinction you need to justify the improvements you have suggested and say how they will improve the skills that you felt needed improving.

Further reading

Crisfield, P. (2001) *Analysing Your Coaching*, Coachwise.

Gordon, D.A. (2009) *Coaching Science*, Exeter: Learning Matters.

Martens, R. (2004) *Successful Coaching*, Champaign, Il.: Human Kinetics.

Miles, A. (2004) *Coaching Practice*, Coachwise.

Useful websites

www.brianmac.co.uk/coachsr.htm

A good introduction to coaching and its principles, with links to related topic areas

www.nspcc.org.uk/Inform/cpsu/resources/disability/disability_wda62080.html

An online list of publications relating to coaching young people, particularly those who are disabled, in sport

http://news.bbc.co.uk/sport1/hi/academy/4354156.stm

A short online article from BBC's Sports Academy on what makes a good sports coach

www.footy4kids.co.uk/planning-a-soccer-coaching-training-session.htm#

Excellent article with lots of advice on organising a coaching session for young footballers

6: Sports development

6.1 Introduction

Sports development, as we understand the term today, has been evolving over the last 25 years. It now has a wider national importance, which is demonstrated in its positive links with other important national issues such as health, crime reduction, lifelong learning and economic regeneration.

This unit starts by looking briefly at the background to the evolvement of sports development. Models of sports development and their uses will be considered, as will the use of target groups within sports development work. An understanding of the barriers to sports participation that exist will be provided and the difference between provision and enablement in sports development will be discussed. The key providers of sports development are then explored, and the structures and functions they use to deliver their work are discussed. The many different roles that exist for sports development workers will also be examined.

Methods often used to measure quality in sports development are discussed, together with the purpose of these quality measures along with their relative advantages and disadvantages. Finally, sports development in practice will be looked at. The importance of working in partnership will be demonstrated, as will some examples of current initiatives and the overall effectiveness of sports development will be discussed.

By the end of this chapter you should:

- know key concepts in sports development
- know the key providers of sports development
- understand how quality is measured in sports development
- know about sports development in practice.

Assessment and grading criteria

To achieve a PASS grade the evidence must show that the learner is able to:	To achieve a MERIT grade the evidence must show that, in addition to the pass criteria, the learner is able to:	To achieve a DISTINCTION grade the evidence must show that, in addition to the pass and merit criteria, the learner is able to:
P1 describe three examples of the sports development continuum, from three different sports	**M1** compare and contrast three examples of the sports development continuum, from three different sports, identifying strengths and areas for improvement	
P2 describe barriers to participation for individuals from three different target groups at different levels of the sports development continuum	**M2** explain barriers to participation for individuals from three different target groups at different levels of the sports development continuum	**D1** analyse the barriers to participation for individuals from three different target groups at different levels of the sports development continuum, providing effective and realistic solutions
P3 describe the structures and roles of three sports development providers in the UK		
P4 explain two methods of measuring quality in sports development	**M3** evaluate two methods of measuring quality in sports development	
P5 describe two different sports development initiatives.	**M4** compare and contrast two different sports development initiatives, identifying strengths and areas for improvement.	**D2** analyse two different sports development initiatives, offering realistic recommendations for improvement.

6.2 Key Concepts in Sports Development

P1 P2 M1 D1

Sports development can be defined as:

> Ultimately about provision of more and better quality opportunities for people, irrespective of age, gender or level of ability/disability, to access sport.
>
> (Eady, 1993)

Sports development is a broad term that has developed over time. It is used to describe the work undertaken by a range of organisations that try to ensure a positive change in sporting behaviour or physical activity throughout the community.

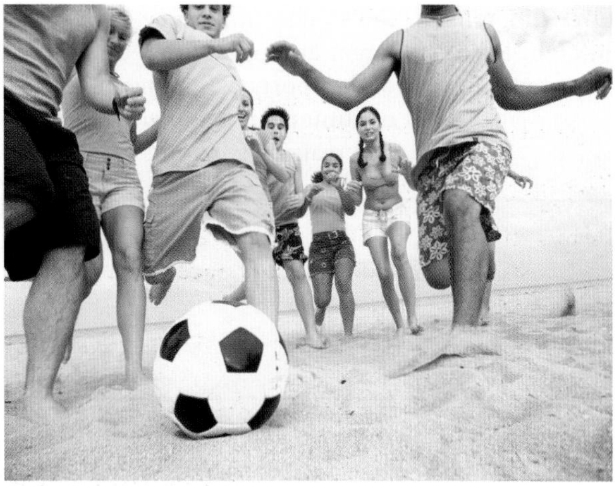

Fig 6.1 Enjoying sport

Sports development was first accepted as a term in the Wolfenden Report of 1960. The recommendations of the Wolfenden Report led to more sports facilities being developed in the UK and to financial support being given to governing bodies for sport. It also led to government funds being used for sporting initiatives and for national councils for sport. In essence, the outcomes of the report provided the principal framework for sports development until 1998. The scope of sports development was then widened by 'New Labour'. This will be considered in more detail later.

Key term

Wolfenden Report: the Central Council for Physical Recreation (CCPR) set up a committee to commission a report in 1957 called 'Sport in the Community'. As this committee was chaired by Sir John Wolfenden, the report has since been commonly known as 'the Wolfenden Report'.

Sports development continuum

The sports development continuum is used widely by many sporting organisations in the UK to help inform strategies and policies on sports development. It locates the development of sport on a hierarchical basis from foundation, through participation and performance to excellence (see Figure 6.2).

- **Foundation:** encouraging young people into the exercise habit and developing basic movement and sports skills (for example, throwing, catching and hand-to-eye coordination) to provide a foundation for personal development and future participation in the sport of their choice
- **Participation:** opportunities for all members of the community to take part in a sport, whether for reasons of enjoyment, fitness, social contact or simply to get involved in the sport for its own sake
- **Performance:** opportunities for those already participating to improve their performance from whatever base they start, where the desire to improve is the key factor for involvement
- **Excellence**: opportunities for those with the interest and ability to achieve publicly measured levels of excellence.

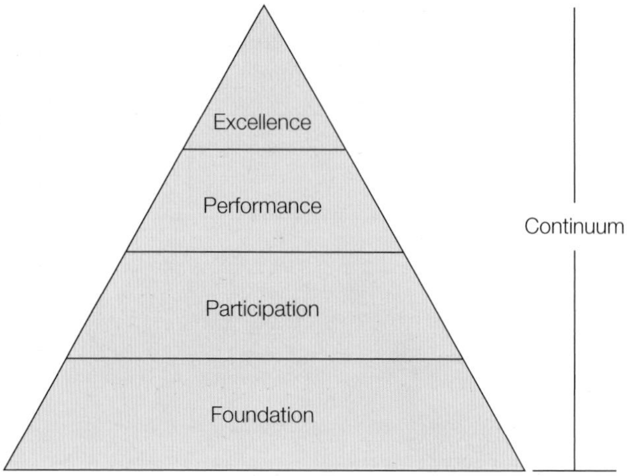

Fig 6.2 Traditional sports development continuum

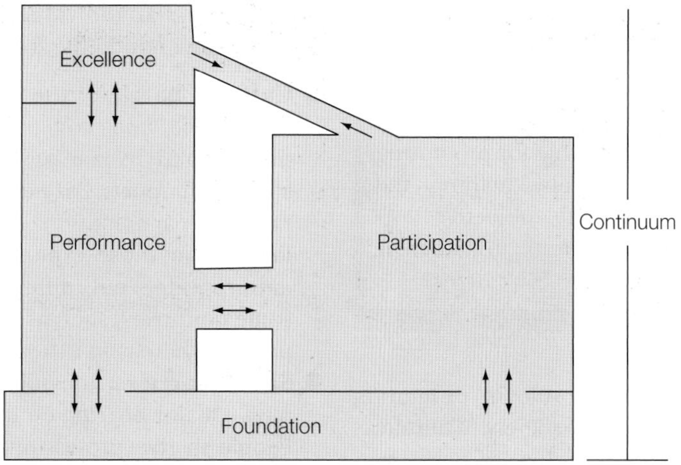

Fig 6.3 Model 2 of the sports development continuum (*Source*: Sport England)

The model implies that individuals move upwards through the continuum until they find their preferred level or the limit to their ability. It is a simple but useful model as it demonstrates the integration of different forms of involvement in sport.

This traditional model has been refined over time to take into account the rather more complex methods via which an individual may move along the continuum (see Figure 6.3).

The final model (see Figure 6.4) is flexible enough to allow an individual to remain at a particular level of performance for the time being if they choose, or to allow the individual to leave and re-enter the sport (and the level at which they participate) over time.

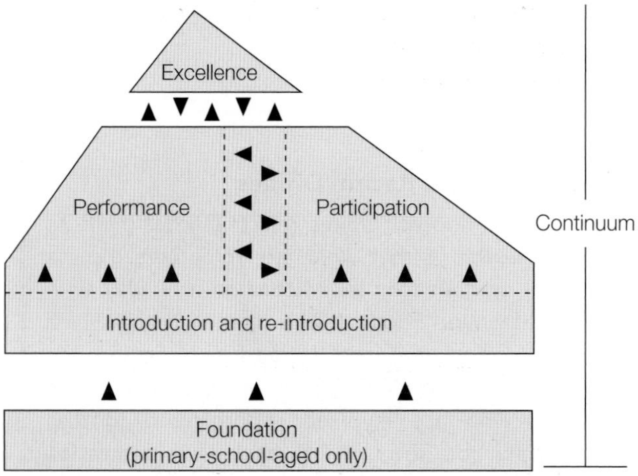

Fig 6.4 Revised model 2 of the sports development continuum

In addition to these models of the sports development continuum, other stages have sometimes been added. For example, a stage has often been added after 'participation' to show that many participants become 'committed participants' before they move on to become performers:
[display text begins]

Foundation → participation → committed participation → performance → excellence

Target groups

Inequalities have traditionally existed within sport, particularly in relation to gender, race and disability.

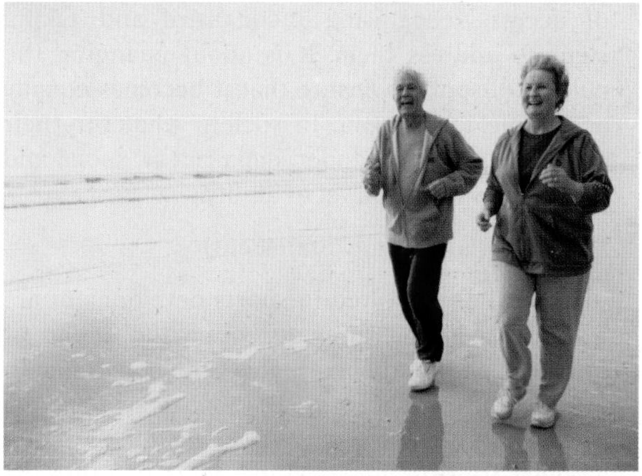

Fig 6.5 Older people are often under-represented in sport

In the 1980s Sport England identified a number of 'target groups' in sport. These were groups of people who were under-represented in terms of participation in sport. These target groups included:

- women
- people aged 5+
- people with a disability
- young people
- black and minority ethnic groups.

Key term

Sport England (the brand name of the English Sports Council): established by Royal Charter in 1972, Sport England is responsible for promoting and investing in sport, thereby helping the government meet its sporting objectives. At present it is the principal deliverer of government and Lottery funding to sport.

Sport can and does play a big role in promoting the inclusion of all groups in society. Therefore, many different campaigns and activities have been organised across the UK in order to try to increase the number of people from these target groups participating in sport and physical activity. See **Case Study Football Unites Racism Divides** and **Case Study Inclusive Fitness Initative**, which demonstrate initiatives aimed at target groups.

In sport these target groups are not the only population groups that are under-represented. In society in general, many population groups may feel discriminated against. Today the main organisations involved in sports development have moved away from using the term 'target groups' and instead use the term 'sports equity'.

> Sports equity is about fairness in sport, equality of access, recognising inequalities and taking steps to address them. It is about changing the culture of sport to ensure that it becomes equally accessible to everyone in society, whatever their ethnic origin, age, gender, impairment, social and economic status or level of ability.
>
> (Sport England Equity Statement)

All organisations involved in sports development are now encouraged to ensure equal opportunities are at the heart of all their policies. This is demonstrated in Sport England's publication *The Framework for Sport in England* (2004), which sets out the strategic direction and policy priorities for sport in England. Within the framework, sports equity and variations in access are given a high priority. Visit the Sports England website to find out more (see **Useful websites**).

Barriers to participation

Even though there has been a huge growth in the number of sports facilities open for public use since the 1970s, there has not been the same increase in participation. Some barriers have been identified that can affect an individual's ability to participate in sport. These include the following.

- **Cultural barriers:** the beliefs and knowledge of individuals and communities about sport and physical activity may prevent them participating in some or all sports. For example, in England women's rates of participation in sport are consistently lower than those experienced by men. Different cultures also put different values on sport. In some countries, such as the USA, sport has a high profile, whereas in others it is not valued.
- **Social barriers:** the social class of a person can have a major bearing on their sports participation. People in the 'professional' social class are three times more likely to participate in sport than those in the 'unskilled manual' group.
- **Economic barriers:** sports participation for many people is out of reach because they simply cannot afford the membership fees, equipment or clothing required. Also, they may unable to reach the sporting facility of their choice because they do not own a car or cannot afford public transport.
- **Historical barriers:** many sports have been around for a long time and have often been played by predominantly one type of population group. It is, therefore, often hard to change these sports.
- **Fitness/health barriers:** some people who do not participate in sport do have genuine health reasons why they should not. Health professionals try to encourage most people to participate in sport for the many associated physical and mental health benefits. However, many people do not take part in sport because they think they will not be any good at it, or because they are simply too embarrassed.

CASE STUDY

Football Unites Racism Divides

In Sheffield, Football Unites Racism Divides (FURD), in partnership with Millennium Volunteers, runs a football academy for four hours on a Sunday with Sheffield United Football Club. This academy, which has been running since 1995, has increased the number of people from black and minority ethnic groups who are involved in organised football at a grassroots level. It has been very successful, attracting well over 100 youngsters aged from six upwards each week. It has also attracted a number of volunteers, from very diverse backgrounds, who help to deliver the football programme each week.

> **CASE STUDY**
>
> **Inclusive Fitness Initiative**
>
> In 1998 the English Federation of Disability Sports piloted the Inclusive Fitness Initiative with the aim of including equipment in gyms that could be used by people with a disability. The pilot was successful so Sport England awarded the initiative £5m of Lottery funds to extend it further. There are now 150 'inclusive' gyms all across England.

Cross-cutting agendas

The focus of sports development was widened in the late 1990s when Labour was elected to government. In particular, the government wanted to use the wider benefits of sports participation to tackle 'social exclusion'.

> There are so many reasons to invest in sport. It helps our children become fit and healthy. It diverts many young people from crime and disorder. They do better at school.
>
> (Tessa Jowell MP, Secretary of State for Culture, Media and Sport, 2004)

> **Key term**
>
> **Social exclusion:** when people are prevented from taking up opportunities because of socio-economic reasons; mainly occurs when people or areas suffer from a combination of linked problems such as unemployment, poor skills, low incomes, poor housing, high crime, bad health and family breakdown.

> **CASE STUDY**
>
> **Positive Futures programme**
>
> Targeted at 10–16 year olds at risk. Its aim is to reduce youth offending and drug use, and increase regular participation in sport and physical activity.
>
> The programme has operated in over 20 locations, one of which is on the Gascoigne estate in Barking, London. Here this programme has worked in partnership with Leyton Orient Football Club's community sports programme to set up a football scheme that has mushroomed into a community sports club for teenagers. Police statistics show that the number of offences in this ward had decreased by 77 per cent in June to August 2001 compared with the same quarter in 2000 immediately prior to the start of this programme.

The wider benefits of sporting participation include the following.

- **Improving the health of the nation:** By participating in sport and physical activity certain mental and physical health problems can be reduced. For example, 30 minutes of moderate activity five times a week can reduce the risk of cardiovascular diseases, some cancers, strokes and obesity.
- **Reduction of crime and drug use:** There has been some evidence that sports participation has a positive effect on crime reduction and drug use.
- **Raising educational standards**
- **More cohesive, sustainable communities.**

Provision and enabling

There are many different ways of providing sports development activities.

- Many organisations directly provide courses on specific sports. For example, swimming lessons are run by many different organisations including schools, local authority sports centres and private/commercial providers. These organisations may

> **Key learning points 1**
>
> - Sports development is a broad term used to describe the work undertaken by a range of organisations that try to ensure a positive change in sporting behaviour or physical activity throughout the community.
> - There are four main stages in the sports development continuum: foundation, participation, performance and excellence.
> - The key target groups that have been highlighted as being under-represented in terms of participation in sport are:
>   - women
>   - people aged 50+
>   - people with a disability
>   - young people
>   - black and minority ethnic groups.
> - Sports equity is the 'in vogue' term used today to describe how all sports should be accessible to everyone.
> - There are a number of barriers to people participating in sport. These include social, economic, cultural, historical and health barriers.
> - There are different ways of providing sports development activities, including directly providing an activity, enabling another organisation to provide an activity or working in a partnership.

run 'taster sessions' to encourage participants to try out a sport before they commit to paying for more sessions.

- Some organisations in sports development, such as sports coach UK, do not directly provide sports development activities. Instead, they enable and facilitate the activities being run by other organisations by providing, for example, coach education courses. Many sports development organisations may also give grants or help with the provision of sports equipment or facilities to enable sports development activities to take place.
- Partnership working (two or more organisations working together) in sports development is very common. This may include, for example, a local authority sports development department joining forces with a Primary Care Trust to deliver initiatives such as a GP referral scheme.

Quick quiz 1

Give short answers to the following questions:

1 Briefly describe each of the main stages of the sports development continuum.

2 Name four target groups for sports development.

3 List four barriers to participation in sport.

Student activity 6.1

90 minutes P1 P2 M1 M2 D1

Task 1

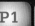

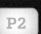

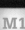

Research and then describe the sports development continuum in three different sports, then compare and contrast the examples identifying strengths and areas for improvement in the development of each sport.

Task 2

Complete the following table to show your knowledge of the barriers to sports participation that performers experience at different levels of the sports development continuum.

Target group	Describe the barriers at different levels of the sports development continuum	Explain the barriers at different levels of the sports development continuum	Analyse the barriers at different levels of the sports development continuum and offer solutions
Women	Foundation Participation Performance Excellence	Foundation Participation Performance Excellence	Foundation Participation Performance Excellence
Disabled people	Foundation Participation Performance Excellence	Foundation Participation Performance Excellence	Foundation Participation Performance Excellence
Black and ethnic minorities	Foundation Participation Performance Excellence	Foundation Participation Performance Excellence	Foundation Participation Performance Excellence

6.3 Key Providers of Sports Development

P3

There are many different organisations involved in the provision of sports development today. These include national organisations such as UK Sport and voluntary organisations such as sports coach UK. Most local authorities have a sports development unit or department. There are also a number of professional and private-sector sports development providers. Let's look at some of these in more detail.

National organisations

UK Sport

UK Sport was established by Royal Charter in 1996. It has a strategic role in sports development. It focuses on high-performance sport in the UK, with the aim of achieving sporting excellence on the world stage. It works in partnership with the sports councils (i.e. Sport England, Sport Wales and Sport Scotland) and other agencies. It is responsible for managing and distributing public funds (approximately £29 million annually) and is a distributor of funds raised by the National Lottery.

UK Sport is responsible to the Department for Culture, Media and Sport (DCMS). Its work is directed by a board, to which the DCMS appoints members. This board meets every two months. It also has various committees that report to the board on different matters. For more details on its work visit the UK Sport website.

> **Key term**
>
> **Department of Culture, Media and Sport (DCMS):** the DCMS is the government department responsible for policy direction in sport (as well as tourism and creative industries). It aims to improve the quality of life for its people through cultural and sporting activities and through the strengthening of the sport, tourism and creative industries. Visit the DCMS website for more details of its work.

Sport England

Sport England also has a strategic role in sports development. It is responsible for promoting and investing in sport and helping the government meet its sporting objectives in England.

Sport England's vision is to make England an active and successful sporting nation. It aims to achieve this by getting people to:

- **start in sport:** to improve the health of the nation, particularly for disadvantaged groups
- **stay in sport:** through a thriving network of clubs, coaches and volunteers, and a commitment to equity
- **succeed in sport:** via an infrastructure capable of developing world-class performers.

Since 1994 the organisation has invested £2bn in sport in England. This money comes from the Lottery and from government funds.

The main board of Sport England has overall responsibility for its performance. It deals with strategy, finance, major projects and performance management. Its board members are appointed by the DCMS. Its chief executive is responsible to the main board for the day-to-day running of Sport England. It also has a number of committees that focus on specific tasks, strategies or policies. They report back to the main board.

Sport England works through nine regional offices, along with their regional sports boards. It also funds County Sports Partnerships throughout England. Visit the Sport England website for more details of its work (see **Useful websites**).

> **Key term**
>
> **County Sports Partnership (CSP):** across England there are 49 CSPs, whose core funding comes from Sport England. Each CSP is a partnership of agencies that seek to make the connections between national planning and local delivery. They aim to provide 'one voice for sport' in each county. Their main goals are to:
>
> - put together pathways for young people to move on in sport
> - help club development in their area
> - develop the workforce involved in sport.

Voluntary organisations

There are a number of voluntary, independent agencies that are outside the influence of the government organisations mentioned above. They also have a great influence on policies and strategies for sport, though. These include:

- the Central Council for Physical Recreation (CCPR)
- the Youth Sport Trust (YST)
- sports coach UK (SCUK).

The Central Council for Physical Recreation

The Central Council for Physical Recreation (CCPR) has existed since 1944. It is the 'umbrella organisation' for the national governing and representative bodies of sport and recreation in the UK. It works on behalf of:

- 270 national governing and representative bodies of sport and recreation
- 150,000 voluntary sports clubs
- millions of individuals who participate in sport and recreation.

Independent of any form of government control, the CCPR speaks and acts to **promote, protect and develop** the interests of sport and physical recreation at all levels. The CCPR is at the **forefront** of sports politics, providing support and services to those who participate in and administer sport and recreation. For further details, visit the CCPR website.

Sports National Governing Bodies

All major sports in Britain have a national governing body (NGB). For example, the Football Association is the NGB for football, the All England Netball Association is the NGB for netball, and the Lawn Tennis Association is the NGB for tennis. There are over 265 national governing bodies in the UK.

Teams and clubs normally pay a subscription to their sport's governing body, which administers the sport nationally and organises competitions and the national team.

Most sports governing bodies receive funding and resources from Sport England. To receive this funding each NGB has to produce a whole sport plan.

The NGB for each sport may also receive funding and resources for its elite athletes from UK Sport.

Key term

Whole sport plan: these are plans for the whole of a sport from grassroots to performance (at a county level). These plans identify the help and resources they need to deliver their plans; for example, partners such as county sports partnerships, and programmes such as PE, School Sport and Club Links (PESSCL).

The Youth Sport Trust

The Youth Sport Trust was established in 1994 as a registered charity to support the education and development of all young people through physical education (PE) and sport. It believes that all young people have the right to:

- experience and enjoy PE and sport
- a quality introduction to PE and sport suited to their own level of development
- the best teaching, the best coaching and the best resources
- experience and benefit from positive competition
- develop a healthy lifestyle
- progress along a structured pathway of sporting opportunities
- fulfil their sporting potential.

Sports coach UK

Originally named the National Coaching Foundation, sports coach UK was established in 1983 as a sub-committee of the Sports Council, becoming a separate charitable organisation in 1989. It works at a strategic level, its main aim being to guide the development and implementation of a coaching system for all coaches at every level in the UK. Its main activities include:

- providing coaching resources
- running coaching courses
- administering coaching qualifications
- working with governing bodies to raise the quality of coaching schemes.

A board of directors who are responsible for policy direction runs sports coach UK. The management team implements these policies on a day-to-day basis. The organisation also has a network of Coach Development Officers (one per county) who work on these activities at a local level.

Local authorities

Local authorities are extremely important to the sports development industry. They spend approximately £1bn per year on sport and leisure – more than 50 per cent of the total resources available to sport. They follow the national lead in developing sport.

> There is a need for all local authorities to 'take the lead' individually or in partnership with neighbouring authorities for overseeing the strategic planning for structured sport, physical education and lifelong learning through sport .
> (Sport England, 2004)

Local authorities recognise the benefits of developing sport for their population. Most local authorities employ at least one Sports Development Officer, while many will have a whole team. They will tend to focus on sports participation trends within their area and will then target their resources at any apparent inequalities that exist.

Local authorities in the UK directly provide many public leisure facilities, including sports halls, swimming pools, golf courses and football pitches. They, therefore, provide most of the facilities used to facilitate sports development activities. Many operate concessionary schemes or special initiatives within these facilities in order to encourage as many of their population to use their facilities as possible. They also have important links to schools in terms of sporting facilities and policies on sport.

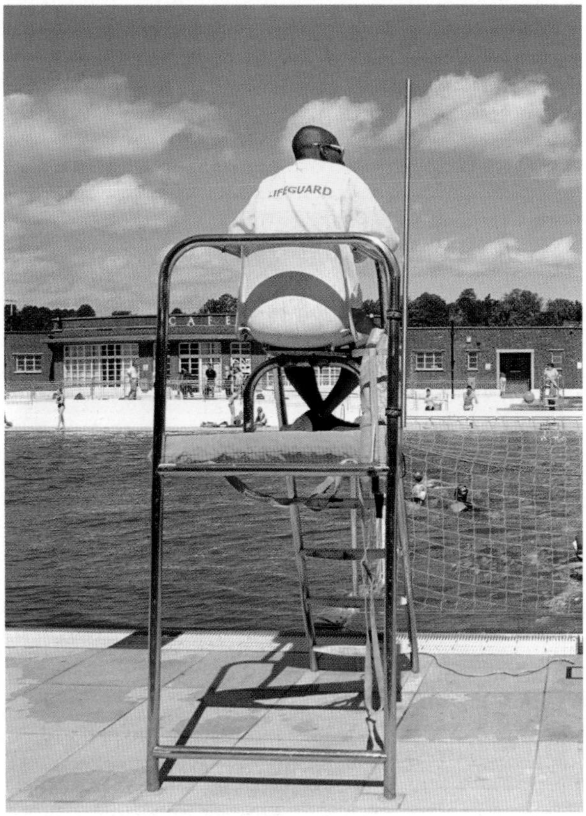

Fig 6.6 Local authority-owned swimming pool

Many local authorities also support local organisations in their development of sports facilities, sometimes with financial help, but mainly with advice on strategy and building regulations.

Private and professional organisations

There are many private organisations involved in directly providing sports development activities. For example, many private leisure or health clubs run activities for their paying members, such as swimming, golf or tennis lessons.

There are also many small businesses within the sports development industry that run sports coaching sessions for a fee. They may provide, for example, football coaching sessions for children.

Sport development roles

Sports development is one of the fastest-growing areas of the sports industry and just as there are many different organisations involved in sports development, there are also many different roles. The decision to award the 2012 Olympics to London means that there is likely to be an increase in opportunities for Sports Development Officers (SDOs) over the coming years.

SDOs aim to improve access to sport and physical activity for people of all ages and ability. They may promote sport in general, working for a County Sports Partnership or local authority, or may be Sports Specific Development Officers (SSDOs), concentrating on a specific sport and working for an NGB.

Generally the work of an SDO can include anything from organising events for communities, devising and implementing sports programmes, ensuring people can get access to activities, linking into local and regional sports initiatives, as well as speaking to schools, clubs, governing bodies and individuals. They may work with the local community, liaising with clubs and schools, as well as agencies such as the police and sports' national governing bodies.

They may also work closely with specific groups, including those who may not have had access to sporting opportunities before, such as the socially excluded, young people, disabled people, or people from disadvantaged backgrounds.

Much of their work involves formulating and implementing strategies aimed at increasing participation and improving standards.

There are currently approximately 100,000 paid SDOs working in the UK. There are, however, many more people working in sports development who are volunteers, i.e. working in a non-paid capacity. A recent study by Sport England (Sport Volunteering in England, 2002) estimated that there are 5.8 million volunteers in sport. Their roles range from coaching and officiating in local clubs to sitting on regional sports boards.

> ... 47% of young people's volunteering takes place in sport. The sport sector accounts for 26% of all volunteers and volunteers are vital to the success of our national sporting life – the London Marathon relies on 6000 volunteers. The Manchester Commonwealth Games involved 10,000 volunteers and the role of volunteers will be integral to the 2012 Olympics ... [and Paralympic Games]
>
> (Russell Commission, 2005)

Many sports clubs are run entirely by volunteers. Volunteers are now recognised by the main organisations involved in sports development as making an extremely important contribution. As a result, a number of initiatives have been set up to try to encourage more people to volunteer in sport, e.g. Sport England's 'Step into Sport' initiative.

CASE STUDY

London Borough of Enfield: free swims for young people

As part of its target to increase the number of attendances at leisure centres by young people (aged 0–18), the London Borough of Enfield, in partnership with Enfield Leisure Centres Ltd (ELCL), the operator of the Council's leisure facilities, agreed a free swims programme during public swimming sessions for several weeks during school holidays in 2006. The cost to the Council was £18,000.

The free swims were located in council-owned facilities in the eastern corridor of the borough, which is one of the more deprived areas in Enfield and where many young people are not currently taking part in sporting activities. The scheme was extremely successful, with approximately 20,000 extra swims by young people taking place during this period in comparison with similar periods in 2005.

The aim is that the free swims initiative will encourage the young people who have taken part to continue to take part regularly in swimming or other physical activity in the future and to make physical activity a habit in their lives.

Key learning points 2

- There are several key providers in sports development including:
  - national organisations such as UK Sport and Sport England
  - voluntary organisations such as sports coach UK and National Governing Bodies of sports
  - local authorities
  - private and professional organisations.
- There are currently approximately 100,000 people in paid employment in the sports development industry. They are employed in a variety of roles but are collectively known as sports development officers.
- There are many volunteers (i.e. non-paid) working in the sports development industry. They have a variety of roles, ranging from coaching at a local club to sitting on a regional sports board.

Q Quick quiz 2

Match the organisation to the brief description of their role.

Organisation	Description of role
Department of Culture, Media and Sport	Responsible for promoting sport and investing in its development
UK Sport	Responsible for the development of sports policy.
Sport England	Represents the interests of the national governing bodies
CCPR	Focuses on high performance sport with the aim of achieving sporting excellence

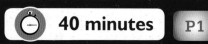

Student activity 6.2 40 minutes **P1**

Present a poster that describes the roles and structures of three of the sports development providers.

6.4 Quality Measurement in Sports Development

P4 **M3**

Key term

Quality: displaying excellence in an organisation.

Methods of quality measurement in sports development

Traditionally many different methods have been used to try to measure quality in sports development, such as attendances at sporting activities or local participation levels. These methods have not provided consistency across the sports development industry because not all organisations have measured the same outputs or used the same methods to do so. As a result of this, and to gain the benefits listed below, a number of schemes have been developed to measure quality in sports development. The main idea behind these schemes is that by putting together a clear set of quality standards that are appropriate to the industry sector, performance in the sector can be measured more realistically. The main quality measures that have been developed, and are appropriate to sports development, include those described below.

Towards an Excellent Service (TAES)

This quality scheme was originally developed by Sport England for local authority sport and recreation services. An additional modified version was created to be used by County Sports Partnerships (CSPs) within the sports development industry. This scheme is based on good practice taken from other quality schemes used across the sports industry. TAES aims to provide a clear measurement of the present and future health of 'how' a CSP is functioning through an assessment that defines its strengths and areas for improvement.

In practice, each CSP has to complete a self-assessment on different areas of its work and grade itself as either poor, fair, good or excellent. External assessors then carry out their own assessment of the CSP. The results of these two assessments are combined to create an improvement plan where the CSP identifies its improvement priorities. It will then measure its progress towards these priorities over a specified time period.

Quest

This quality management system is aimed at sports development units in local authorities, governing bodies and voluntary organisations. The Quest quality management system defines what the industry standards in sports development are and what good practice is. It encourages organisations to apply and develop these standards in all areas of their work: management, operations, customer relations and staffing, etc.

To achieve Quest accreditation organisations must have both a self-assessment improvement programme and the opportunity for an independent external assessment. Here is an example.

1. To complete a self-assessment improvement programme an organisation must look at all the work it currently does and assess how well it thinks it is doing. It then has to put together an action plan of how and when it is going to improve on certain areas. This action plan has to be monitored and evaluated regularly so that the organisation is constantly striving for improvement. This promotes continuous improvement within its work.
2. External assessment/audits are completed by an industry professional who carries out an independent audit of the organisation's work.

There are a number of other quality awards that are used within the sports development industry, such as:

- ISO 9001:2000
- Investors In People
- Charter Mark
- Green Flag (for grass pitches).

National Governing Body schemes

Many sports' national governing bodies have themselves developed their own quality schemes or quality marks that are open for their members to achieve. One good example is the Amateur Swimming

Association's (ASA) Swim 21 Accreditation scheme, which is its own 'quality mark' scheme. It recognises nationally and regionally the swimming clubs that are committed to providing safe, effective and high-quality services for the benefit of their members.

To gain this quality mark, swimming clubs must work towards attaining a series of outcomes. These are seen as essential if the right level of support is to be provided at each stage of a swimmer's development.

The Swim 21 scheme is really a planning tool, based on the principles of Long Term Athlete Development (see below), enabling swimming clubs to help athletes, teachers, coaches and administrators to achieve their full potential. It focuses mainly on the needs of swimmers – looking to provide them with the best possible support and environment. Other examples of quality marks or schemes used by sports' governing bodies include the Football Association's Charter Standard and the Amateur Athletic Association of England Clubmark award.

An added benefit of gaining a quality mark or award is that many are recognised by Sport England as a Clubmark accredited scheme. Swim 21 is one such award and therefore all clubs gaining Swim 21 accreditation will automatically receive Clubmark status. Clubmark is a Sport England quality accreditation scheme, which will eventually be accessible to all sports. It seeks to ensure that young people are participating within a safe and friendly environment.

Key term

Long Term Athlete Development (LTAD): the principle used to achieve optimal training, competition and recovery throughout an athlete's career.

Why measure quality in sports development?

There are a number of important reasons why quality should be measured in sports development. These include the following.

1. All organisations should be constantly striving to improve their service – this is known as 'continuous improvement'. For example, by being involved in Quest or TAES, organisations are having to continually evaluate how they are performing and put in place systems to measure their performance. This can bring many benefits to organisations, such as:
   - increasing their customer focus
   - improving their consultation with users
   - improving their staff morale
   - developing better internal systems of work and procedures
   - developing more effective service delivery
   - an improvement in complaints handling
   - delivering more cost-effective services.
2. Recognition: by achieving a quality mark sports development organisations can use this to promote the service they provide.
3. When sports development organisations apply for additional funding, external agencies will be able to tell by the quality marks the organisation holds that it provides a successful service. This is looked upon favourably by most funding bodies.
4. Standardisation: it is easier to measure the performance of one sports development organisation against another when they achieve a quality accreditation.

There are some disadvantages in measuring quality in any sports development organisation. Applying for and then going through the process of achieving quality accreditation can be both costly and time-consuming. This is mainly because most organisations will need to pay for some expert help in order to achieve the quality accreditation. They will also have to spend a great deal of time collecting evidence themselves from within their organisation.

Key learning points 3

- Quality is about displaying excellence in an organisation.
- Traditional methods of measuring quality in sports development have been inconsistent and difficult to compare from one organisation to another.
- Quality awards such as TAES and Quest are used by many sports development organisations.
- There are many benefits to a sports development organisation of gaining a quality award, such as continuous improvement in its service.
- The process of gaining a quality award can be both time consuming and costly to sports development organisations.

Q Quick quiz 3

Using the list of words/phrases given in the box below, complete the following paragraph:

Quality is a measure of __________ in an organisation. There are quality _________ such as TAES and _____ that can be gained through _____ _________ of the quality of their service. Measuring quality can bring continuous ____________ in _________ focus, staff _______ and in _________ handling.

quest	morale	complaints	self assessment
excellence	customer	improvements	awards

Student activity 6.3 — 30 minutes — P4 M3

Complete the table below to explain two methods of measuring quality in sports development.

Method of measuring quality in sports development	Explain the methods of measuring quality in sports development	Evaluate the methods of measuring quality in sports development
1		
2		

6.5 Sports Development in Practice

P5 M4 D2

We have already looked at some of the key providers in sports development, ranging from national organisations at one end of the spectrum to local sports clubs at the other. The way that these key providers operate in practice and their effectiveness will now be considered.

Sports development organisations working in partnership

The interaction of sports development organisations has been the subject of a number of recent Sport England documents. In the past, many sports development organisations have worked in isolation and as a result there has been a lot of duplication of effort. This duplication has wasted valuable resources.

As a result of this, all the main organisations involved in the delivery of sport are now committed to supporting the new Delivery System for Sport (see Figure 6.7).

The Delivery System for Sport has two aims: to increase the number of people taking part in sport and recreation, especially amongst the hard-to-reach; and to build clear pathways for people with sporting talent to achieve their full potential. Figure 6.7 shows the relationship between the key components of the system and how the national and regional partners connect to the sub-regional and local components of the system. The two key elements of the Delivery System at the local levels are the County Sport Partnerships (CSPs) and the Community Sport Networks (CSNs).

> The ambition of Sport England is to lead and support the development of a holistic, coherent and quality-assured delivery system that ensures everybody, no matter where they live or their personal circumstances, is able to access high quality sporting opportunities that truly meet their personal needs.
> (Sport England, 2006)

Key term

Community Sports Network (CSN): these are locally coordinated networks of organisations with an interest in sport. They identify local sporting needs and develop a shared vision for sport and physical activity in their area. A CSN's geographical boundaries are often the same as those of a local authority.

Partnerships in practice

As mentioned before, sports development organisations often work together in partnerships with other sports development organisations or with other types of organisation. For example, in Case Study: Football Unites Racism Divides, the Millennium Volunteers organisation worked with Sheffield United Football Club and the Football Unites Racism Divides organisation, to offer football to girls and boys from black and minority ethnic groups.

Working in partnerships can have a number of benefits to all those involved, including the pooling of resources so that more can be achieved than if the organisations were working alone. Inevitably, there are often a number of barriers to be overcome in partnership working. For example, differing opinions or ideas as to how a project should be set up or delivered. However, joint strategies can be devised so that the partners adopt a coordinated approach. This often informs others about the targets of the partnership and how they expect to achieve these targets. This then enables the partnership to measure its level of success.

Local authority sports development in practice

Each local authority provides sports development work in different ways. For example, many local authorities will have a small section within a Leisure Department devoted to sports development. This may consist of only one Sports Development Officer or many Sports Development Officers. Some local authorities have 'contracted out' their sports development work along with the management of their sport and leisure facilities.

CASE STUDY

Manchester City Council

Established in 1992, Manchester Leisure is the department within Manchester City Council responsible for sports development and parks. The Sports Development Team employs over 60 people. This includes:

- Sports Development Managers such as a Strategic Sports Development Manager and administrative staff
- Sports Specific Development Officers who represent 13 sports including badminton, cricket and swimming
- Community Sports Development Officers who work within specific communities citywide
- Sports Officers with a remit to work with targeted sectors of the community such as refugees, disabled people and people aged over 50.

Manchester Leisure's team of Sports Development Officers has two main objectives. These are to:

- maximise participation in sport by all sectors of the community within Manchester
- provide pathways to excellence that enable every person to fulfil their real sporting potential.

The sports development team has put together a number of strategies and action plans to guide its work. It also provides advice and guidance on funding issues, hosts both national and local events and runs a coach education scheme in the City of Manchester. It works in partnership with many other organisations, such as NGBs.

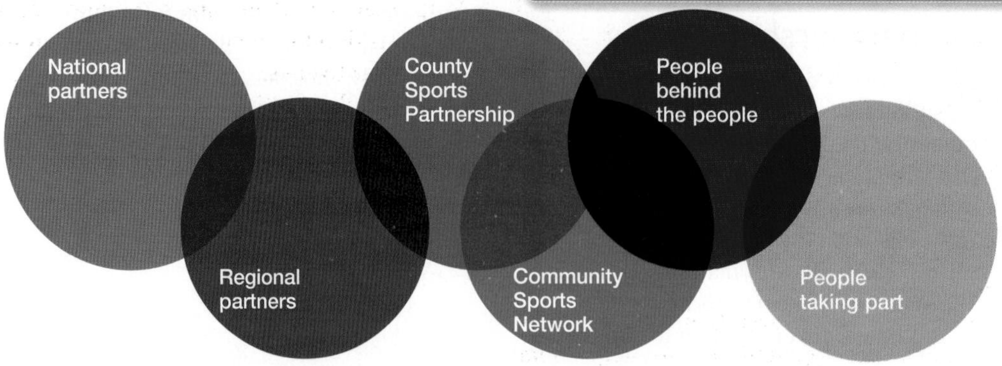

Fig 6.7 The delivery system for sport (Sport England, 2006)

CASE STUDY

Herts Sports Partnership

The Herts Sports Partnership (HSP) was established in 2004 as one of 49 County Sport Partnerships in England, as part of the Sport England delivery system. The HSP is led by a voluntary representative executive board and has a core team of full- and part-time paid sports development officers.

The core team works alongside partners bringing together knowledge, ideas and expertise from the sports world in Hertfordshire; providing a central and coordinated 'sports authority' for the county. Its key purposes for Hertfordshire are to:

- increase the number of people taking part in sport and physical activity
- develop the sports infrastructure
- increase the quality of provision.

The HSP offers services and support at all levels to those who:

- take part in sport or physical activity
- deliver sport or physical activity
- are involved with the strategic development of sports and physical activity.

Examples of the services and support offered include: planning schemes to increase participation, such as school–club link programmes and 'Get Active' campaigns; workshops for clubs, coaches, officials, administrators and volunteers; providing advice and guidance on writing funding applications, and coordinating countywide projects.

Sport can also contribute to the improvement of a number of community priorities such as healthier communities, safe, strong and sustainable communities, economic vitality and workforce development, and meeting the needs of children and young people. The HSP forges partnerships across a range of industries and organisations to create sport schemes designed, for example, to tackle anti-social behaviour and the fear of crime.

More information about this partnership can be found by visiting the Sports in Herts website (see **Useful websites**).

The effectiveness of sports development organisations in practice

There are a number of criteria that organisations involved in sports development use to help them measure their effectiveness.

- **Quality measures (as detailed above):** can be used to measure the effectiveness of organisations.
- **Achievement of stated aims and objectives:** most organisations involved in sports development produce a business or development plan. This should clearly set out the aims and objectives that the organisation wants to achieve. It will then state how these aims and objectives are going to be achieved, i.e. what resources are going to be needed and how long it will take to achieve them.
- **Customer feedback:** this may take many forms, i.e. customer complaints cards, questionnaires, interviews or mystery visit results. The results will give a good indication of whether the customer is satisfied with an organisation.
- **Value for money:** this can be hard to quantify because not all benefits of sports participation can be reliably measured. However, generally a cost/benefit analysis based on human and financial resources can be carried out.
- **Consultation:** valuable feedback can be gained from those involved in delivering sports development, i.e. SDOs and other organisations and partners.

Good-quality monitoring and evaluation is necessary so that delivery organisations, partners and funders know whether sport and physical activity projects have been efficiently run and effective in achieving their aims.

Key learning points 4

- Most sports development organisations, in practice, work in partnership with other organisations.
- In practice, Sport England, along with other key sports development organisations, is committed to providing a single delivery system for sport.
- Each local authority, in practice, will provide its sports development work in a different way.
- In practice, there are a number of ways a sports development organisation can measure its effectiveness, e.g. by achieving its stated aims and objectives.

Student activity 6.4

90 minutes **P5** **M4** **D2**

Prepare a presentation to present to your tutor about two different sports development initiatives.

To achieve **P5**, describe two different sports development initiatives; to achieve **M4**, compare and contrast two different sports development initiatives and identify strengths and areas for improvement, and to achieve **D2**, analyse two different sports development initiatives and offer realistic recommendations for improvement.

References

Eady, J. (1993) *Practical Sports Development*. London: Pitman.

Houlihan, B. and White, A. (2002) *The Politics of Sports Development*. London: Routledge.

Hylton, K., Bramham, P., Jackson, D. and Nesti, M. (2001) *Sports Development: Policy, Process and Practice*. London: Routledge.

Joint DCMS/Strategy Unit Report (2002) 'Game Plan: a strategy for delivering Government's sport and physical activity objectives'.

Russell Commission (2005) 'A National Framework for Youth Action and Engagement'.

Sport England (1996) 'The value of sport to Local Authorities'.

Sport England (2004) 'The Framework for Sport in England'.

Further reading

Bill, K. (2009). *Sport Management*. London: Learning Matters.

Collins, M. (2006). *Examining Sports Development*. London: Routledge.

Houlihan, B. and White, A. (2002). *The Politics of Sports Development*. London: Routledge.

Useful websites

www.sportdevelopment.info/

An online library with a wealth of reports, articles and academic papers relating to sports development in the UK; offers a 'student zone', but registration required for full access

www.authorstream.com/Presentation/eddie23081940-173616-sport-development-sportdevelopment-lecture1-sports-ppt-powerpoint/

A brief PowerPoint presentation on what sports development involves

7: Fitness testing for sport & exercise

7.1 Introduction

The ability to conduct fitness testing is a vital skill for the sport scientist to possess. All athletes and people starting exercise need to know where they are at any point in time so they can work out how close they are to where they want to be.

This unit will start by looking at a battery of fitness tests that can be used with athletes and people taking exercise, and will consider any advantages or disadvantages with these methods. Then we will look at screening techniques and health-monitoring tests that are used to identify whether a person is healthy enough to perform these fitness tests, which can push an individual to the limits of their fitness. Once we have knowledge of the tests, we will look at how these tests can be administered safely and how the data you gain from the tests can be interpreted.

By the end of this unit you should:

- know a range of laboratory-based and field-based fitness tests
- be able to use health-screening techniques
- be able to administer appropriate fitness tests
- be able to interpret the results of fitness tests and provide feedback.

Assessment and grading criteria		
To achieve a PASS grade the evidence must show that the learner is able to:	**To achieve a MERIT grade the evidence must show that, in addition to the pass criteria, the learner is able to:**	**To achieve a DISTINCTION grade the evidence must show that, in addition to the pass and merit criteria, the learner is able to:**
P1 describe one test for each component of physical fitness, including advantages and disadvantages	**M1** explain the advantages and disadvantages of one fitness test for each component of physical fitness	
P2 prepare an appropriate health-screening questionnaire		
P3 devise and use appropriate health-screening procedures for two contrasting individuals		
P4 safely administer and interpret the results of four different health-monitoring tests for two contrasting individuals	**M2** describe the strengths and areas for improvement for two contrasting individuals using information from health-screening questionnaires and health-monitoring tests	**D1** evaluate the health screening-questionnaires and health-monitoring test results and provide recommendations for lifestyle improvement
P5 select and safely administer six different fitness tests for a selected individual, recording the findings	**M3** justify the selection of fitness tests, commenting on suitability, reliability, validity and practicality	
P6 give feedback to a selected individual, following fitness testing, describing the test results and interpreting their levels of fitness against normative data.	**M4** compare the fitness test results to normative data and identify strengths and areas for improvement.	**D2** analyse the fitness test results and provide recommendations for appropriate future activities or training.

7.2 Laboratory-based and field-based fitness tests

P1 M1

Tests are conducted to assess each different component of fitness. It is important to choose the components of fitness relative to the person you are working with. This will depend on their own goals and the activities they are involved in, be it sport or exercise.

Performance-related fitness

Performance in sport and exercise is dependent on a range of components of fitness. These are shown in Figure 7.1.

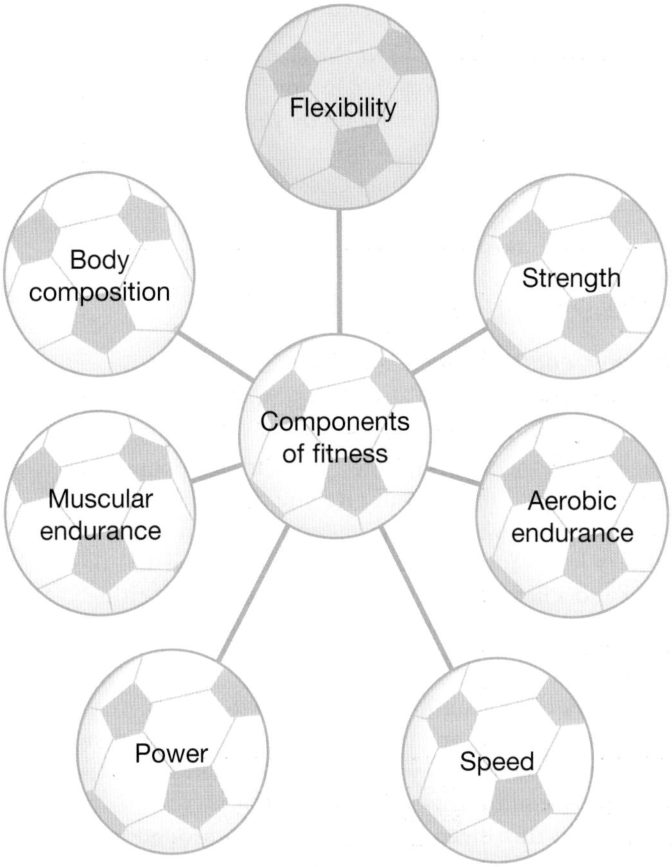

Fig 7.1 Components of fitness

Test protocols

The following is a list of test protocols:

- sit and reach
- one repetition maximum
- grip strength dynamometer
- multi-stage fitness test
- step test
- 40-metre sprint
- vertical jump
- Wingate test
- one-minute press-up test
- one-minute sit-up test
- skinfold assessment
- bioelectrical impedance
- hydro-densitometry.

We will now look at each of these in turn.

Flexibility

The **sit and reach test** measures the flexibility of the muscles in the lower back and hamstrings. This test is safe to perform unless the athlete has a lower back injury, particularly a slipped disc. The test is performed in the following way:

1. Warm the athlete up with five minutes' jogging or cycling.
2. Ask the athlete to take off their shoes and any clothing that will limit movement.
3. The athlete sits with their legs straight and their feet against the board. Their legs and back should be straight.
4. The client reaches as far forward as they possibly can and pushes the marker forward.
5. Record the furthest point the marker reaches.

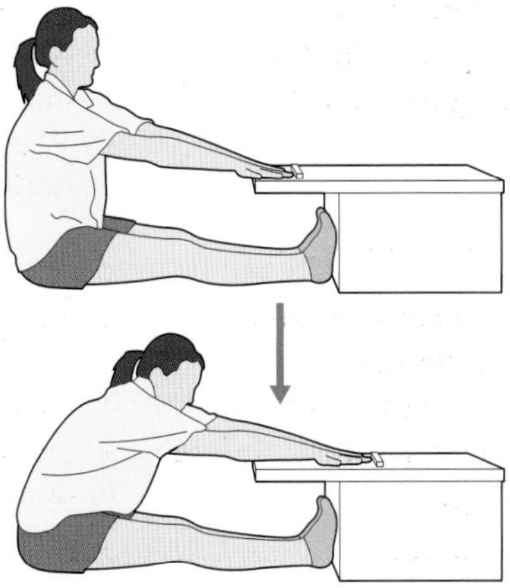

Fig 7.2 Sit and reach test

This test is quick and easy to administer and perform; however, it is a fairly non-specific test as it tells us something about the range of movement in the back, hamstrings and calves, but we may not be able to identify where there are restrictions or tight muscles. Also it tells us nothing about the range of movement in other important muscle groups, such as the chest, quadriceps or hip flexors.

Category	Males (cm)	Females (cm)
Elite	>27	>30
Excellent	17 to 27	21 to 30
Good	6 to 16	11 to 20
Average	0 to 5	1 to 10
Fair	–8 to –1	–7 to 0
Poor	–9 to –19	–8 to –14
Very poor	<–20	<–15

Table 7.1 Categories for sit and reach scores (adapted from Franklin, 2000)

Strength

The **one repetition maximum** (1 RM) is a measure of absolute strength and is the maximum weight that can be moved once with perfect technique.

This is clearly a dangerous test to perform unless the client is of an advanced skill level and is very well conditioned. The test will also require a thorough warm-up prior to its performance.

The test is performed in the following way:

1. Choose an exercise requiring the use of large muscle groups, such as a bench press or a leg press.
2. Warm up with a light weight for ten repetitions.
3. Give one minute rest.
4. Estimate a resistance that can be used for three to five repetitions.
5. Give two minutes' rest.
6. Estimate a load that can be used for two to three repetitions.
7. Give two to three minutes' rest.
8. Decide on a load that can be used for one repetition.
9. If successful, then give two to four minutes' rest.
10. Add a little more weight and complete one repetition.
11. Weight is gradually added until the client fails.
12. 1 RM is the last weight that can be completed successfully.

There are no normative tables for 1 RM tests as they are used to monitor progress and strength gains. They can also be used to decide on training loads for the individual.

The **grip strength dynamometer** is a static test to assess muscular strength in the arm muscles. Unfortunately, it will give no indication as to the strength of other muscle groups. The test involves squeezing a hand-grip dynamometer as hard as possible. The test is conducted in the following way:

1. Adjust the handle to fit the size of your hand.
2. Hold the dynamometer in your strongest hand and keep the arm hanging by your side with the dynamometer by your thigh.
3. Squeeze the dynamometer as hard as you can for around five seconds.
4. Record the results and repeat after about a minute.
5. Take your best recording.

Aerobic endurance

The **multi-stage fitness test** was developed at the University of Loughborough and is known as the 'bleep' test because athletes have to run between timed bleeps. The test will give you an estimation of your VO_2max, which is the measure of your aerobic fitness level. You will need the pre-recorded CD or tape and a flat area of 20 metres, with a cone at either end. This test can be used with large groups, as all the athletes will run together. The procedure is as follows:

1. Mark out a length of 20 metres with cones.
2. Start the tape and the athletes run when the first bleep sounds. They will run the 20 metres before the second bleep sounds.
3. When this bleep sounds, they turn around and run back.
4. They continue to do this and the time between the bleeps gets shorter and shorter, so they have to run faster and faster.
5. If an athlete fails to get to the other end before the bleep on three consecutive occasions, they are out.
6. Record at what point the athlete dropped out.
7. Using Table 7.2, you can find out the athlete's predicted VO_2max.

This is an excellent field-based test which can be used to assess and monitor the fitness levels of individuals and groups of people. The results are dependent on the motivation level of the participants and how willing they are to drive themselves to their limits.

The **Canadian step test** is a simple and straightforward test to perform, and measures how heart rate increases with steady-state exercise.

You need a step 30 cm high, a heart-rate monitor and a stopwatch. This test is carried out in the following way:

1. The client steps up and down for three minutes while you monitor their heart rate.
2. You keep the client at a steady state by saying 'up, up, down, down' at a normal speech rate. The client should complete 24 steps per minute.
3. At the end of the third minute, record their heart rate.
4. Compare the result to the normative data for males and females shown in Tables 7.3 and 7.4.

Category	Males (mm/O2/kg/min‴ l)	Females (mm/O2/kg/min‴ l)
Extremely high	>70	>60
Very high	63–69	54–59
High	57–62	49–53
Above average	52–56	44–48
Average	44–51	35–43

Table 7.2 Categories for predicted VO_2max scores (adapted from Baechle and Earle, 2008)

Age	Excellent	Good	Above average	Average	Below average	Poor	Very poor
18–25	<79	79–89	90–99	100–105	106–116	117–128	>128
26–35	<81	81–89	90–99	100–107	108–117	118–128	>128
36–45	<83	83–96	97–103	104–112	113–119	120–130	>130
46–55	<87	87–97	97–105	106–116	117–122	123–132	>132
56–65	<86	86–97	98–103	104–112	113–120	121–129	>129
65+	<88	88–96	97–103	104–113	114–120	121–130	>130

Table 7.3 The classification for males measured in b.p.m. (adapted from Franklin, 2000)

Age	Excellent	Good	Above average	Average	Below average	Poor	Very poor
18–25	<85	85–98	99–108	109–117	118–126	127–140	>140
26–35	<88	88–99	100–111	112–119	120–126	127–138	>138
36–45	<90	90–102	103–110	111–118	119–128	129–140	>140
46–55	<94	94–104	105–115	116–120	121–129	130–135	>135
56–65	<95	95–104	105–112	113–118	119–128	129–139	>139
65+	<90	90–102	103–115	116–122	123–128	129–134	>134

Table 7.4 The classification for females measured in b.p.m. (adapted from Franklin, 2000)

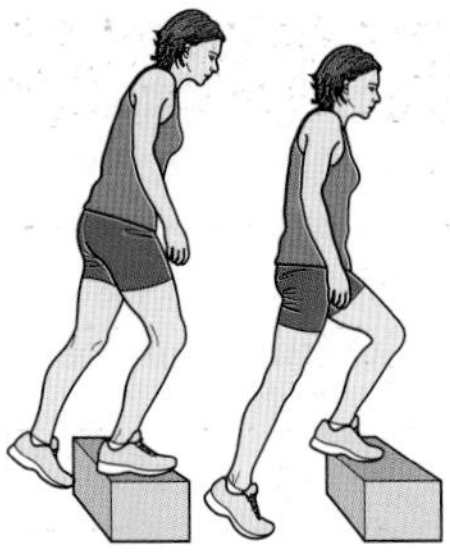

Fig 7.3 Canadian step test

This is a safe test to use with clients and provides a useful means to monitor progress. It will not provide any information regarding their maximal aerobic capacity.

Speed

The **40-metre sprint** is a test for pure speed. You will need a flat running surface and a tape measure to ensure the distance is correct. You also require a stopwatch and a person who can time the run. The test is conducted in the following way:

1. The athlete warms up for several minutes.
2. They then do the 40-metre run at a speed less than their maximum.
3. The athlete starts the test behind the line, with one or two hands on the ground.
4. The starter will shout 'go' and the athlete sprints the 40 metres as quickly as possible.
5. This run should be repeated after two or three minutes and the average of the two runs taken.

This test is a good, accurate test of pure speed; it is dependent on the competence of the testers to accurately record the times of the performers.

Power

The **vertical jump** is a test of power, with the aim being to see how high the athlete can jump. It is important that you find a smooth wall, with a ceiling higher than the athlete can jump. A sports hall or squash court is ideal. The test is conducted in the following way:

1. The athlete rubs chalk on their fingers.
2. They stand about 15 cm away from the wall.
3. With their feet flat on the floor, they reach as high as they can and make a mark on the wall.
4. The athlete then rubs more chalk on their fingers.
5. They then bend their knees to 90 degrees and jump as high as they can up into the air.
6. At the top of their jump they make a second chalk mark with their fingertips.
7. The trainer measures the difference between their two marks – this is their standing jump score.
8. This test is best done three times, so the athlete can take the best of their three jumps.

Category	Males (seconds)	Females (seconds)
Elite	<4.6	<5.5
Excellent	4.6–4.7	5.5–5.7
Good	4.8–5.0	5.8–6.3
Average	5.1–5.5	6.4–6.7
Below average	>5.6	>6.7

Table 7.5 Categories for the 40-metre sprint test (adapted from Franklin, 2000)

Rating	Males (cm)	Females (cm)
Excellent	>70	>60
Very good	61–70	51–60
Above average	51–60	41–50
Average	41–50	31–40
Below average	31–40	21–30
Poor	21–30	11–20
Very poor	<21	<10

Table 7.6 Ratings for males and females in the vertical jump test (adapted from Franklin, 2000)

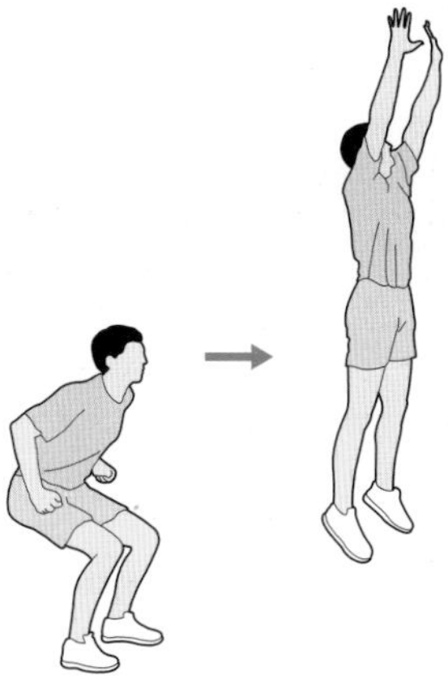

Fig 7.4 Vertical jump test

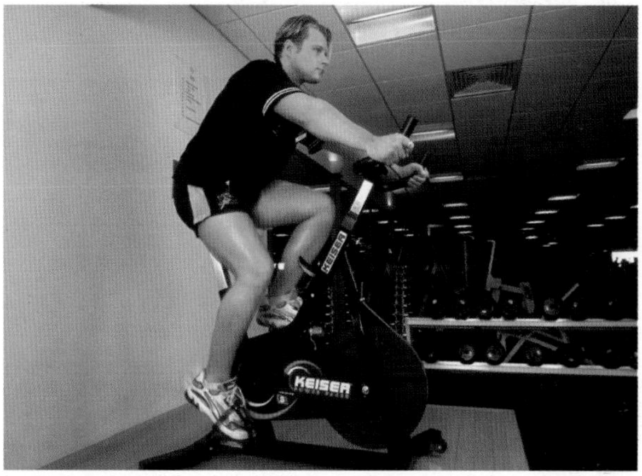

Fig 7.5 Wingate test

Anaerobic Capacity

The **Wingate test** is a maximal test of anaerobic capacity and is thus suitable only for highly conditioned clients. It is used to measure peak anaerobic power and anaerobic capacity. It is carried out in the following way:

1. The client warms up for around two to three minutes at increasing intensities until their heart rate is 180 b.p.m.
2. Once they are ready, the client cycles as fast as they can for 30 seconds at a calculated load. The load is calculated for use on the Monark cycle ergometer. For a person aged under 15 years, the load is their body weight in kilograms × 0.35 g. For an adult, it is their body weight in kilograms × 0.75 g. A 70 kg adult's workload would be worked out in the following way: 70 × 0.75 = 52.5 kg.
3. The client is instructed to start and then given two seconds to achieve their maximum speed, at which point the workload is added.
4. The client pedals for 30 seconds as fast as they can, and the tester needs to count the number of revolutions of the flywheel every five seconds.
5. There needs to be a second tester who records the scores as they are called out for each five seconds.
6. At the end of the 30 seconds, the client cools down at a light workload.

To work out the power for each five-second interval, you need to use the following equation:

Power = load (kg) × revolutions of flywheel in five seconds × radius of flywheel × 12.33

This score is then divided by their body weight in kilograms to calculate the power per kilogram of body mass.

To analyse the results you need to do the following:

- Plot a graph with power in watts (y-axis) against time in seconds (x-axis).
- The peak anaerobic power is the highest power score in a five-second period.

- The minimum anaerobic power is the lowest score in a five-second period.
- The power decline can be calculated in the following way:

$$\text{Power decline} = \frac{\text{Peak power} - \text{Minimum power}}{\text{Peak power} \times 100}$$

You will need to use Table 7.7 to record the results and then work out the power achieved.

This is a test of maximal aerobic capacity and should be used only with advanced, well-conditioned performers. Again, its accuracy is dependent on the motivation of the individual to push themselves to their maximum capacity.

Muscular endurance

The **one-minute press-up test** is a test of muscular endurance in the chest and arms. You will need a mat and a stopwatch.

It is carried out in the following way:

1. This test involves the male starting in the press-up position, with their hands facing forwards and below the shoulders, back straight and pivoting on their toes. Females will perform the test from their knees, with their knees, hips and shoulders all in line and their lower legs resting on the ground.
2. The subject will go down until their chest is 2 cm off the floor and push up to a straight elbow. They must maintain a straight back.
3. The number of press-ups performed in one minute without rest is recorded.
4. If a client is unable to maintain good technique or shows undue fatigue, the test must be stopped.

Time (s)	Number of revolutions of flywheel	Power (watts)	Power per kg of body mass
0–2			
2–7			
7–12			
12–17			
17–22			
22–27			
27–32			

Table 7.7 Recording the information from the Wingate test

Age	Excellent	Very good	Good	Fair	Needs improvement
20–29	36	29–35	22–28	17–21	<17
30–39	30	22–29	17–21	15–20	<15
40–49	25	17–24	13–16	8–12	<8
50–59	21	13–20	10–12	7–9	<7
60–69	18	11–17	8–10	5–7	<5

Table 7.8 Categories for males measured in the number of completed press-ups (adapted from Franklin, 2000)

Age	Excellent	Very good	Good	Fair	Needs improvement
20–29	30	21–29	15–20	10–14	<10
30–39	27	20–26	13–19	8–12	<8
40–49	24	15–23	11–14	5–10	<4
50–59	21	11–20	7–10	2–6	1
60–69	17	12–16	5–11	2–4	1

Table 7.9 Categories for females measured in the number of completed press-ups (adapted from Franklin, 2000)

Age	High	Above average	Average	Below average	Low
17–19	>49	44–48	37–43	24–36	<24
20–29	>44	39–43	32–38	20–31	<20
30–39	>39	34–38	27–33	16–26	<16

Table 7.10 The classification for males measured in the number of completed sit-ups (adapted from Franklin, 2000)

Age	High	Above average	Average	Below average	Low
17–19	>42	32–41	25–31	19–24	<19
20–29	>36	27–35	21–26	15–20	<15
30–39	>30	22–29	17–21	11–16	<11

Table 7.11 The classification for females measured in the number of completed sit-ups (adapted from Franklin, 2000)

The **one-minute sit-up test** is a test of muscular endurance in the abdominals. You will need a mat and a stopwatch.

The test procedure is as follows:

1. The athlete lies on the floor with their fingers on their temples and their knees bent.
2. On the command of 'go', the athlete sits up until their elbows touch their knees.
3. They then return to the start position, with the back of their head touching the floor. That will be one repetition.
4. The athlete does as many repetitions as they can in one minute.

Body composition

In very simple terms, a person's body weight or mass can be split into two categories: fat mass and lean body weight (all that is not fat).

- Fat mass is made up of fat (adipose tissue).
- Lean body weight consists of:
  - muscle
  - water
  - bone
  - organs
  - connective tissue.

This shows that you can lose weight by reducing any of the components of the body. However, lean body weight could be seen as healthy weight, as it contributes to the performance of the body. Fat weight in excess would be unhealthy weight, as it would cause a loss in performance as it requires oxygen without giving anything back to the body.

It is necessary to take a body fat measurement to show that the weight loss is fat and not muscle.

It is impossible to turn muscle into fat or fat into muscle. This is because they are completely different types of tissue in the body. A good training programme will produce a loss of fat or excess fat and a gain in muscle tissue. So while it may look like one is turning into the other, this is not the case. This happens particularly when an athlete does weight training.

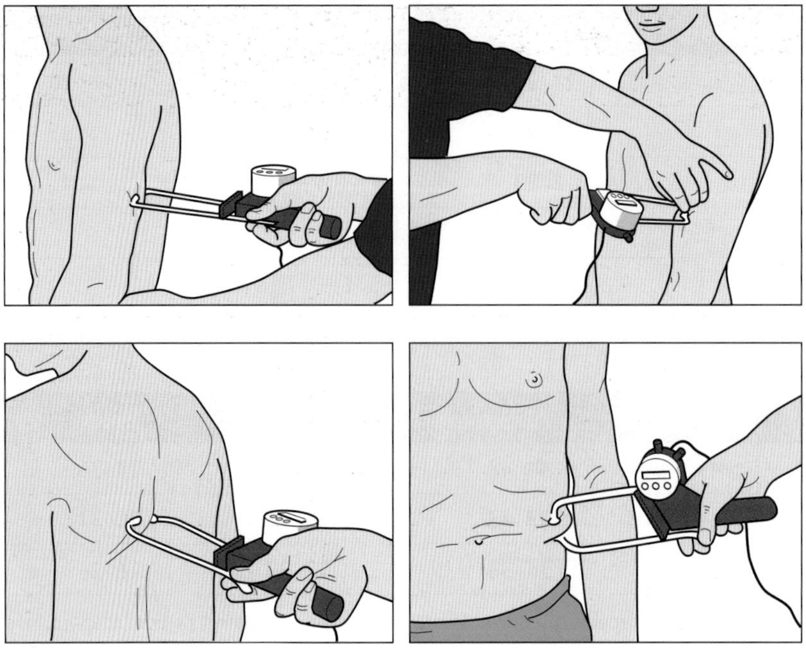

1. **Triceps brachii** With the client's arm hanging loosely, a vertical fold is raised at the back of the arm, midway along a line connecting the acromion (shoulder) and olecranon (elbow) processes.

2. **Biceps brachii** A vertical fold is raised at the front of the arm, opposite the triceps site. This should be directly above the centre of the cubital fossa (fold of the elbow).

3. **Subscapular** A fold is raised just beneath the inferior angle of the scapula (bottom of the shoulder blade). This fold should be at an angle of 45 degrees downwards and outwards.

4. **Anterior suprailiac** A fold is raised 5–7 cm above the spinale (pelvis), at a point in line with the anterior axillary border (armpit). The fold should be in line with the natural folds downwa and inwards at up to 45 degrees.

Fig 7.6 Body fat measurement

Area	Description of site
Triceps	This is taken halfway between the shoulder and elbow on the back of the arm. It is a vertical pinch.
Biceps	This is taken 1 cm above the site for the triceps on the front of the arm. It is a vertical pinch.
Subscapular	This is taken 2 cm below the lowest point of the shoulder blade. It is taken at a 45-degree angle.
Suprailiac	This is taken just above the iliac crest (hip bone), directly below the front of the shoulder.

Table 7.12 Description of four sites for measuring body composition

The **skinfold assessment** test is carried out using skinfold calipers. It is conducted using the Durnin and Wormsley sites, and is carried out as follows:

1 Take the measurements on the left-hand side of the body.
2 Mark up the client accurately.
3 Pinch the skin 1 cm above the marked site.
4 Pull the fat away from the muscle.
5 Place the calipers halfway between the top and bottom of the skinfold.
6 Allow the calipers to settle for one or two seconds.
7 Take the reading and wait 15 seconds before repeating for accuracy.
8 Add up the total of the four measurements.
9 Calculate body fat percentage using Table 7.13.

This test has proved to be an accurate method of assessing and monitoring body composition; however, it is very dependent on the tester's competence to correctly identify the skinfold sites and then to take the measurement accurately. This does involve a fair amount of skill and practice.

The **bioelectrical impedance** technique involves placing electrodes on one hand and one foot and then passing a very small electrical current through the body. The theory is that muscle will conduct the electricity, while fat will resist the path of the electricity. Therefore, the more electricity that comes out of the body, the more muscle a person has, and the less electricity that comes out, the more fat a person has.

This technique has benefits over skinfold measurement because it is easier to do and does not mean that the client has to remove or adjust any clothing. However, it has been shown to be not such an accurate measure of body fat percentage, as it is dependent on how well hydrated the individual is at any point.

Hydro-densitometry, or underwater weighing, is a technique based on the Archimedes principle.

Males		Females	
Sum of skinfolds	Body fat %	Sum of skinfolds	Body fat %
		14	9.4
		16	11.2
		18	12.7
20	7.1	20	14.1
22	9.2	22	15.4
24	10.2	24	16.5
26	11.2	26	17.6
28	12.1	28	17.6
30	12.9	30	19.5
35	14.7	35	21.6
40	16.3	40	23.4
45	17.7	45	25.0
50	19.0	50	26.5
55	20.2	55	27.8
60	21.2	60	29.1
65	22.2	65	30.2
70	23.2	70	31.2
75	24.0	75	32.2
80	24.8	80	33.1
85	25.6	85	34.0
90	26.3	90	34.8
95	27.0	95	35.6
100	27.6	100	36.3
110	27.8	110	37.7
120	29.9	120	39.0
130	31.0	130	40.2
140	31.9	140	41.3
150	32.8	150	42.3
160	33.6	160	43.2
170	34.4	170	44.6
180	35.2	180	45.0

Table 7.13 Body fat measurements for males and females (adapted from Franklin, 2000)

It involves a person being weighed on land and then when fully submerged in water. Muscle and bone are denser than water, while fat is less dense. A person with more bone and muscle will weigh more in water, have a higher body density and therefore less fat. Once the weight on land and weight in water are taken, a formula is used to work out percentage body fat.

This technique involves the use of a large pool of water and significant amounts of equipment. It is impractical for use outside a sport science laboratory.

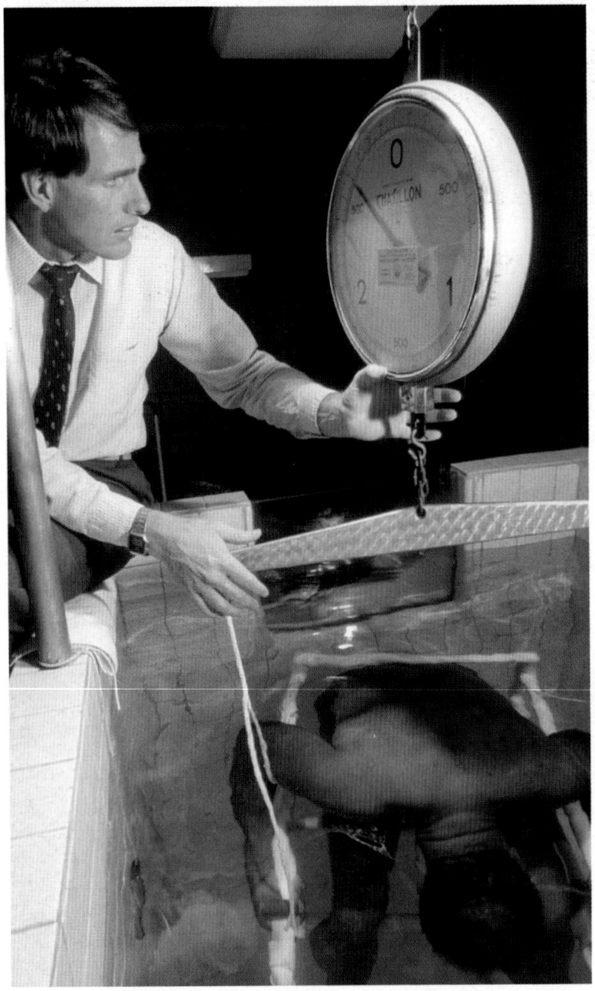

Fig 7.7 Underwater weighing

Key learning points 1

- Blood pressure, resting heart rate, lung function, body mass index and hip-to-waist ratio are all static tests which are performed to see if the client is healthy enough to perform the dynamic fitness tests.
- Performance-related fitness is made up of the following components: flexibility, strength, aerobic endurance, speed, power, muscular endurance and body composition.
- Flexibility is measured by a sit and reach test.
- Strength is measured by one repetition maximum and grip strength dynamometer.
- Aerobic endurance is measured by the multi-stage fitness test and the step test.
- Anaerobic capacity is measured by the Wingate test.
- Speed is measured by the 40-metre sprint test.
- Power is measured by the vertical jump test.
- Muscular endurance is measured by the one-minute press-up test and the one-minute sit-up test.
- Body composition is measured by skinfold assessment, bioelectrical impedance and hydro-densitometry tests.

Classification	Males (% body fat)	Females (% body fat)
Under-fat	<6	<14
Athletes	6–13	14–20
Fitness	14–17	21–24
Acceptable	18–25	25–30
Overweight	26–30	31–40
Obese	>30	>40

Table 7.14 Calculating your body fat percentage (adapted from Franklin, 2000)

Student activity 7.1

45 minutes P1 M1

Fill in the following table to demonstrate your knowledge of the tests for the different components of fitness and their advantages and disadvantages.

Component of fitness	Description of a test for component of fitness	Description of test's strengths and weaknesses	Explanation of test's strengths and weaknesses
Flexibility	Sit and reach test – where the person sits with their feet against a board and slowly bends forwards to see how far they can reach.	It is an easy-to-use test for flexibility, but it does not give us very specific scores.	The test is easy to explain and easy for the participant to perform. It is safe and we can get the results quickly. However, it gives us a score that measures flexibility in the back, hamstrings and calves, but cannot be used to identify range of movement specifically in one of the areas or any other joint/muscle in the body. It gives us a general measure of flexibility but lacks specificity.
Strength			
Aerobic endurance			
Speed			
Anaerobic endurance			
Muscular endurance			
Body composition			

Quick quiz 1

Match each fitness test in the table below to the component of fitness that it tests, choosing from the following:

- flexibility
- strength
- aerobic endurance
- speed
- anaerobic capacity
- muscular endurance
- body composition.

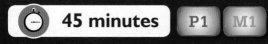

Name of test	Component of fitness tested
Wingate test	
Bioelectrical impedance	
1 RM	
One-minute press-up test	
40-metre sprint	
Sit and reach test	
Multi-stage fitness test	

7.3 Using health-screening techniques

P2 P3 P4 M2 D1

Before you start to conduct fitness tests with an athlete or a person who wants to start exercising, you will need to conduct a detailed fitness consultation. This will consist of the following:

- health-screening questionnaire
- informed consent form
- identification of coronary heart disease risk factors
- identification of any causes for medical referral.

Health-screening questionnaire

You will need to have prepared a detailed questionnaire to cover areas such as medical conditions, illnesses and injuries, as well as history of exercise and lifestyle factors. A sample questionnaire is shown here.

Section 1: Personal Details

Name ______________________________

Address ______________________________

____

____

____

Home telephone ______________

Mobile telephone ______________

Email ______________________________

Occupation ______________________________

Date of birth ______________________________

Section 2: Sporting Goals

1 What are your long-term sporting goals over the next year or season?

____

____

2 What are your medium-term goals over the next three months?

____

____

____

3 What are your short-term goals over the next four weeks?

Section 3: Current Training Status

1 What are your main training requirements?

(a) Muscular strength.
(b) Muscular endurance.
(c) Speed.
(d) Flexibility.
(e) Aerobic fitness.
(f) Power.
(g) Weight loss or gain.
(h) Skill-related fitness.
(i) Other (please state).

2 How would you describe your current fitness status?

3 How many times a week will you train?

4 How much time do you have available for each training session?

Section 4: Your Nutritional Status

1 On a scale of 1 to 10 (1 being very low quality and 10 being very high quality), how would you rate the quality of your diet?

2 Do you follow any particular diet?

(a) Vegetarian.
(b) Vegan.
(c) Vegetarian and fish.
(d) Gluten-free.
(e) Dairy-free.

3 How often do you eat? Note down a typical day's intake.

4 Do you take any supplements? If so, which ones?

Section 5: Your Lifestyle

1 How many units of alcohol do you drink in a typical week? __________

2 Do you smoke? _______ If yes, how many a day? _____________

3 Do you experience stress on a daily basis? ____________

4 If yes, what causes you stress (if you know)?

____

____

____

5 What techniques do you use to deal with your stress?

____

Section 6: Your Physical Health

1 Do you experience any of the following?

(a) Back pain or injury.

(b) Knee pain or injury.

(c) Ankle pain or injury.

(d) Swollen joints.

(e) Shoulder pain or injury.

(f) Hip or pelvic pain or injury.

(g) Nerve damage.

(h) Head injuries.

2 If yes, please give details.

____

____

____

____

3 Are any of these injuries made worse by exercise?

____

4 If yes, what movements in particular cause pain?

____

____

5 Are you currently receiving any treatment for any injuries? If so, what?

____

Section 7: Medical History

1 Do you have or have you had any of the following medical conditions?

(a) Asthma.

(b) Bronchitis.

(c) Heart problems.

(d) Chest pains.

(e) Diabetes.

(f) High blood pressure.

(g) Epilepsy.

(h) Other.

____

2 Are you taking any medication? If yes, state what, how much and why.

Section 8: Informed Consent

Name | Signature

Trainer's name | Trainer's signature

Date

Notes

1 **Explanation of the tests.**
You will perform a series of tests which will vary in their demands on your body. Your progress will be observed during the tests and stopped if you show signs of undue fatigue. You may stop the tests at any time if you feel unduly uncomfortable.

2 **Risks of exercise testing.**
During exercise certain changes can occur, such as raised blood pressure, fainting, raised heart rate and, in a very small number of cases, heart attacks or even death. Every effort is made through screening to minimise the risk of these occurring during testing. Emergency equipment and relevantly trained personnel are available to deal with any extreme situation that occurs.

3 **Responsibility of the participant.**
You must disclose all information in your possession regarding the state of your health or previous experiences of exercise, as this will affect the safety of the tests. If you experience any discomfort or unusual sensations, it is your responsibility to inform your trainer.

4 **Benefits to expect.**
The results gained during testing will be used to identify any illnesses and the types of activities that are relevant for you.

5 **Freedom of consent.**
Your participation in these tests is voluntary and you are free to deny consent or stop a test at any point.
I have read this form and understand what is expected of me and the tests I will perform. I give my consent to participate.

Client's signature | Trainer's signature

Print name | Print name

Date | Date

Informed consent

An informed consent form lets a client know what to expect during the exercise test, and the associated risks involved in exercise or training. It also stresses that any participation in the tests is voluntary and that they have the choice to stop at any point.

An example of an informed consent form is shown at the end of the health-screening questionnaire above.

Risk of coronary heart disease

Coronary heart disease (CHD) is a leading cause of death in all industrialised countries. It is caused by a narrowing of the coronary arteries, which limits the amount of blood flowing through the arteries.

Key term

Coronary arteries: blood vessels that bring oxygenated blood to nourish the muscle cells of the heart muscle.

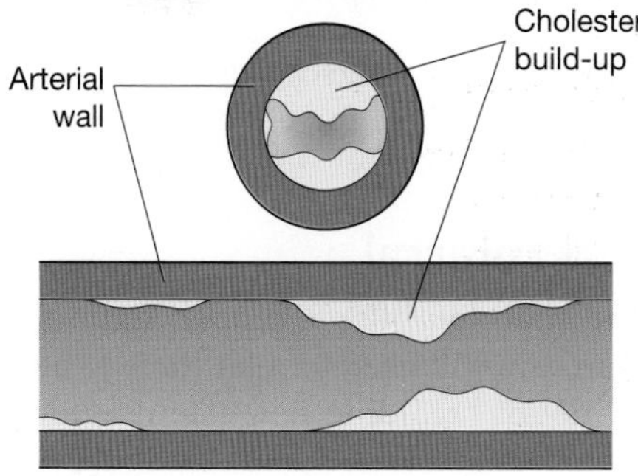

Fig 7.8 Build-up of cholesterol in an artery

Arteries losing their elasticity is part of the ageing process. However, there are many lifestyle factors that cause damage or narrowing of the arteries. Obstructions are created as cholesterol and fatty plaques are laid down in the artery, causing a narrowing of the artery space.

The coronary arteries are found only in the heart and they supply the heart with oxygen to enable it to pump. When these arteries narrow or become blocked, the blood supply to the heart is reduced. As a result, carbon dioxide builds up in the heart muscle and this causes pain, which is called angina. Angina feels like a crushing pain on the chest. If this pain becomes a shooting pain into the left arm and the neck, the person is having a heart attack.

The following lifestyle factors will increase an individual's chance of having CHD:

- diet high in fat (particularly deep-fat fried foods)
- diet high in table salt (sodium chloride)
- obesity (particularly abdominal fat)
- smoking
- excess alcohol consumption
- older age
- male gender
- high blood pressure
- type 2 diabetes.

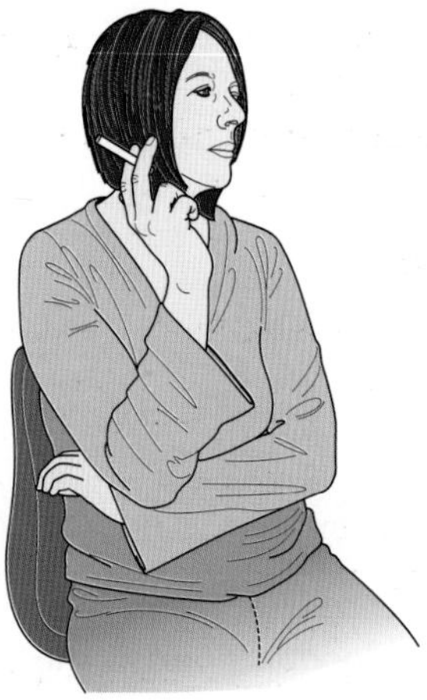

Fig 7.9 Smoking will increase an individual's chance of having CHD

If you consider that a person has a high risk of CHD, it is best to refer them for GP clearance before you start to train them.

Medical referral

To ensure that you offer a proper 'duty of care' to your client, you will need to refer them to a GP if you have any doubt regarding how safe it is for them to exercise. If your client has any of the following, they must be referred to their GP:

- high blood pressure (over 160/100)
- poor lung function
- excess body fat (40 per cent or more for a female, 30 per cent or more for a male)
- high resting heart rate (100+ b.p.m.)
- medication for a heart condition (e.g. beta blockers).

Likewise, if they experience any of the following, they must also be referred to their GP:

- Muscle injuries
- Chest pain or tightness
- Light-headedness or dizziness
- Irregular or rapid pulse
- Joint pain
- Headaches
- Shortness of breath.

Health-monitoring tests

Tests can be split into two clear categories: those that measure health and those that measure fitness. Health tests are carried out to see if the individual is healthy enough to do the fitness tests or whether they need to receive GP clearance. Health tests will be static in nature while fitness tests will be dynamic and involve bodily movement and exertion.

The health tests conducted are:

- heart rate
- blood pressure
- lung function
- waist-to-hip ratio
- body mass index (BMI).

Resting heart rate

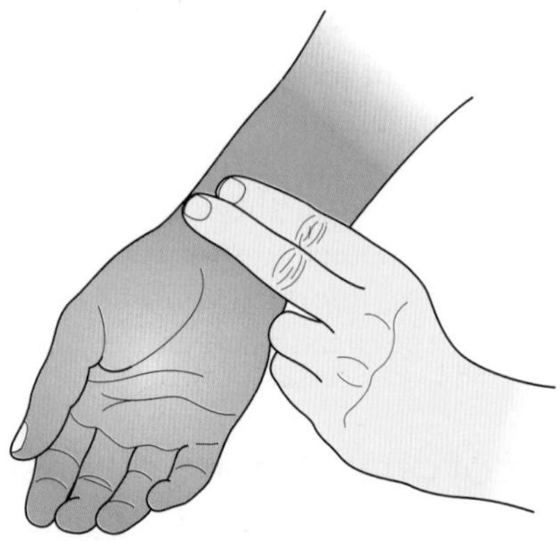

Fig 7.10 Taking a pulse rate

To measure the resting heart rate, you can use a heart rate monitor or do it manually. The best time to take a person's resting heart rate is before the person gets out of bed and experiences the stresses of the day. To perform it manually, complete the following steps:

1 Let your client sit down and rest for about five minutes.
2 Find their radial pulse (wrist) or brachial pulse (front of elbow).
3 Place your middle and index fingers over the pulse. The thumb has a pulse of its own and will produce an inaccurate reading.
4 Count the pulse for 60 seconds and record the result before repeating for another 60 seconds.
5 If there is a large variation in readings you should take a third reading.

Here is a reference for resting heart rates for men and women:

Category	Males (b.p.m.)	Females (b.p.m.)
Normal	60–80	60–80
Average	70	76
Proceed with caution	90–99	90–99
GP referral	100+	100+

Table 7.15 Heart rate reference tables for males and females (adapted from Franklin, 2000)

Blood Pressure

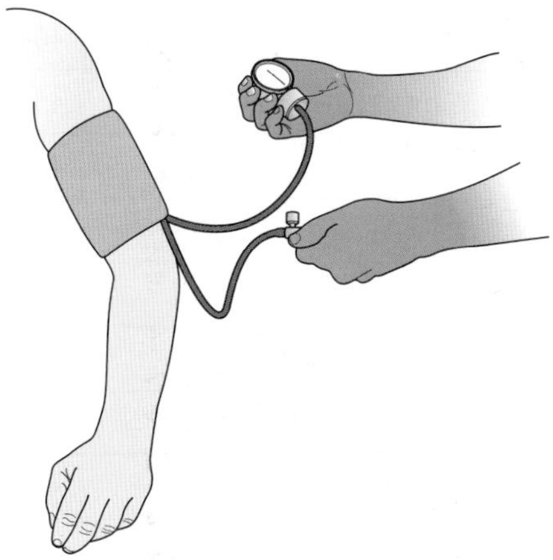

Fig 7.11 Taking a blood pressure reading

Blood pressure is the pressure blood exerts on the artery walls and is a clear indication of general health. It is vital to measure blood pressure before a client exercises, because it will tell you whether they are at risk of having a heart attack.

We need to split this up into the short-term and long-term. Short-term means the blood pressure rises for a period and then falls again, while long-term means that the blood pressure remains high all the time.

Blood pressure is taken by a blood pressure meter and stethoscope, or it can be done using an electronic blood pressure meter.

1 Allow the client to be relaxed for about five minutes.
2 Ask the client to sit down, with their left arm resting on a chair arm. Their elbow should be at 45 degrees, with the palm of the hand facing up.
3 Find the brachial pulse – it should be on the inner side of the arm, just under the biceps muscle.
4 Place the cuff just clear of the elbow (about 2–3 cm above the elbow). The bladder of the cuff (the part which inflates) should be directly over the pulse.
5 Place the earpieces of the stethoscope in your ears and place the microphone over the brachial pulse.
6 Inflate the cuff up to 200 mmHg.
7 Slowly open the valve by turning it anticlockwise and release the pressure.
8 Listen out for the first time you hear the thud of the heart beat and make a mental note of it. This is the systolic blood pressure reading.
9 Keep deflating the cuff, and when the heart beat becomes muffled or disappears, this is your diastolic reading.
10 Keep deflating the cuff and, if necessary, repeat after around 30 seconds.

Lung function

We need to assess lung function to see whether the airways between the mouth and the alveoli are clear and conducive to good air flow. Poor lung function will limit the amount of oxygen that can be delivered to the bloodstream and the tissues.

Lung function can be measured using a micro-spirometer or a hand-held peak flow meter.

To use a peak flow meter, work through the following steps:

1 Ask the client to hold the peak flow meter directly in front of their mouth.
2 Ask them to turn their head to the side and take three deep breaths.
3 On the third breath, ask them to put their mouth around the end of the tube and, ensuring a good lip seal, blow as hard as they can into the tube.
4 Say that it should be a short, sharp blow, as if they were using a pea shooter.
5 Repeat twice more and take the highest reading. This is called their peak expiratory flow rate (PEFR).

Age	1.55 m	1.60 m	1.65 m	1.70 m	1.75 m	1.80 m	1.85 m	1.90m
25	515	534	552	570	589	607	625	644
30	502	520	539	557	576	594	612	632
35	489	508	526	544	563	582	600	619
40	476	495	513	531	550	568	586	606
45	463	482	501	519	537	556	574	593
50	450	469	487	505	524	543	561	580
55	438	456	475	493	511	530	548	567
60	424	443	462	480	498	517	535	545
65	412	430	449	460	486	504	522	541
70	399	417	436	454	472	491	509	528

Table 7.16 PEFR for males (adapted from Franklin, 2000)

Age	1.45 m	1.50 m	1.55 m	1.60 m	1.65 m	1.70 m	1.75 m	1.80m
25	365	383	400	416	433	449	466	482
30	357	374	390	407	423	440	456	473
35	348	365	381	398	414	431	447	464
40	339	356	372	389	405	422	438	455
45	330	347	363	380	397	413	429	446
50	321	338	354	371	388	404	420	437
55	312	329	345	362	379	395	411	428
60	303	320	336	353	370	386	402	419
65	294	311	327	344	361	377	393	410
70	285	302	318	335	352	368	384	401

Table 7.17 PEFR for females (adapted from Franklin, 2000)

The PEFR is a measurement of the power of the lungs. It is a hypothetical figure which tells us how much air would pass through our lungs if we breathed in and out at our maximum power for one minute. It is hypothetical because it cannot really be measured, as we would faint after about 15 seconds of breathing at maximum power.

You will need to know the gender, age and height of the client to work out their acceptable score.

The PEFR for males and for females are shown in Tables 7.16 and 7.17.

If your client's score is 100 below the acceptable figure, this is classified as poor lung function and they should be referred to their GP before they exercise.

Body mass index

Body mass index is used to give us an idea of whether a client is obese. It then gives the extent of their obesity.

This is worked out by using the following formula:

Body mass index (BMI) = weight in kilograms divided by height in metres squared.

For a male who weighs 75 kg and is 1.80 m tall: $75 \div 1.80^2 = 23.1$. Thus his body mass index will be 23.1 kg/m^2.

What does this mean? Table 7.18 shows the classification for overweight and obesity.

The body mass index has serious limitations because it does not actually measure body composition. It can be used as a quick measure to see if a person is over-fat, but it is inaccurate because it does not make a distinction between muscle and fat. Thus, someone with a lot of muscle may come out as fat!

Hip-to-waist ratio

Hip-to-waist ratio is taken as an indicator of the health risks associated with obesity, and in particular the risk of coronary heart disease. Fat stored in the abdominal area is a greater risk factor for CHD because it is closer to the heart and can more easily be mobilised and taken to the heart.

Hip-to-waist ratio is calculated in the following way, using a tape measure.

- Waist measurement is taken at the level of the navel, with the stomach muscles relaxed and after a normal expiration. The tape measure is put around the waist and a horizontal reading is taken.
- Hip measurement is taken with the client standing up and is the widest measurement around the hips. It is usually taken at the level of the greater trochanter, which is at the top of the femur.

The ratio is worked out by dividing the waist measurement by the hip measurement. For a male with a 26" waist and 30" hips, this would be: $26 \div 30 = 0.87$.

What do these scores mean? Table 7.19 shows the classification for hip-to-waist ratio.

A male with a score above 0.90 and a female with a score above 0.80 will have an increased risk of developing CHD.

	Obesity class	BMI (kg/m2)
Underweight		< 17.5
Normal		17.5–24.9
Overweight		25–29.9
Obesity	I	30–34.9
Obesity	II	35–39.9
Extreme obesity	III	>40

Table 7.18 BMI classification of overweight and obesity

	Hip-to-waist ratio	Classification
Males	> 1.0	High risk
	0.90–0.99	Moderate risk
	< 0.90	Low risk
Females	> 0.85	High risk
	0.80–0.85	Moderate risk
	< 0.80	Low risk

Table 7.19 CHD risk classification from hip-to-waist ratio scores

Key learning points 2

- Before a fitness test is conducted, a health-screening form and an informed consent form must be completed.
- A client must be screened for risk of CHD. Risk factors include poor diet, obesity, smoking, excess alcohol intake, male gender and type 2 diabetes.

Student activity 7.2

90 minutes P2 P3 P4 M2 D1

- Using the health-screening questionnaire provided as a template (see pages 128–131), design your own questionnaire that covers personal details, goals, current activity levels, lifestyle factors and medical history.
- Use the health-screening questionnaire for two individuals who have different goals and a different health status (e.g. conditioned and unconditioned).
- Use the following table to record and analyse the results of four health-related tests for the two individuals:

Name of test	Result of test	Interpretation of test: fit and healthy/proceed with caution/ GP referral
Resting heart rate		
Blood pressure		
Lung function		
Body mass index		
Strengths:		
Areas for improvement:		

Evaluate the information gained from the health-screening questionnaire and the fitness tests and make recommendations on how each individual could improve their lifestyle.

Q Quick quiz 2

1 Describe why coronary heart disease develops.
2 State three occasions when you would refer someone to the GP before letting them start exercising.
3 What is the difference between a static test and a dynamic test?
4 A high hip-to-waist ratio may indicate a raised risk of which medical condition?

7.4. Administering Appropriate Fitness Tests

P5 M3

In order to administer fitness tests safely and effectively, you need to follow certain procedures. The test protocols have been described in Section 7.2, but you also need to ensure that the tests are valid and reliable, and that the individual being tested is appropriately prepared. You also need to be aware of any signs that would suggest that you ought to terminate the test.

Validity and reliability

These two terms must be considered before a test is conducted. The two questions you must ask yourself are:

1. Does this test actually test what I say it tests?
2. If this test were to be repeated, would I get the same results?

The first question tests validity. For example, a speed test using a shuttle run may actually test a person's ability to turn, which is more about agility than speed.

The second question tests its reliability. The conditions of the test must always be identical, making it most likely that the same results will be produced. However, there are many factors that may change, such as the temperature of the environment, the physical state of the athlete and the technique of the tester. All these may alter the results produced.

The purposes of fitness testing

The purposes of fitness testing are to:

- ensure that the person is safe to exercise
- find out their current position in terms of the components of fitness
- identify the strengths and weaknesses of each of their components of fitness
- gain information to allow a specific training programme to be written
- be able to monitor any changes in fitness
- provide an opportunity to educate individuals about health and fitness.

Pre-test procedures

When testing people, it is important that the tests are safe for the client, and also that the conditions the tests are performed in are consistent and stable.

The following should be taken into consideration in relation to the client:

- They should have medical clearance for any health conditions.
- They should be free of injuries.
- They should be wearing appropriate clothing.
- They should not have had a heavy meal within three hours of the test.
- They should have had a good night's sleep.
- They should not have trained on the day and should be fully recovered from previous training.
- They should have avoided stimulants such as tea, coffee or nicotine for two hours before the test.

The following should be taken into consideration regarding the environment:

- Heating in the area should be at room temperature (around 18 °C).
- The room should be well ventilated.
- The room should be clean and dust-free.

Test sequence

The order in which tests are conducted must be considered because it may change the accuracy of the results you produce. You may even have to do different tests on different days to produce the best results.

Your knowledge of sport science can help you to decide which tests should be done first and for how long the athlete will have to rest between tests. For example, a test that requires effort over a long period of time or works to failure will require one to two hours of recovery. A test requiring a high level of skill or coordination needs to be done first because skill level decreases when a person is tired. The correct order to follow would be:

- sedentary tests – height, weight, body composition, flexibility
- agility tests
- maximum power and strength tests
- sprint tests
- muscular endurance tests
- aerobic endurance tests.

Reasons to terminate a fitness test

There will be occasions when it becomes unsafe to continue with a test due to physiological changes within the client. The following is a list of specific situations when a test should be stopped:

- chest pains or angina-like symptoms
- excessive increase in blood pressure (250/115)
- shortness of breath and wheezing
- leg cramps or pain
- light-headedness, nausea or pale, clammy skin

- heart rate does not rise with exercise intensity
- irregular heart beat
- client requests to stop
- signs and symptoms of severe exhaustion
- equipment fails.

Key learning points 3

- Tests can be split into two types: those which test health and are static in nature and those which test fitness and are dynamic in nature.
- Before conducting a test, you must consider whether both the client and the environment are in an appropriate state for the test to take place.
- A valid test is one that tests what it says it will test.
- A reliable test is one that would yield the same results if it were to be repeated.

Q Quick quiz 3

Fill in the blank spaces to complete the following sentences, choosing from the list of words below.

- Safe
- Reliable
- Sedentary
- Strengths
- Valid
- Coordination
- Maximal
- Weaknesses.

When administering a fitness test, you must make sure it is _________ by considering whether it tests what it says it is testing, and also how to make it ________, which means that if you did the test again you would get the same results. Fitness testing is done to make sure the person is ______ to exercise and to identify their ________ and ________. It is important to do the _______ tests first and then tests requiring _______, and finally tests requiring _________ effort.

7.5. Interpreting the Results of Fitness Tests and Providing Feedback

P6 M4 **D2**

Once you have completed a fitness test, it is important to give detailed feedback to the individual. Before you conduct a test, you need to say what you are testing and explain how the test will be conducted. Feedback is given once you have conducted the test, written down the result and then worked out how the result compares with the normative tables.

Feedback should be given in the following format:

- Repeat the component of fitness that has been tested.
- Tell the individual what the result of the test was.
- Explain what you have tested and what the score represents.
- Tell the individual where they fit within the population norms.
- Tell the individual what the implications of the result are in terms of their health and fitness.
- Discuss what recommendations you would make for the future.

If you have carried out a blood pressure test, for example, you would give feedback in this specific way:

- 'I have just taken your blood pressure.'
- 'Your blood pressure was 120/80 mmHg.'
- 'Blood pressure is the pressure of blood in the arterial system. 120 mmHg is the pressure during the contraction phase of the heart beat, and 80 mmHg is the pressure during the relaxation phase of the heart beat.'
- 'This score is within the normal healthy range.'
- 'It means you are healthy enough to take part in sport and exercise.'

The scores of all fitness tests must be recorded in writing to ensure you have the information available in the future when you come to retest.

Recommendations

Once you have completed all the tests, you will be able to write an action plan or a report on the individual. This should cover the following information:

- current situation, highlighting strengths and weaknesses
- client's aims and objectives
- changes to be made, with options
- actions – a step-by-step guide to achieving aims.

Key learning points 4

- When giving feedback, you must let the individual know what you were testing, what score they achieved, what their score means and any implications this score may have.
- Once fitness tests have been completed, you can write an action plan for the individual, with recommendations for them to improve their health and fitness.

Student activity 7.3

3 hours | P5 | P6 | M3 | M4 | D2

Task 1

- Choose six fitness tests specifically identified for the individual that you have selected to test.
- Justify why you chose these six tests for this individual (think about choosing tests specific to the goals and fitness needs of that individual).
- Develop a table and record the scores for each of the six tests.

Task 2

- Once your selected individual has done the fitness tests and you have recorded their results, you should prepare and then present feedback to the individual in the form of a consultation. You should have worked out how their score fits into the normative data for each test, and what the implications of the results are.
- As part of the consultation, summarise by identifying the individual's strengths and weaknesses and then provide recommendations for their future training activities.

Further reading

Baechle, T. and Earle, R. (2008) *Essentials of Strength Training and Conditioning*, Champaign, Il: Human Kinetics.

Coulson, M. (2007) *The Fitness Instructor's Handbook*. London: A & C Black.

Sharkey, B.J. and Gaskill, S.E. (2006) *Fitness and Health*, Champaign, Il: Human Kinetics.

Useful websites

www.brianmac.co.uk/eval.htm

Provides details of how to evaluate and test sports performance

www.pponline.co.uk/encyc/sports-performance-analysis-coaching-and-training-39

Article detailing how sports analysis can help coaching and training

www.topendsports.com/testing/tests.htm

Over 100 fitness tests to try, all divided into different fitness categories

References

Baechle, T. and Earle, R. (2008) *Essentials of Strength Training and Conditioning*, Human Kinetics.

Davis, R., Bull, C., Roscoe, J. and Roscoe, D. (2005) *Physical Education and the Study of Sport*, Elsevier Mosby.

Franklin, B. (2005) *American College of Sports Medicine's (ACSM) Guidelines for Exercise Testing and Prescription*, 6th edn, Lippincott, Williams and Wilkins.

8 & 9: Practical Team & Individual Sports

8.1 Introduction

Sport and sports participation are on the increase in the UK. Sport has many purposes: to improve health, for enjoyment and the natural human urge to compete among others. There are many different types of sports, and this unit includes details of how to improve your performance in sport and your knowledge of the rules and regulations, as well as the ways in which you can measure and assess performance.

By the end of this unit you should:

- be able to use a range of skills, techniques and tactics in selected team and/or individual sports
- understand the rules and regulations of selected team and/or individual sports
- be able to assess your own performance in selected team and/or individual sports
- be able to assess the performance of a team in two selected team sports or other individuals in selected individual sports
- be able to use a range of skills, techniques and tactics in selected team and individual sports.

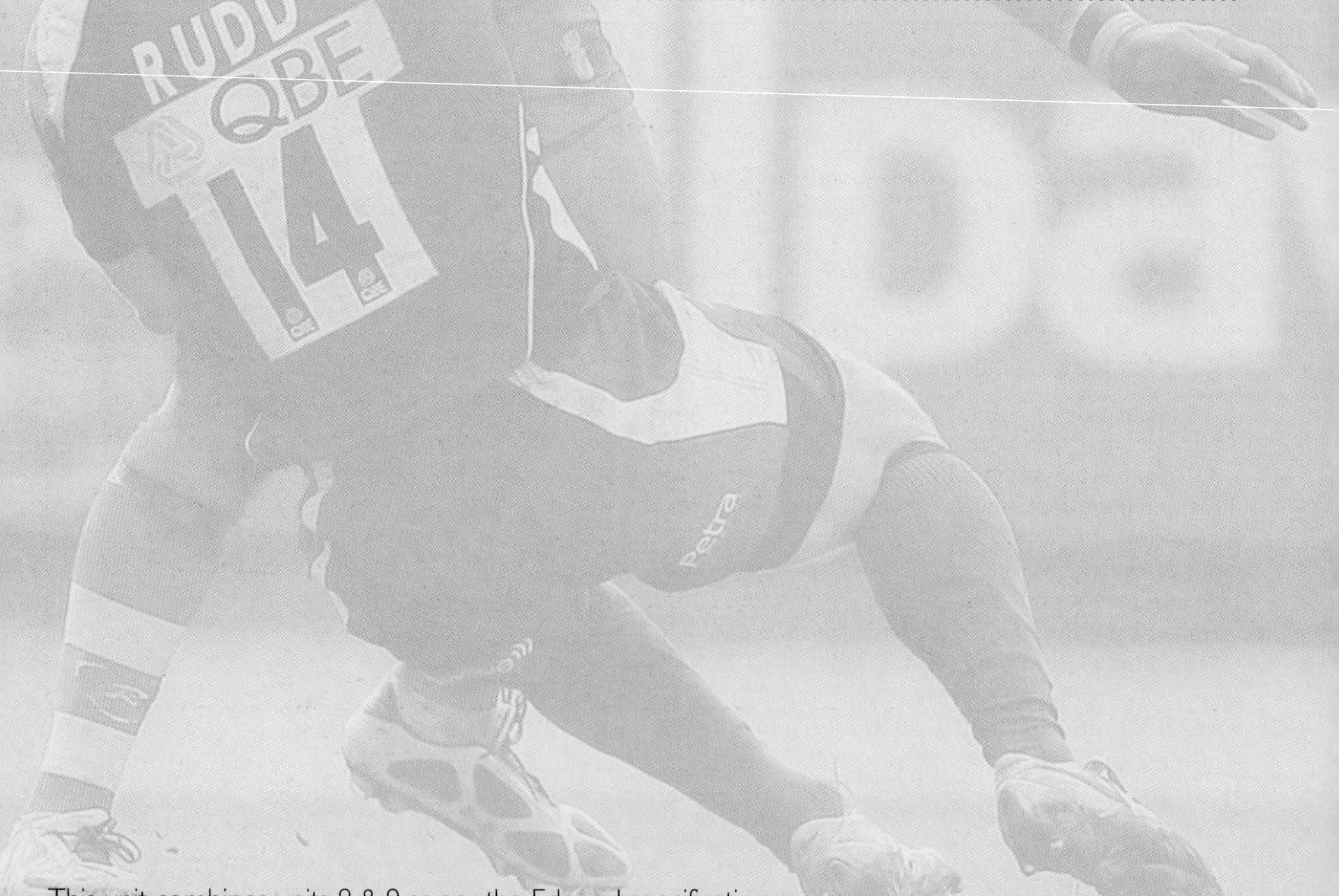

This unit combines units 8 & 9 as per the Edexcel specification

Assessment and grading criteria		
To achieve a PASS grade the evidence must show that the learner is able to:	**To achieve a MERIT grade the evidence must show that, in addition to the pass criteria, the learner is able to:**	**To achieve a DISTINCTION grade the evidence must show that, in addition to the pass and merit criteria, the learner is able to:**
P1 describe skills, techniques and tactics required in two different team/ individual sports	**M1** explain skills, techniques and tactics required in two different team/ individual sports	
P2 describe the rules and regulations of two different team/individual sports, and apply them to three different situations for each sport	**M2** explain the application of the rules and regulations, of two different team/individual sports, in three different situations for each sport	
P3 demonstrate appropriate skills, techniques and tactics in two different team/individual sports		
P4 carry out a self-analysis using two different methods of assessment, identifying strengths and areas for improvement in two different team/individual sports	**M3** explain identified strengths and areas for improvement in two different team/individual sports, and make suggestions relating to personal development	**D1** analyse identified strengths and areas for improvement in two different team/individual sports, and justify suggestions made
P5 carry out a performance analysis using two different methods of assessment, identifying strengths and areas for improvement in the development of a team/an individual in a team/individual sport.	**M4** explain identified strengths and areas for improvement in the development of a team/an individual in a team/individual sport, and make suggestions relating to development of a team.	**D2** analyse identified strengths and areas for improvement in the development of a team/an individual in a team/individual sport, and justify suggestions made.

8.2 Team and Individual Sports

P1 P3 M1

Team sports are those in which two or more players compete together with a single aim. They include sports such as football, rugby, netball and lacrosse.

Individual sports are those in which the competitor usually competes on their own and is solely responsible for their own actions. These include sports such as gymnastics, judo, trampolining and golf.

Sports can be further classified as follows:

- **Invasion sports**: games such as football, netball, basketball and rugby, where the object of the sport is to invade the opponent's territory

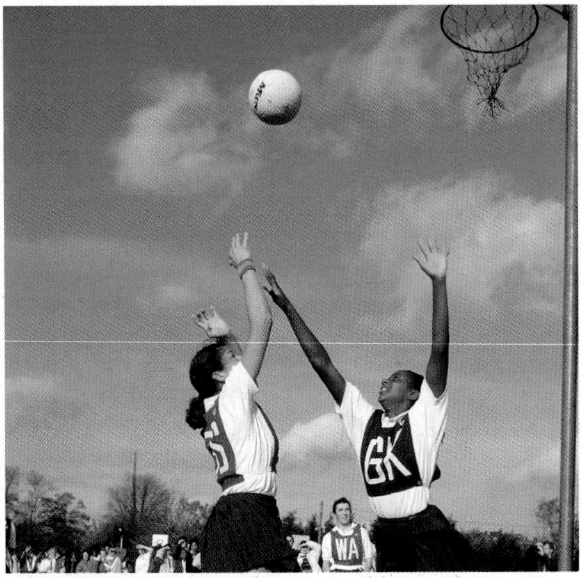

Fig 8.1 Netball is an example of an invasion sport

- **Court sports**: non-contact sports because opponents are normally on opposite sides of a net, such as badminton, volleyball and tennis
- **Target sports**: involve the use of marksmanship and include golf and archery
- **Striking/fielding**: games with a batting and a fielding team, and include cricket, baseball and rounders
- **Martial arts**: these come from different ancient fighting methods, many of which originated in the Far East, such as judo, taekwon do and karate
- **Water sports**: activities undertaken on or in water, including swimming, sailing and water polo
- **Athletic sports**: activities that take place on the field or track
- **Field sports**: hunting sports associated with the outdoors, such as shooting and fishing.

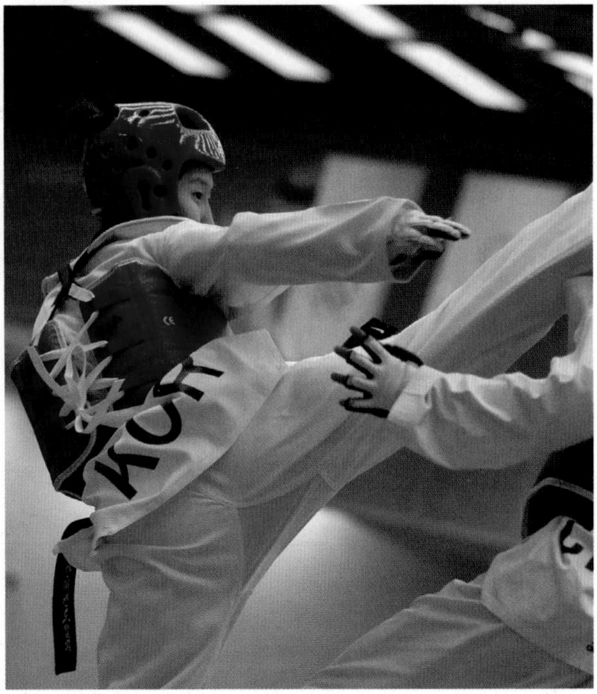

Fig 8.2 Taekwon do – an example of a martial art

Skills and Techniques in Team and Individual Sports

A skill is the ability to do something well and requires lots of practice. Technique is a way of undertaking a particular skill. If a basketball player is able to perform a jump-shot well, it is said that they have a good technique in playing the shot.

There are many shared skills in different team sports, and having the awareness and ability to undertake them will be an advantage to your team. They include:

- Passing – moving the ball around your teammates
- Receiving – being able to receive a pass from a teammate
- Shooting – aiming at a specific target, such as a goal or a basket
- Dribbling – moving around with the ball
- Throwing – there are many ways of throwing an object, normally specific to the sport being played
- Intercepting – this is where a player stops the ball from reaching its intended place; this could be through a block or a tackle
- Creating space – this means moving away from opponents so that you are in a position in which you can receive a pass or create a shooting opportunity.

In addition to the skills and techniques required of a sport, players may also be judged on other criteria, such as their performance over the duration of a game.

All sports are made up of a range of specific skills. In tennis there are a number of different shots that you can play at different times during a game. Playing these effectively will allow you to win points. They include:

- Forehand drive with spin variation
- Forehand volley
- Service
- Lob
- Smash
- Return of service.

Tactics

Key term

Tactic: a plan of action to achieve a goal.

Tactics in sport are usually focused directly or indirectly on winning. Tactics can depend on the opposition, players of the other team or opponents, the importance of the competition and maybe the weather.

Tactics can be:

- Pre-event tactics – a particular plan before the event
- In-event tactics – a plan implemented during the game, such as switching from man-to-man to zone defence in basketball.

Tactics can fail if the opposition work them out too easily, if the tactic is employed too late or if the player or players are simply not able to understand or execute the necessary tactic(s).

Consider the range of options that a tennis player has at their disposal. First, where should they stand while waiting for their opponent's return? If the ball is likely to come over the net in the middle and low, then the player might consider standing close to the net to make a volley. In this way, the player has selected a tactical position and shot selection. The same player might also consider serving the ball to the forehand or backhand of their opponent, some with spin, some without and some faster than others. This is known as variation.

If the conditions of the match are that the player is losing, that player might start to play defensive shots in an attempt to prevent them from falling further behind.

Tactics can include playing precise formations against specific opponents. Football teams may play more defensively away from home and opt to play with more defending players rather than strikers. In certain sports, opposing players may be marked to stop them having a positive effect for their team.

Other tactics may include working on specific set plays, such as line-outs in rugby, and corners and free kicks in football.

In order to improve your performance, it is a good idea to actually watch yourself perform the skill. Ask a friend or coach to video you while you perform a set skill. You can then analyse your performance and see what you are doing. You may be surprised and realise your body is not doing what you thought it was! You will then need to amend the skill, practise it and video yourself again, to check that you are now performing the skill properly.

Key learning points 1

- Sports can be classified as:
  - Invasion games
  - Court sports
  - Target sports
  - Striking/fielding
  - Martial arts
  - Water sports
  - Field sports.
- A skill is the ability to perform something well.
- Techniques are a way of undertaking a particular skill.
- A tactic is a plan of action to achieve a goal.
- Team and individual sports are different, not just in terms of numbers, but also in terms of the skills and techniques to be developed and assessed.

Q Quick quiz 1

1 Place the following sports into their correct classification:
   (a) Tennis.
   (b) Judo.
   (c) Clay-pigeon shooting.
   (d) Windsurfing.
   (e) 400 m running.
   (f) Shot put.
   (g) Squash.
   (h) Lacrosse.
   (i) Curling.
   (j) Mountain biking.
2 What skills do you need to perform well for your favourite sport?
3 Name three different tactics used in your favourite sport.

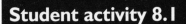

Student activity 8.1 60 minutes P1 M1

Select two individual or two team sports for the following tasks.

Task 1

Draw a spidergram for two sports which illustrates the skills, techniques and tactics required for each.

Task 2

Write a report that describes and explains the skills, techniques and tactics for each of your two selected sports.

Task 3

Take part in your two selected sports and demonstrate appropriate skills, techniques and tactics in each sport.

8.3 Rules and Regulations

P2 M2

The rules and regulations of any sport are normally set and amended by its national governing body (NGB) and international sports federations (ISFs). These are set to ensure that the sport is played fairly and that the opponents are aware of how to win.

International sports federations and national governing bodies may change the rules and regulations periodically, as they look to improve the sport. For example, FIBA, the international governing body for basketball, meets every four years at a world congress, with a view to changing or clarifying rules to the benefit of the sport.

Time

Many team sports have time constraints and are split into periods of play:

- Ice hockey has three periods of 20 minutes.
- Basketball has four periods of 10 minutes.
- Rugby union has two halves of 40 minutes.

Usually the team with the most points or goals is declared the winner, and if the scores are tied, the game is normally declared a draw. For sports like rugby and football, the timing is described as real time, since the start and finish times are exact (except for added time), whereas basketball and ice hockey are played in artificial time, because the game clock is stopped on a regular basis for a variety of reasons, meaning that the whole of the running game time is spent on the court/field of play.

In some sports, a winner can be declared before the allocated time has elapsed. Often in test match cricket, a team will have bowled out a team twice and scored the required number of runs before the five days are completed.

Few individual sports are constrained by time, the outcome of the event usually being determined by the success of the competition, and usually by accruing points to a critical point.

Scoring

Each sport has a different scoring system, with the team or individual with the most points usually being declared the winner. An exception to this is golf, where the player who has taken the fewest strokes is the winner. Scoring may include putting the ball into a goal in football and handball.

Facilities and Equipment

Specific sports require certain facilities to enable play to take place. Different surfaces can be used for different sports, and often sports are played on a range of surfaces. Tennis is a good example, as it can be played on grass, clay and hard surfaces, and can be played inside or outdoors. Occasionally, rules may be adapted for sports played on different surfaces.

Many sports require the participants to wear or use specialist equipment. In football, the laws of the game insist that all players must wear shin guards to protect their lower legs. In sports such as hockey, rugby and cricket, players may wear specific equipment to reduce the risk of injury. This could include arm guards, helmets and padding.

You can find the rules and regulations of each sport via its national governing body. The NGB looks after many aspects of a sport, including organising major competitions, running coaching schemes and dealing with the development of the sport at all levels.

Unwritten Rules and Etiquette

Unwritten rules cover those situations in sports where the normal rules of the sport are unclear or require the discretion or cooperation of the competitors. Examples include the following:

- **Football**: when a player appears to be injured, the opposition often put the ball out of play, and in an act of fair play the other team returns the ball to its generous opponents.
- **Fencing**: points in fencing are scored when an opponent strikes another. In a fast-moving sport, the electronic scoring apparatus can misinterpret an inaccurate contact, such as the blade contacting the floor. Sporting opponents often either concede the point or suggest that the contact was not eligible for scoring.
- **Cricket**: a batsman can choose to 'walk' on appeal. In other words, if a fielder appeals for a dismissal decision, the batsman can choose to walk from the field of play, effectively admitting that they were out.
- **Golf**: players can 'give' competitors shots, usually when their opponent's ball is very close to the hole. In doing so, they allow them to score that shot without actually playing it.

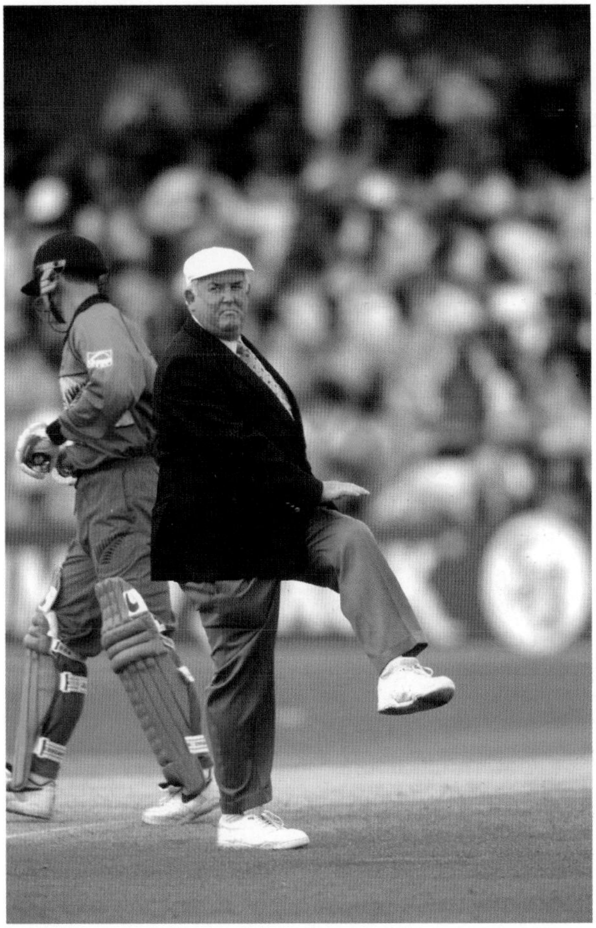

Fig 8.3 A cricket umpire indicating a leg bye during a match

Officials

Officials in sport have wide-ranging roles and duties, including football fourth officials, trampoline judges, athletics markers, cycle marshals, netball umpires and cricket third umpires. The role of these officials varies in terms of their physical nature, their proximity to the event and the support that they receive from their co-officials.

Playing Surfaces

The amount and type of surfaces played on in sports are many and varied. While some surfaces can be used for a variety of sports, others are more specialised. The level of competition can also have a bearing. Artificial surfaces come in many varieties – with rubber crumbs or sand drainage.

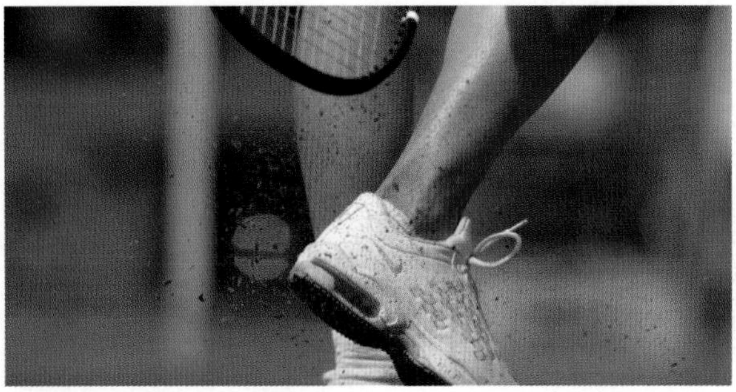

Fig 8.4 Playing tennis on clay

Situations

Rules and regulations are often used to describe what should be done in certain situations, such as what to do if a player handles the ball in football, or when a ball is out of bounds in golf. Where rules are broken, officials have a predetermined course of action and a penalty may follow.

Football Rules

Football rules are known as the 'laws of the game'. There are 17 laws, which have changed marginally over the years. The international sports federation, FIFA, adapts them as it considers necessary. Recent examples of this include changing the offside law to encourage more attacking football.

The following is a summary of the 17 laws:

- **Field of play**: this law looks at the surface, dimensions, layout and markings of the football pitch.
- **Ball**: the shape and dimensions of the football are covered, as well as replacing the ball should it burst during a match.

- **Number of players**: there should be 11 players at the start of a match, including a designated goalkeeper; the use of substitutions is also looked at.
- **Players' equipment**: the health and safety considerations of what players wear is mentioned. No jewellery should be worn and all players must wear shin guards. The goalkeeper must also wear a top that distinguishes him from the other players.
- **Referee**: this law looks at the responsibilities of the referee, which include enforcing the laws, taking responsibility for the safety of the players, acting as a timekeeper, punishing serious offences and providing a match report to the relevant authority.
- **Assistant referees**: assistant referees assist the referee to control the game, signalling when the ball goes out of play and any offences that the referee may miss.
- **Duration of the match**: a football match is played over two equal periods of 45 minutes. This time may be reduced for youth football. Time can be added for substitutions, injuries and time wasting, at the referee's discretion.
- **Start & restart of play**: the team that wins the toss of a coin can choose which goal they want to attack. The game starts with a kick-off, where all players must be in their own half of the pitch; this method is also used after a goal has been scored.
- **Ball in & out of play**: the ball is out of play when the whole ball crosses one of the perimeter lines or when the referee blows his whistle to stop play.
- **Method of scoring**: the rule states that a goal is scored when the ball crosses the line between the posts and under the crossbar. The team with the most goals wins.
- **Offside**: a player is offside if 'he is nearer to his opponent's goal line than both the ball and the second last opponent' and receives a pass from one of his teammates. The player also needs to be in his opponent's half and interfering with the game. However, you cannot be offside if you receive the pass from a goal kick or throw-in.
- **Fouls & misconduct**: fouls and misconduct are penalised by either a direct or indirect free kick. There are ten offences that result in a direct free kick, including kicking, tripping or pushing an opponent. Indirect free kicks are given for infringements such as a goalkeeper picking up a back pass or throw-in, or for impeding an opponent. Direct free kicks are given for offences that are committed by a player in their own penalty box and are awarded as a penalty kick.
- **Free kicks**: following a foul, a free kick is awarded, which will be either direct or indirect. Opponents must be a minimum of ten yards away from the ball. A direct free kick shot directly into the opponent's goal will be awarded a goal, while a goal can be scored from an indirect free kick only if it has touched another player before going into the goal. A referee will signal an indirect free kick by raising one arm into the air above their head.
- **Penalty kick**: awarded when an offence is committed by a player in their own penalty area. The goalkeeper must remain on their line until the ball has been kicked. A penalty taker cannot touch the ball until it has touched another player if they miss.
- **Throw-in**: the ball is thrown back on to the pitch when the ball goes out of play on either side of the pitch. A throw-in is taken with two hands on the ball and the ball must be released from behind the player's head.
- **Goal kick**: the ball is kicked back into play from within the goal area when the ball crosses the goal line and was last touched by an attacking player. The ball must leave the penalty area before it can be played again.
- **Corner kick**: a corner is awarded when the ball crosses the goal line and was last touched by a defending player. The kick is taken from within the corner arc. A goal can be scored direct from a corner kick.

The FA has set a number of regulations to help the running of football in England. Regulations are rules controlled by the organising bodies. The FA has included regulations on:

- The control of youth football
- The doping control programme
- Disciplinary procedures.

Key learning points 2

- Rules are established and controlled by national governing bodies (NGBs), such as the Rugby Football Union (RFU).
- Sports can be played in real time, like one-day cricket, or in artificial time, like basketball.
- Unwritten rules are situations that can occur when players and officials can choose to demonstrate fair play.
- Governing bodies are responsible for any necessary changes to rules or changes to interpretations of rules.

Student activity 8.2 60–90 mins P2 M2

Select two team or two individual sports of your choice to carry out the following:

- List the rules and regulations of each of your selected sports.
- Describe and explain the rules and their application for each of your two selected sports.
- Demonstrate your ability to apply these rules in three different situations for each of your selected sports.

Q Quick quiz 2

1 Name three sports that take more than one day to complete.
2 Name three sports that can be completed in two hours.
3 Describe why sports need rules.
4 Give four examples of where you have witnessed fair play.
5 Name six different types of playing surfaces.
6 Give the name for the leading official(s) in the following sports (e.g. for football, it is referee).
   (a) Tennis.
   (b) Netball.
   (c) Athletics.
   (d) Gymnastics.

8.4 Assessing Own and Other People's Performance in a Team or Individual Sport

P4 P5 M3 M4 D1 D2

Performance Assessment

Performances can all be assessed. Assessment should always be conducted with a view to improve future performances.

Some assessors try to correct errors in performance by simply shouting instructions, like 'You are not trying hard enough' or 'Get more aim on your shot' in basketball. These instructions give the sportsperson an idea of what they should be doing, but not how to achieve this. To analyse techniques from a coach's viewpoint, it is important to:

- Sort the effective techniques from the less effective
- Break down complete movements into simple parts
- Concentrate on the techniques that need the most improvement, in the right order.

There are many different factors to consider when evaluating a team's or individual's performance:

- How well do they perform specific skills?
- Are they using the correct techniques?
- Are they using appropriate tactics?
- Are they successful at employing these tactics?

There are several ways in which to assess performance:

- Assessment can be completed by the individual, known as self-assessment.
- Peer assessment is the assessment of an individual or a group of individuals on performance.
- Other observers could be teachers, coaches or judges.

Here are some key terms in assessing performance:

- **Observation** – watching sporting performances
- **Analysis** – deciding what has happened
- **Evaluation** – the end-product of observation and analysis, where decisions are made and feedback is given to the performer
- **Qualitative analysis** – largely subjective, meaning that it is open to personal interpretation and is therefore subject to bias or error; the more knowledge the observer has, the more valid the observations
- **Quantitative analysis** – more involved and scientific, and involves the direct measurement of a performance or technique; match statistics recorded while the game is in progress are called 'real-time', while match statistics recorded after the events are called 'lapsed-time' analysis.

There are a number of methods of assessment that can be used to assess performance.

Video Analysis

Video gives the person who watches it an objective record of a performance. The greatest benefit of video is the playback feature, including slow motion, which can be used to demonstrate skill execution, tactical efficiency or a more general generic performance evaluation.

Here are some guidelines on the use of video analysis:

- Do not try to film your performers and coach them at the same time. Ask someone reliable to do the filming, and brief them on what you want – follow the player or the ball, try to capture tactics or specific techniques, and so on.
- Try to pick up all the sound, as it can provide useful feedback.
- Start the recording before the action and end it well after, judging players' body language before and after performance.
- Label and date the film immediately to keep a record.

Table 8.1 is an example of a match analysis sheet for a team sport. This could be filled in by the performer, a peer or a neutral observer, scoring 1 to 10 for both achieved and target scores.

Notation

Notation is a way of collecting data and can be done by hand or with a computer.

Hand notation is a system of recording detailed analysis of a sport and literally noting the data on a sheet of paper using a predefined set of symbols. Systems like this exist for many sports, such as tennis, archery and football.

The advantage of these systems is that they are inexpensive and, if completed by a skilful recorder, produce quick information in real time, so that the coach or performer can have instant access to detailed information. The main disadvantages of this system are that it is open to human error, can be difficult to interpret and can be difficult in certain conditions, such as bad weather.

Figure 8.5 gives an example of a profile of a hockey player's skills and techniques. The darker column is the assessment of the level of performance by the performer, and the lighter column is the assessment of the level of performance as identified by the coach.

If you look at the results, it is clear that there are differences in opinion as to level of performance. It is important that, if there are such differences, the coach and performer discuss the issues and decide on what needs development in practice and game situations and how that can be achieved.

Technology in Performance Analysis

As video and sound technology improve, new software packages have been developed that can analyse all physical activities. Packages such as Kandle and Dartfish are capable of producing a range of exciting analysis tools, including:

- Video delay systems
- Distance and angle measurement
- Overlays and comparators that compare other performances
- Multi-frame sequencing that breaks down complex skills
- Drawing and annotation tools.

Date	Opponent	Result	
		Mark	Target
Analysis area			
Positional play			
Tactical awareness/decision-making			
Fitness levels			
Skills/techniques			
Cooperation/teamwork			
Concentration/psychological factors			
Diet/nutrition			

Table 8.1 Match analysis of an individual sport

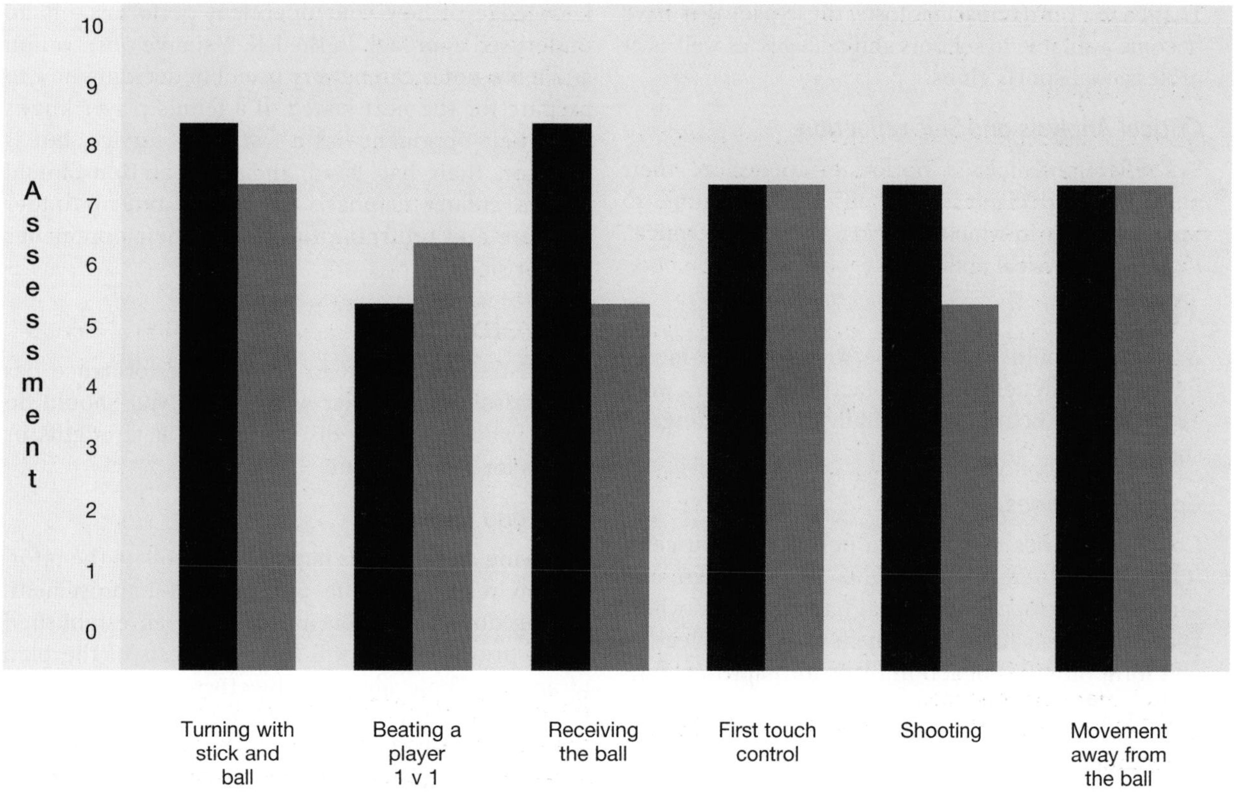

Fig 8.5 Profile of hockey player's skills & techniques

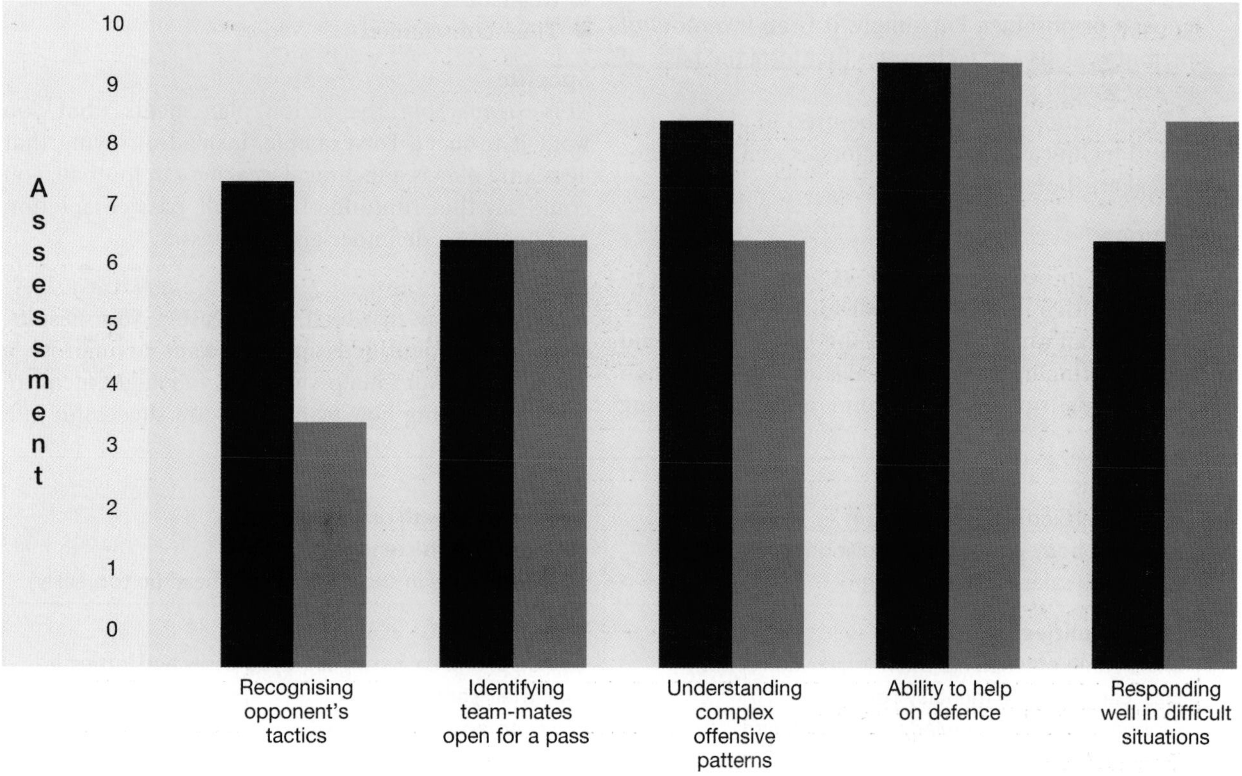

Fig 8.6 Profile of basketball player's skills & techniques

Thanks to ever decreasing costs, these packages have become available in schools and colleges, as well as at professional sports clubs.

Critical Analysis and Self-reflection

Self-reflection allows a performer to explore their perceptions, decisions and subsequent actions, to work out ways in which they can improve technical, tactical or physical ability.

A Mentor

A mentor should be someone who is a role-model figure, who can help provide practical solutions, work as a sounding board and generally provide a range of support.

Coaching Diaries

Coaching diaries can act as a permanent source of information to record thoughts and feelings, and serve as a true account of what happened and when. Diaries or logs can certainly help with self-reflection and form the basis of action plans for improvement.

SWOT Analysis

An example of a SWOT analysis carried out on a golfer is shown in Table 8.2.

Performance Profiling

Performance profiling is a method that can be used by a performer or, more typically, applied by a coach or observer. Put simply, it is an inventory of attributes, skills and techniques that form the basis of an assessment grading model.

Performance profiling can be used to analyse and record technical or tactical factors as well as psychological attributes.

Scouting

This is a process where an expert observer can identify either a talented individual or produce a report about an opponent. In the first case it could result in bringing a new player to a team to strengthen the existing squad. The second aspect – gaining knowledge of how your opponent performs – is an underused approach in the UK. A simple observation and a few notes can be very useful in deciding how to prepare for the next match. If a tennis player knows that their opponent has a fast, hard service, but is poor on their backhand, their preparation should have a greater emphasis on service returns under pressure and returning the ball to their opponent's weaker side.

Development

The last stage is what to do once performance has been assessed. In other words, what you should do about what you have discovered, be it strengths or points for improvement.

Aims and Objectives

Following analysis, it is important to collate the information relating to the performance improvement. Having done this, there needs to be an established set of priorities that will form the basis of the plan of action. These aims or objectives need to be the foundation of the targets to be set.

It is a good idea to use the SMART principle in designing an action plan. SMART stands for:

- **S**pecific
- **M**easurable
- **A**chievable
- **R**ealistic
- **T**ime-constrained.

Specific
This means that the action plan meets what you want it to meet. For example, instead of saying that attacking play is a technical weakness in football, you could say that running off the ball, pass completion and beating a defender are weaknesses.

Measurable
This is the way in which you measure your results. If you have identified that you want to improve a basketball player's jump-shooting, you might measure this by counting how many shots are successful in a

Strengths A good relaxed swing Excellent body positioning in relation to the ball A low-risk safety-first approach	**Weaknesses** Not accurate with driving clubs Putting is inconsistent Poor technique in short iron game (head up too early)
Opportunities Short game practice has been improved recently Has learnt how to mentally rehearse Opponent has no knowledge of the course	**Threats** Can be prone to getting annoyed easily and letting it spoil their game Environment – windy day Opponent is a better player

Table 8.2 An example of a SWOT analysis

training or game situation, and then measure again after additional training sessions.

Achievable
What you set out to improve must be possible. It would not be fair to ask a beginner in trampolining to complete a complicated routine with multiple somersaults.

Realistic
It must be possible and realistic to achieve what we intend to achieve.

Time-constrained
There should be a reasonable amount of time to complete an action plan or achieve a goal.

Key learning points 3

- Performances can be analysed by the performer themselves, their peers and observers such as coaches.
- Video capture and analysis is a very effective performance assessment tool, especially features like slow motion, freeze frame and video playback.
- SMART goals should be used to establish action points for the improvement of performance.

Student activity 8.3

90–120 mins P4 P5 M3 M4 D1 D2

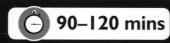

Task 1

Select two different methods of self-analysis, then carry out this self-analysis for two different individual or team sports of your choice.

Task 2

Write a report based on your self-analysis that identifies, explains and analyses identified strengths and areas for improvement. Where possible, try to make justified suggestions on your own personal development.

Task 3

Select two different methods of performance analysis, then carry out this analysis for an individual who is taking part in either two team or two individual sports.

Task 4

Write a report based on your performance analyses that identifies, explains and analyses identified strengths and areas for improvement. Where possible, try to make justified suggestions on the individual's personal development.

Further reading

Crisfield, P. (2001) *Analysing your Coaching*, Coachwise.

Galligan, F., Crawford, D. and Maskery, C. (2002) *Advanced PE for Edexcel, Teacher's Resource File*, Heinemann.

Miles, A. (2004) *Coaching Practice*, Coachwise.

Stafford-Brown, J., Rea, S., Janaway, L. and Manley, C. (2006) *BTEC First Sport*, Hodder Arnold.

Useful websites

www.kidsexercise.co.uk/TeamSports.html

Online article that explains the benefits of playing team sports; also links to wider site that offers advice such as sports nutrition and free exercises (downloadable) for young people

http://news.bbc.co.uk/sport1/hi/academy/default.stm

Access to information and resources on a wide range of sports and sports skills

11: Sports nutrition

11.1 Introduction

As we seek to gain an extra edge in our sporting performances and to maximise the effects of our training, so the spotlight has fallen on areas other than training. Nutrition has been shown to be an area of increasing interest. We know that training brings benefits and we know that eating properly brings benefits. So if we combine the correct training with the correct nutritional strategy, the gains are multiplied. Nutrition is as important for people who are seeking to improve their sporting performance as it is for those seeking fitness gains or weight-management objectives.

By the end of this unit you should:

- know the concepts of nutrition and digestion
- know energy intake and expenditure in sports performance
- know the relationship between hydration and sports performance
- be able to plan a diet appropriate for a selected sports activity.

Assessment and grading criteria

To achieve a PASS grade the evidence must show that the learner is able to:	To achieve a MERIT grade the evidence must show that, in addition to the pass criteria, the learner is able to:	To achieve a DISTINCTION grade the evidence must show that, in addition to the pass and merit criteria, the learner is able to:
P1 describe nutrition, including nutritional requirements, using recommended guidelines from public health sources associated with nutrition		
P2 describe the structure and function of the digestive system		
P3 describe energy intake and expenditure in sports performance	**M1** explain energy intake and expenditure in sports performance	
P4 describe energy balance and its importance in relation to sports performance	**M2** explain the importance of energy balance in relation to sports performance	**D1** analyse the effects of energy balance on sports performance
P5 describe hydration and its effects on sports performance		
P6 describe the components of a balanced diet	**M3** explain the components of a balanced diet	
P7 plan an appropriate two-week diet plan for a selected sports performer for a selected sports activity.	**M4** explain the two-week diet plan for a selected sports performer for a selected sports activity.	**D2** justify the two-week diet plan for a selected sports performer for a selected sports activity.

11.2 Nutrients

P1

Key term

Nutrients: chemical substances obtained from food and used in the body to provide energy, as well as structural materials and regulating agents to support growth, maintenance and repair of the body's tissues.

Nutrients can be divided into two main groups: macronutrients and micronutrients. The three macronutrients are:

- carbohydrate
- protein
- fat.

Macronutrients are needed in large amounts in the diet and all provide energy for the body. They are also used to build the structures of the body and produce functions needed to sustain life.

The two micronutrients are:

- vitamins
- minerals.

They are needed in smaller amounts in the diet and contain no energy themselves. They work in conjunction with the macronutrients to produce life-sustaining functions and are needed to unlock the energy present in the macronutrients.

There are other food groups such as water and fibre. Water is not usually regarded as a nutrient because it has no nutrient value despite being highly important in sustaining life. Fibre is a type of carbohydrate so it would be part of that food group.

Carbohydrate

Almost every culture relies on carbohydrate as the major source of nutrients and calories – rice in Asia, wheat in Europe, the Middle East and North Africa, corn and potato in the Americas.

Carbohydrate should provide between 50 and 60 per cent of calorie intake and its main role is to supply energy to allow the body to function. The energy content of carbohydrate is that 1 g provides 4 kcals.

There are many sources of carbohydrate, such as bread, rice, pasta, potatoes, fruit, vegetables, sweets and biscuits. They all differ in form slightly but are all broken down into glucose because that is the only way the body can use carbohydrate.

The functions of carbohydrate are to provide energy for:

- the brain to function
- the liver to perform its functions
- muscular contractions at moderate to high intensities.

When carbohydrate foods are digested they are all broken down into glucose which is then absorbed in the small intestine and enters the bloodstream. From the bloodstream it can either be used immediately as energy or stored in the liver and muscles. Glucose is stored in the form of glycogen, which is bound to water (1 g of glucose needs 2.7 g of water) for storage. However, the glycogen molecule is bulky and difficult to store in large amounts. The body can store around 1600 kcals of glycogen, which would enable us to run for around two hours.

Key terms

Glucose: the smallest unit of a carbohydrate.

Glycogen: stored glucose in the muscles and liver attached to water molecules.

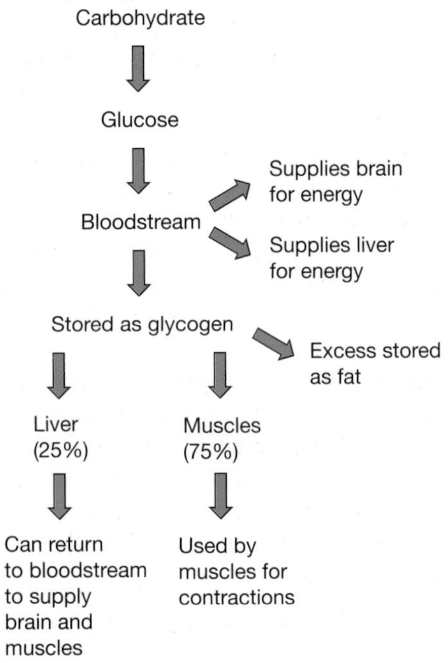

Fig 11.1 What happens to carbohydrate when it is digested

Forms of carbohydrate

Carbohydrates come in a variety of forms, but they are all made up of molecules of sugar. These molecules of sugar are called saccharides; they come in different forms depending upon the foods in which they are found. Eventually through the process of digestion they all become glucose. These saccharides are found as one of the following:

- monosaccharides
- disaccharides
- polysaccharides.

Monosaccharides are one saccharide molecule on its own. There are three types of monosaccharide:

- glucose – occurs naturally in most carbohydrate foods
- fructose – occurs in fruit and honey
- galactose – does not occur freely but is a component of the sugars found in milk products.

Disaccharides are two saccharide molecules joined together by a bond:

- sucrose = glucose + fructose – most commonly found as table sugar
- lactose = glucose + galactose – found in milk and milk products
- maltose = glucose + glucose – found in malt products, beers and cereals.

Mono- and disaccharides are commonly known as simple carbohydrates because they are in short simple chains – existing as individual molecules.

Polysaccharides are long, complex chains of glucose molecules containing ten or more molecules. Due to their complicated structures they are called 'complex carbohydrates'.

To digest polysaccharides, the bonds need to be broken down through the process of digestion so that they can become individual glucose molecules and be absorbed into the bloodstream. If a complex carbohydrate is processed or cooked in any way these bonds will start to be broken down before they enter the digestive system.

Polysaccharides or complex carbohydrates can come in either their natural or refined forms. Wheat and rice are naturally brown in colour due to their high levels of fibre, vitamins and minerals. Therefore, the brown varieties of bread, rice and pasta are of greater nutrient value than the white, refined varieties.

Good sources of polysaccharides:

- wholemeal, wholegrain or granary breads
- wholemeal pasta
- wholegrain rice
- potatoes
- sweet potatoes
- vegetables
- pulses.

Poorer choices of polysaccharides:

- white bread
- white pasta
- white rice
- rice cakes.

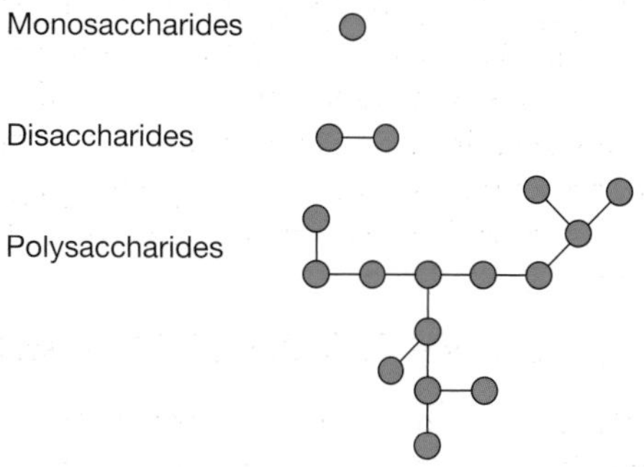

Fig 11.2 Structure of saccharides

Glycaemic index

The rate at which carbohydrate foods are broken down and how quickly they raise blood glucose levels is measured via the glycaemic index (GI). It is a ranking system that shows how quickly the carbohydrate is broken down and enters the blood as glucose in comparison with the speed at which glucose would enter the blood if consumed. Foods with a high glycaemic index break down quickly and rapidly increase blood glucose levels. Table sugar is a good example. Pasta would have a lower glycaemic index, breaking down into glucose more slowly. It would also have less of an immediate effect on blood glucose levels, causing a slower increase over a longer period.

The glycaemic index is one of the most important principles in nutrition currently. We deal best with foods of a low glycaemic index that release their energy slowly and over time. Foods of a high glycaemic index cause a rapid release of glucose into the bloodstream, followed by a rapid drop in blood glucose, causing hunger and fatigue. The person who eats high glycaemic index foods will experience fluctuating blood glucose levels and be tempted to overeat the wrong type of food. High glycaemic index foods, such as sweets, cakes, biscuits, fizzy drinks, white breads and sugary cereals, are linked to obesity and the development of type 2 diabetes. If a person eats low glycaemic index foods they will find that their stable blood glucose levels give them energy and enable them to concentrate throughout the day.

In the glycaemic index foods are either high, moderate or low.

High	Moderate	Low
Above 85	60–84	Below 60

Table 11.1 Glycaemic index for foods

The speed at which a food is broken down and enters the bloodstream is dependent on a range of factors. The following will lower the speed at which glucose enters the bloodstream:

- the presence of fibre in the food
- the presence of fat in the food
- the presence of protein in the food
- the type of saccharides present in the food
- the amount of carbohydrate eaten.

The following will increase the speed at which glucose enters the bloodstream:

- the length of the cooking process
- the amount the food has been refined or processed
- the riper the fruit has become.

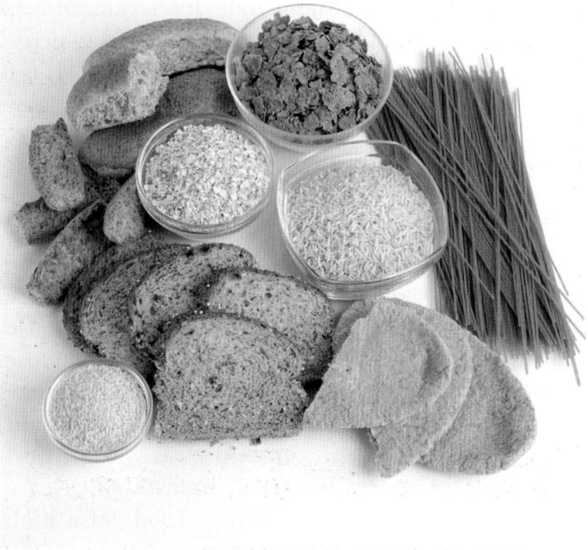

Fig 11.3 Unrefined brown foods

Fibre

Dietary fibre is the part of a plant that is resistant to the body's digestive enzymes. It is defined as 'indigestible plant material', and although it is a carbohydrate and contains calories, the digestive system cannot unlock them from the plant. As a result, fibre moves through the gastrointestinal tract and ends up in the stool. The main benefit in eating fibre is that it retains water, resulting in softer and bulkier stools that prevent constipation and haemorrhoids. Research suggests that a high-fibre diet also reduces the risk of colon cancer. All fruits, vegetables and grains provide some fibre.

There are two types of fibre – soluble and insoluble – that perform slightly different functions.

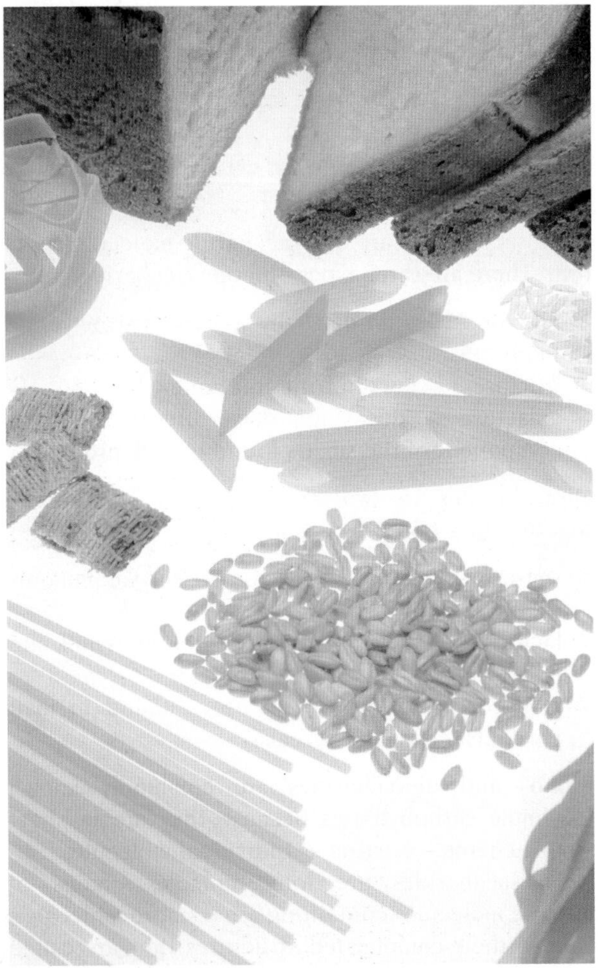

Fig 11.4 Refined white foods

Soluble fibre dissolves into a gel in water and is found in the fleshy part of fruit and vegetables, oats, barley and rice. For example, when you make porridge the oats partly dissolve into a sticky gel and this is the soluble fibre.

Soluble fibre has two main roles to play:

- it slows down how quickly the stomach empties and how quickly glucose enters the bloodstream
- it binds to fat and blood cholesterol, thus decreasing the risk of heart disease.

Insoluble fibre will not dissolve in water and is found in the skin of fruit and vegetables, wheat, rye, seeds and pips of fruit. Insoluble fibre passes through the digestive system without being altered in any way. Its main roles are as follows:

- It adds bulk to faeces and speeds its passage through the large intestine.
- It helps to keep the large intestine clean and prevent bowel disease.
- It stretches the stomach and makes you feel full for longer.

- It slows down the release of glucose into the bloodstream.

It is recommended that we eat around 18 g of fibre a day. This can be done by eating foods in their natural form rather than in their processed or refined states.

Recommended daily intake of carbohydrate

A minimum recommended daily intake of at least 50 per cent of total kilocalories consumed should come from complex carbohydrate sources. The British Nutrition Foundation found that in Britain the average intake of carbohydrate is 272 g for men and 193 g for women, providing just over 43 per cent of the energy in the diet.

As with most nutrients, eating excess amounts can lead to problems. Excessive consumption of sugar (for example sucrose) can lead to tooth decay and is linked to a number of major diseases, such as diabetes, obesity and coronary heart disease. Excess carbohydrate in the diet will be converted to and stored as fat. Thus it is possible to gain body fat even on a low-fat diet.

Key learning points 1

- Carbohydrate provides energy for:
  - brain function
  - liver function and digestion
  - muscular contractions.
- Carbohydrates are made up of saccharides, of which there are three types:
  - monosaccharides – single units of saccharides known as 'simple sugars'
  - disaccharides – two units of saccharides joined by a bond called 'simple sugars'
  - polysaccharides – long chains of saccharides called 'complex carbohydrates'.
- Glycaemic index (GI) is the rate at which a carbohydrate food enters the bloodstream as glucose:
  - high GI = above 85
  - moderate GI = 60–85
  - low GI = less than 60.
- Fibre is 'indigestible plant material' which cannot be digested. It protects against heart disease and diseases of the colon by keeping the colon clean and the waste moving through quickly.

Q Quick quiz 1

Look at the list of carbohydrate-rich foods and put them into the appropriate column (some of them can go into more than one column).

Monosaccharide	**Disaccharide**	**Polysaccharide**	**Fibre**

Apple	Milk	Pasta
Cereal	Rice	All Bran
Bread	Cabbage	Banana
Honey	Potatoes	Cream
Sweetcorn	Beer	

Protein

The word 'protein' is derived from Greek and means 'prime importance'. Proteins are of prime importance because they are the building blocks that make up the structures of the body. Muscle, skin, bones, internal organs, cartilage and ligament all have a protein component. We gain our protein by eating protein-rich foods such as red meat, fish, chicken, eggs and dairy products.

The diet should consist of between 10 and 20 per cent protein depending upon the specific needs of the individual. Protein also provides a source of energy: 1 g of protein provides 4 kcals.

Amino acids

The smallest unit of a protein is an amino acid. Proteins are made up of long chains of amino acids which are formed into structures. Amino acids are the smallest unit of a protein and there are 20 amino acids in total. Amino acids can be seen to be like the alphabet. In the English language we have 26 letters from which we can make up millions of words. The protein alphabet has 20 amino acids from which can be produced approximately 50,000 different proteins present in the body. Just as different words are made up of different orders of letters, so different structures are made up of different orders of amino acids.

They can be split into essential and non-essential amino acids. An essential amino acid is one that must be gained through eating it in the diet, while a non-essential amino acid can be made in the liver if all essential amino acids are present. This means to produce all the structures of the body we must gain all the essential amino acids on a daily basis.

There are eight essential amino acids to be gained from the diet:

- isoleucine
- leucine
- lysine
- methionine
- phenylalanine
- threonine
- tryptophan
- valine.

There are 12 non-essential amino acids which are synthesised in the liver if all eight essential amino acids are gained from the diet:

- cystein
- yrosine
- histidine
- glutamine
- glutamic acid
- glycine
- alanine
- serine
- proline
- aspartic acid
- asparagine
- arginine.

Foods that contain all eight essential amino acids are described as being complete, while a food that is missing one or more essential amino acid is described as being incomplete. Table 11.2 shows sources of complete and incomplete proteins.

With the exception of the soya bean, the sources of complete protein are from animals, while incomplete proteins come from plant sources. To gain all eight essential amino acids from incomplete protein sources you need to eat a range of sources or combine protein sources. This is called 'complementary protein' and examples are:

- wheat and pulses (beans on toast)
- nuts and vegetables (nut roast)
- rice and lentils (vegetarian chilli).

All protein sources contain different amounts of amino acids. The greater the quantity of the essential amino acids in the food, the higher the biological value. Eggs have the highest quality or biological

Complete protein	Incomplete protein
Chicken	Wheat
Eggs	Oats
Fish	Rice
Red meat	Pulses
Dairy products	Nuts
Soya beans	Vegetables

Table 11.2 Complete and incomplete proteins

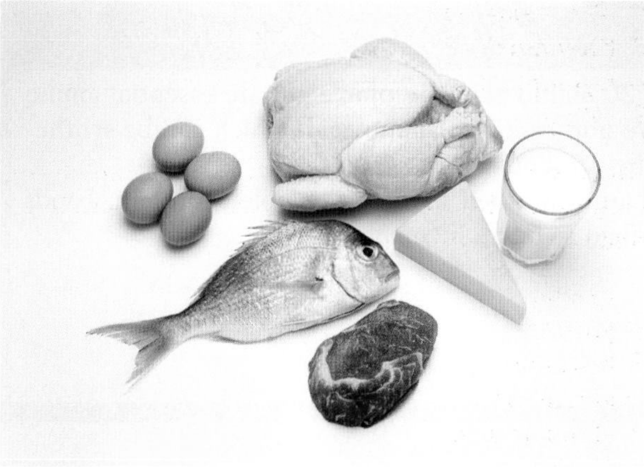

Fig 11.5 Complete protein

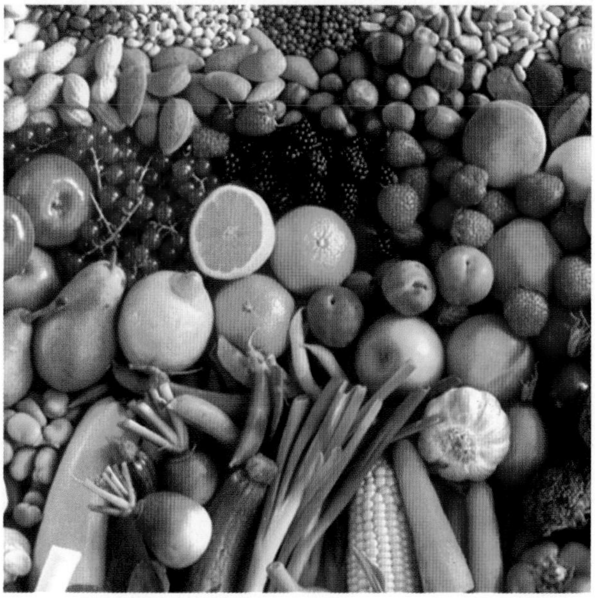

Fig 11.6 Incomplete protein

value of all foods and are given a protein rating of 100. All other proteins are compared with eggs in terms of their quality and quantity of amino acids. This is shown in Table 11.3.

Functions of protein

When we eat protein it is digested in the digestive system and then delivered to the liver as individual amino acids. The liver then rebuilds the amino acids into long chains to make up proteins. The proteins that the liver produces depend upon the needs of the body at that time. If we need to replace muscle the liver will produce the relevant proteins to replace muscle tissue.

Proteins have three specific roles in the body:

- to build structures (structural)
- to perform functions (functional)
- to provide fuel.

Protein forms a part of the following structures:

- muscle (skeletal, smooth and cardiac)
- bone
- internal organs (heart, kidneys, liver)
- connective tissue (tendons and ligaments)
- hair
- nails.

Protein forms part of the following structures which perform specific functions in the body:

- hormones (which send messages to cells – insulin and adrenaline)
- enzymes (biological catalysts which speed up reactions in cells)
- part of the immune system (white blood cells are made partly of protein)
- formation of lipoproteins (these help to transport fats around the body).

Protein is not the body's first choice of fuel but it can be used as energy. It is heavily used during endurance training and events, or at times of starvation.

Food	Protein rating
Eggs	100
Fish	70
Beef	69
Cow's milk	60
Brown rice	57
White rice	56
Soya beans	47
Wheat	44
Peanuts	43
Beans	34

Table 11.3 Protein ratings of different foods
Source: Adapted from McArdle *et al.* (2009)

Recommended intakes of protein

The average daily intake of protein in the UK is 85 g for men and 62 g for women. The recommended daily amount of protein for healthy adults is 0.8 g per kilogram of body weight, or about 15 per cent of total kilocalories. Protein needs are higher for children, infants and many athletes.

Key learning points 2

- Proteins are long chains of amino acids. There are 20 amino acids in total: eight are essential amino acids which need to be eaten in the diet, and 12 are non-essential amino acids which can be synthesised by the liver if all eight essential amino acids are present.
- Foods containing all eight essential amino acids are described as being complete protein. Foods missing one or more essential amino acid are described as being incomplete.
- Protein has the following main functions:
  - to build structures of the body
  - to perform specific functions
  - to provide fuel.

Quick quiz 2

Liver	Isoleucine	20	Nuts	8
Muscle	Aspartic acid	Soya bean	Eggs	Hormone

Choose the correct word or words to match the following descriptions.

1 This is an essential amino acid.
2 This is a complete protein.
3 This is an incomplete protein.
4 This body structure contains protein.
5 There are this number of amino acids in total.
6 There are this number of essential amino acids.
7 This is a non-essential amino acid.
8 This organ rebuilds amino acids into long chains.
9 This food has a very high protein rating.
10 Protein forms part of this structure.

Fats

Fats are often perceived as being bad or a part of the diet to be avoided. In fact, fats are vital to health and perform many important functions in the body. The intake of certain fats does need to be minimised and excess consumption of fats will lead to health problems.

The functions of fat are as follows:

- formation of the cell membrane
- formation of the myelin sheath which coats the nerves
- a component of the brain and nervous system
- protection of internal organs (brain, kidneys, liver)
- production of hormones (oestrogen and testosterone)
- transportation and storage of vitamins A, D, E and K
- constant source of energy
- store of energy
- heat production.

Fats and oils belong to a family called 'lipids' and they perform a variety of important roles in the body. Predominantly fats supply energy for everyday activities and movement. They are described as being 'energy-dense' because they contain a lot of energy per gram: 1 g of fat provides 9 kcals.

If we compare this figure to the 4 kcals which carbohydrates and protein provide (see Table 11.4) then we can see that it is significantly higher.

The difference between a fat and an oil is that a fat is solid at room temperature while an oil is liquid at room temperature.

The smallest unit of a fat is called a 'fatty acid'. There are different types of fatty acid present in the foods we ingest. In particular, a fatty acid can be

Macronutrient	Kcals per gram
Carbohydrate	4
Protein	4
Fat	9

Table 11.4 Kcalories per gram of macronutrients

saturated or unsaturated; this is important because they will be shaped differently. In chemistry shape matters because it influences the function performed. Therefore, different fatty acids perform different functions in the body.

Triglycerides

Triglycerides are dietary fats in that they are how the fats we ingest are packaged. A triglyceride is defined as 'three fatty acids attached to a glycerol backbone'. Glycerol is actually a carbohydrate which the fatty acids attach to. During digestion the fatty acids are broken off from the glycerol backbone to be used by the body as required. The glycerol is used as all carbohydrates are used, to produce energy.

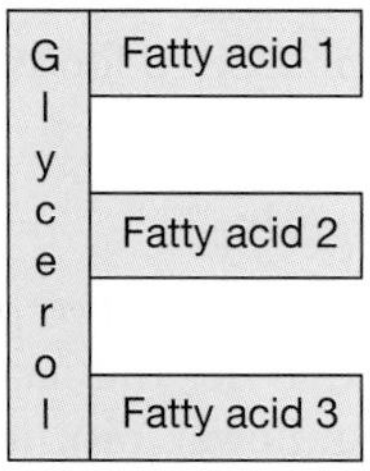

Fig 11.7 Structure of a triglyceride

Types of fatty acid

Fatty acids can be divided into:

- saturated fatty acids
- monounsaturated fatty acids
- polyunsaturated fatty acids.

A fatty acid consists of long chains of carbon atoms with an acid group (COOH) at one end and a methyl group (CH_3) at the other. The structure of the chains of fatty acids attached to the glycerol molecule determines whether the fat is classed as saturated, monounsaturated or polyunsaturated. If you think of different types of fats, such as butter, lard, sunflower oil and olive oil, you will notice that they differ in terms of their colour, texture and taste. This is because of the different types of fatty acids attached to the glycerol backbone.

A saturated fat is one where all the carbon atoms are attached to hydrogen molecules. The chain is said to be saturated with hydrogen.

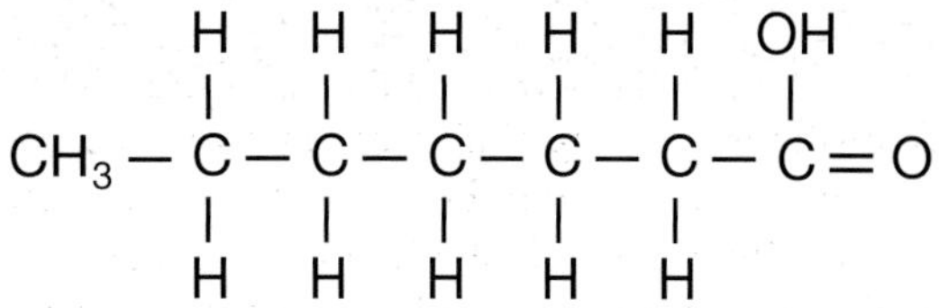

Fig 11.8 Saturated fatty acid

We can see that the carbon atoms each have single bonds between them and each carbon atom has four bonds. The hydrogen atoms possess a very slight charge and gently push away from each other. This has the effect of making the chain straight in shape. In chemistry shape matters as it affects function and it also makes the saturated fat solid at room temperature. This is because the fatty acids can pack tightly together with little space between each one. Saturated fats are also described as being stable or inert. This means that their structure will not change when they are heated. They will melt but the structure of the fatty acid chain stays the same.

The majority of saturated fats come from animal sources (see Table 11.5).

Source	
Animal	Plant
Red meat	Coconut oil
Poultry	Palm oil
Eggs	
Dairy products	

Table 11.5 **Sources of saturated fats**

The Department of Health recommends a person should have a maximum of 10 per cent of daily kilocalories from saturated fat.

An unsaturated fat is one where there are hydrogen atoms missing from the carbon chain, causing the carbon atoms to attach to each other with double bonds. This is because carbon has to have four bonds and if there is no hydrogen present they will bond to each other. In this case the carbon chain is not saturated with hydrogen atoms and is therefore 'unsaturated'.

A monounsaturated fat is one where there is just one double bond in the carbon chain (see Figure 11.9).

Due to the slight charge the hydrogen atoms contain, they push each other away. Now that there are hydrogen atoms missing, it causes the chain to bend and become curved. The curved fatty acids cannot pack so tightly together, so their appearance

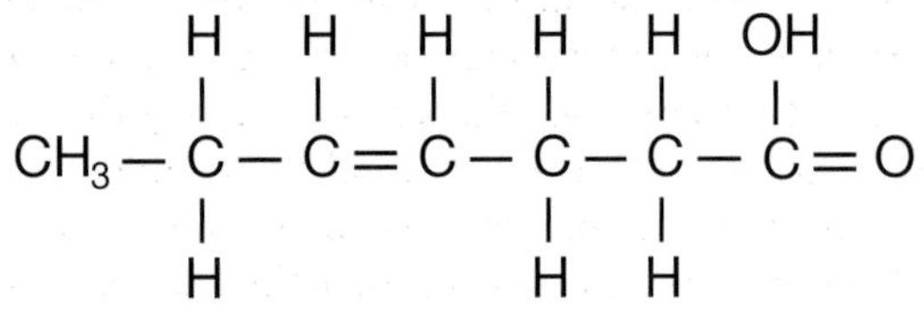

Fig 11.9 Monounsaturated fatty acid

changes and they will be in liquid or oil form. They will also be less stable or more reactive. This is because of the double bonds between the carbon atoms. Carbon attaches to itself only if there is nothing else to be attached to and it will take the opportunity to break off and attach to something else if it can. If monounsaturated fats are heated they change their structure.

Examples of monounsaturated fats are:

- olive oil
- peanut oil
- avocados
- rapeseed oil (canola oil)
- almond oil.

The Department of Health recommends a person should have a maximum of 12 per cent of daily kilocalories from monounsaturated fat.

A polyunsaturated fat is one where there are many double bonds in the carbon chain due to a shortage of hydrogen ions in the chain.

This has the effect of making the fatty acid even more curved and highly reactive in nature. They are also in oil or liquid form. Polyunsaturated fats are highly unstable when heated to high temperatures and will change their structure.

Examples of polyunsaturated fats are:

- sunflower oil
- safflower oil
- corn oil
- fish oils
- nuts
- seeds.

The Department of Health recommends a person should have a maximum of 10 per cent of daily kilocalories from these polyunsaturated fats.

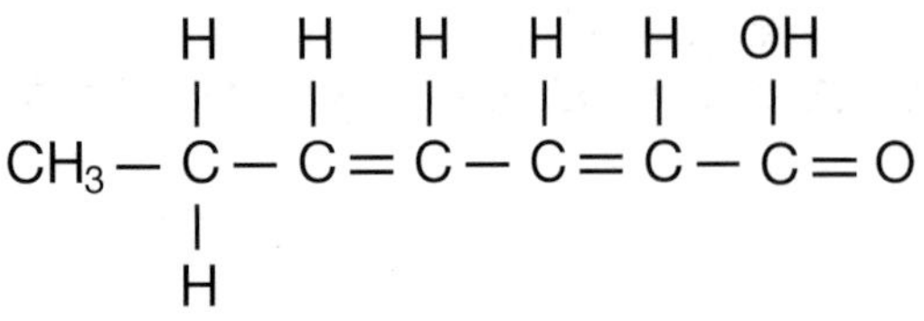

Fig 11.10 Polyunsaturated fatty acid

Saturated versus unsaturated fats

Saturated fats have always received bad press until recently when people realised that they have an important role in the diet. Due to their stable nature they always retain their structure. This is important because when they enter the fat cells, the cells will recognise them and know what to do with them. Saturated fats are always stored as fat in the fat cells.

Naturally occurring unsaturated fats, such as olive oil, have very beneficial effects when they are stored in fat cells – they improve circulation, lower cholesterol levels and improve the health of hair, skin and nails. The problem comes when unsaturated fats are heated or processed in any way because they then change their structure and start to look like saturated fats. They become 'hydrogenated' or altered structurally and when they enter the body they are accepted into the fat cells because they look like saturated fats. Once inside the fat cells, they start to cause damage to the cell and stop positive reactions occurring. The two most dangerous types of fats are:

- hydrogenated vegetable oil
- trans fats.

These have been linked to heart disease and cancer and are present in processed foods and deep-fat-fried foods.

Butter versus margarine?

In terms of fat content these two products are pretty similar. However, due to the margarine being an unsaturated fat (sunflower oil), it would appear to be beneficial to health. Sunflower oil is naturally a liquid and margarine is a solid product, which means it has been processed in some way and thus changed structurally.

The butter will not be changed structurally because it is predominantly saturated fat. For these reasons the butter is a better health choice because it is a more naturally occurring product. In particular, it is the cheap margarines that need to be avoided. If choosing a margarine, check the contents for hydrogenated vegetable oil and trans fats.

Essential fatty acids

The body can make all the fatty acids it needs except for two, the essential fatty acids (EFAs), which must be supplied in the diet. These fatty acids are omega 3 and omega 6.

Sources of omega 3 and 6 are as follows.

Omega 3 fatty acids:

- oily fish (e.g. salmon, mackerel, herring)
- flax oil

- walnuts
- soya beans.

Omega 6 fatty acids:

- sunflower oil
- pumkin seeds
- sesame seeds
- safflower oil.

Research into omega 3, and in particular fish oils, has shown that eating oily fish protects against heart disease. This is because the omega 3s may prevent the formation of blood clots on the artery walls and lower the levels of triglycerides circulating in the bloodstream.

The essential fatty acids are also thought to improve the function of the brain and promote learning as well as being beneficial for arthritics because they reduce swelling in the joints.

Cholesterol

Cholesterol can either be ingested or made in the body. It is found only in animal products and never in plants. It has some useful functions including building cell membranes and helping the function of various hormones.

There are two types of cholesterol: low-density lipoproteins (LDLs) and high-density lipoproteins (HDLs). LDLs are responsible for the deposits lining the walls of arteries and lead to an increased risk of coronary heart disease. HDLs actually reduce this risk by transporting cholesterol away to the liver and so are beneficial to health.

Recommended daily intake of fat

Fat intake should make up no more than 30 per cent of total kilocalories. Only 10 per cent of kilocalories should come from saturated fat. Dietary cholesterol should be limited to 300 mg or less per day.

There are many health problems related to eating an excess of fat, especially saturated fats. These include obesity, high blood pressure and coronary heart disease, although it is important to distinguish between the different types of fat eaten in a person's diet. Consumption of certain fatty acids (omega 3 fish oils found in tuna) is linked to a decreased risk of coronary heart disease.

As fat provides just over twice as much energy per gram as carbohydrate, a diet high in fat can make overconsumption more likely. It is thought that excess dietary fat may be more easily converted to body fat than excess carbohydrate or protein. Research suggests that more people are obese today than ever before. Obese people are more likely to suffer from a range of illnesses including coronary heart disease, adult-onset diabetes, gallstones, arthritis, high blood pressure and some types of cancer. However, most of the health problems associated with obesity are removed once the extra weight is lost.

Key learning points 3

- Fat performs some vital functions in the body:
  - formation of the cell membrane
  - formation of the myelin sheath which coats the nerves
  - a component of the brain and nervous system
  - protection of internal organs (brain, kidneys, liver)
  - production of hormones (oestrogen and testosterone)
  - transportation and storage of vitamins A, D, E and K
  - constant source of energy
  - store of energy
  - heat production.
- Saturated fats occur when all the carbon atoms are saturated with hydrogen. They are solid at room temperature, stable and unreactive. Examples of saturated fats include:
  - animal fats
  - fat of red meat and poultry
  - dairy products
  - eggs
  - coconut oil
  - palm oil.
- Unsaturated fats occur when there is a double bond in the carbon chain due to a shortage of hydrogen. They are liquid at room temperature, unstable and reactive. There are two types of unsaturated fats:
  - monounsaturated fats, which have one double bond in the chain and include olive oil and peanut oil
  - polyunsaturated fats, which have more than one double bond and include sunflower oil and fish oils.

Quick quiz 3

1. Name three functions of fat.
2. What is the name of the family that fats and oils are in?
3. How many kcalories are there in 1g of fat?
4. What is the difference between fats and oils?
5. What is the smallest unit of a fat called?
6. What is a triglyceride?
7. Name the three categories that fatty acids can be placed in.
8. Describe the structure of an unsaturated fat.
9. What are the problems associated with saturated fats?
10. What is an essential fatty acid? Give three examples of one.

Vitamins

Vitamins are organic substances that the body requires in small amounts. The body is incapable of making vitamins for its overall needs, so they must be supplied regularly by the diet.

Vitamins are not related chemically and differ in their physiological actions. As vitamins were discovered, each was identified by a letter. Many of the vitamins consist of several closely related compounds of similar physiological properties.

Vitamins may be subdivided into:

- water soluble – C and B (complex)
- fat soluble – A, D, E and K.

The water-soluble vitamins cannot be stored in the body so they must be consumed on a regular basis. If excess quantities of these vitamins are consumed, the body will excrete them in the urine. Fat-soluble vitamins are stored in the body's fat so it is not necessary to consume these on such a regular basis. It is also possible to overdose on fat-soluble vitamins, which can be detrimental to health.

Varying amounts of each vitamin are required. The amount needed is referred to as the recommended daily allowance (RDA).

Fat-soluble vitamins

Vitamin A

- **Function:** to help maintain good vision, healthy skin, hair and mucous membranes, and to serve as an antioxidant; also needed for proper bone and tooth development
- **Source:** liver, mackerel and milk products
- **RDA:** 1.5 mg

Vitamin D (calciferol)

- **Function:** essential for calcium and phosphorus utilisation; promotes strong bones and teeth
- **Source:** sunlight, egg yolk, fish, fish oils and fortified cereals
- **RDA:** 0.01 mg

Vitamin E

- **Function:** antioxidant, helps prevent damage to cell membranes
- **Source:** wheat germ, nuts, whole grains and dark green leaf vegetables
- **RDA:** 15 mg

Vitamin K

- **Function:** used in the formation of blood clots
- **Source:** leafy green vegetables
- **RDA:** 70 mg

Water-soluble vitamins

B vitamins are not chemically related, but often occur in the same foodstuff. Their main function is to aid in the metabolism of food.

Vitamin B1 (thiamine)

- **Function**: helps convert food to energy and aids the nervous and cardiovascular systems
- **Source**: rice, bran, pork, beef, peas, beans, wheat germ, oatmeal and soya beans
- **RDA:** 1.5 mg

Vitamin B2 (riboflavin)

- **Function:** aids growth and reproduction, and helps to metabolise fats, carbohydrates and proteins; promotes healthy skin and nails
- **Source:** milk, liver, kidneys, yeast, cheese, leafy green vegetables, fish and eggs
- **RDA:** 1.7 mg

Vitamin B3 (niacin)

- **Function**: helps to keep the nervous system balanced and is also important for the synthesis of sex hormones, thyroxine, cortisone and insulin
- **Source:** poultry, fish, peanuts, yeast extract (for example Marmite), rice bran and wheat germ
- **RDA**: 20 mg

Vitamin B5 (pantothenic acid)

- **Function:** helps in cell building and maintaining normal growth and development of the central nervous system; helps form hormones and antibodies; also necessary for the conversion of fat and sugar to energy

- **Source:** wheatgerm, green vegetables, whole grains, mushrooms, fish, peanuts and yeast extract (for example, Marmite)
- **RDA:** 10 mg

Vitamin B6 (pyridoxine)

- **Function:** helps in the utilisation of proteins and the metabolism of fats; also needed for production of red blood cells and antibodies
- **Source:** chicken, beef, bananas, yeast extract (for example Marmite), eggs, brown rice, soya beans, oats, whole wheat, peanuts and walnuts
- **RDA:** 2 mg

Vitamin C (ascorbic acid)

- **Function:** essential for the formation of collagen; helps to strengthen tissues, acts as an antioxidant, helps in healing, production of red blood cells, fighting bacterial infections and regulating cholesterol; also helps the body to absorb iron
- **Source:** most fresh fruits and vegetables
- **RDA:** 60 mg

Folic acid (folacin)

- **Function**: helps the body form genetic material and red blood cells, and aids in protein metabolism; also acts as an antioxidant; research has shown that if folic acid is taken on a daily basis 30 days before conception, the fetus is less likely to suffer from birth defects such as spina bifida
- **Source**: green vegetables, kidney beans and orange juice
- **RDA**: 400 mg

Minerals

There are several minerals required to maintain a healthy body. Some are needed in moderate amounts, others in only very small amounts; the latter are referred to as trace minerals.

Calcium

- **Function**: needed to build strong bones and teeth, helps to calm nerves and plays a role in muscle contraction, blood clotting and cell membrane upkeep; correct quantities of calcium consumption have been shown to significantly lower the risk of osteoporosis
- **Source**: milk and milk products, whole grains and unrefined cereals, green vegetables and fish bones
- **RDA**: adults 1200 mg
- **Deficiency**: fragile bones, osteoporosis, rickets, tooth decay, irregular heartbeat and slowed nerve impulse response; vitamin D is essential for proper calcium absorption and utilisation

Magnesium

- **Function**: aids the production of proteins and helps regulate body temperature; helps lower blood pressure and assists with the proper functioning of nerves and muscles
- **Source**: whole grain foods, wheat bran, dark green leafy vegetables, soya beans, fish, oysters, shrimp, almonds and peanuts
- **RDA**: 350 mg
- **Deficiency**: decreased blood pressure and body temperature, nervousness, interference with the transmission of nerve and muscle impulses

Phosphorus

- **Function**: essential for metabolism of carbohydrates, fats and proteins; aids growth and cell repair, and is necessary for proper skeletal growth, tooth development, proper kidney function and the nervous system
- **Source**: meat, fish, poultry, milk, yoghurt, eggs, seeds, broccoli and nuts
- **RDA**: 800 mg
- **Deficiency**: bone pain, fatigue, irregular breathing and nervous disorders

Potassium

- **Function:** in conjunction with sodium helps to maintain fluid and electrolyte balance within cells; important for normal nerve and muscle function and aids proper maintenance of the blood's mineral balance; also helps to lower blood pressure
- **Source**: bananas, dried apricots, yoghurt, whole grains, sunflower seeds, potatoes, sweet potatoes and kidney beans
- **RDA**: 2500 mg
- **Deficiency**: decreased blood pressure, dry skin, salt retention and irregular heart beat

Sodium

- **Function**: works in conjunction with potassium to maintain fluid and electrolyte balance within cells
- **Source**: virtually all foods contain sodium, for example celery, cheese, eggs, meat, milk and milk products, processed foods, salt and seafood
- **RDA:** 2500 mg
- **Deficiency**: confusion, low blood sugar, dehydration, lethargy, heart palpitations and heart attack

Trace minerals

Copper

- **Function**: assists in the formation of haemoglobin and helps to maintain healthy bones, blood vessels and nerves
- **Source**: barley, potatoes, whole grains, mushrooms, cocoa, beans, almonds and most seafoods
- **RDA**: 2 mg
- **Deficiency**: fractures and bone deformities, anaemia, general weakness, impaired respiration and skin sores

Iron

- **Function:** required for the production of haemoglobin
- **Source**: liver, lean meats, eggs, baked potatoes, soya beans, kidney beans, whole grains and cereals, and dried fruits
- **RDA**: males 10 mg, females 18 mg
- **Deficiency**: dizziness, iron deficiency anaemia, constipation, sore or inflamed tongue

Selenium

- **Function**: a powerful antioxidant, aids normal body growth and fertility
- **Source**: seafood, offal, bran and wheat germ, broccoli, celery, cucumbers and mushrooms
- **RDA**: 1 mg
- **Deficiency**: heart disease, muscular pain and weakness

Zinc

- **Function**: necessary for healing and development of new cells; an antioxidant, plays an important part in helping to build a strong immune system
- **Source**: beef, lamb, seafood, eggs, yoghurt, yeast extract (for example Marmite), beans, nuts and seeds
- **RDA**: 15 mg
- **Deficiency**: decreased learning ability, delayed sexual maturity, eczema, fatigue, prolonged wound healing, retarded growth and white spots on nails

Water

One of the major chemicals essential to life is water, although it has no nutritional value in terms of energy. Water is used by the body to transport other chemicals. It also plays a major role in maintaining the body at a constant temperature. About 2.5 litres a day are needed to maintain normal functions in adults. This amount depends heavily on environmental conditions and on the amount of energy expenditure. In the heat a greater amount of water is needed, and exercise requires an increased intake of water due to the loss of fluid via sweating.

Only half of the body's water requirement comes in the form of liquid. The other half is supplied from food (especially fruit and vegetables) and metabolic reactions (the breakdown of food results in the formation of carbon dioxide and water).

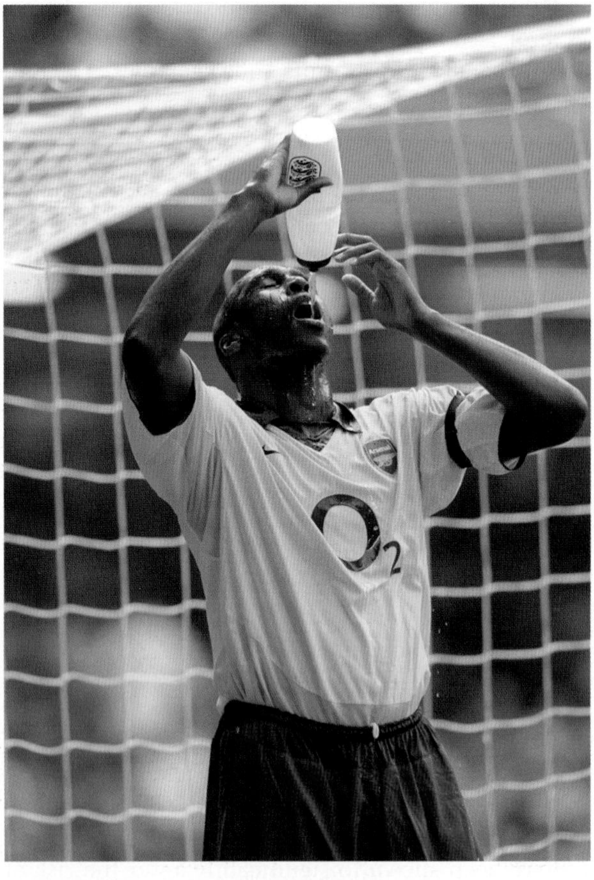

Fig 11.11 Rehydration while performing

Key learning points 4

- Vitamins and minerals play key roles in sustaining life and the health of the body.
- Vitamins B and C are water soluble.
- Vitamins A, D, E and K are fat soluble.

Student activity 11.1 60 minutes P1

Nutrition and nutritional requirements

Good nutrition is important for every person and is even more important for athletes if they want to be able to perform at their optimal level.

Task 1

Design a poster that illustrates a person's normal nutritional requirements. These include:

- carbohydrates
- proteins – including essential and non-essential
- fats – including essential fatty acids
- vitamins
- minerals.

Task 2

Write a leaflet to go with your poster that describes nutrition and the nutritional requirements of people. Include in your leaflet the common terminology used to express how much of each type of macro- and micronutrient we should be consuming, for example RDA, and describe the meaning of each.

11.3 Digestion

P2

The digestive system is where foods are broken down into their individual nutrients, absorbed into the bloodstream and the waste excreted. It works through processes of mechanical and chemical digestion. Mechanical digestion starts before the food enters the mouth as we cook the food and then cut it up or mash it to make it more palatable. In the mouth we chew the food to tear it apart further, then digestive juices continue this process. The chemical digestion of foods occurs through the digestive enzymes which are present in the mouth and the organs the food passes through. Enzymes are defined as biological catalysts that break down the large molecules of the nutrients into smaller molecules which can be absorbed.

The aim of the digestive system is to break down the nutrients into their smallest units (see Table 11.6).

Nutrient	Smallest unit
Carbohydrate	Glucose
Protein	Amino acid
Fats	Fatty acid

Table 11.6 Nutrients and their smallest units

The digestion, absorption and elimination of nutrients take place in the gastrointestinal tract, which is a long tube running from the mouth to the anus. It includes the mouth, oesophagus, stomach, small intestine and large intestine.

Mouth

The technical term for the mouth is the buccal cavity and this is where the food's journey begins. The teeth and jaw produce mechanical digestion through a process of grinding and mashing up the food. The jaw can produce forces of up to 90 kg on the food. Saliva acts to soften and moisten the food, making it easier to swallow and more like the internal environment. Saliva contains the digestive enzyme amylase, which starts the breakdown of carbohydrates. The tongue is also involved in helping to mix the food and then produce the swallowing action.

Oesophagus

When the food has been swallowed it enters the oesophagus, which delivers the food to the stomach through a process of gravity and peristalsis. Amylase continues to break down the carbohydrates.

Stomach

The stomach is situated in the upper left of the abdominal cavity and is behind the lower ribs. The stomach continues the process of chemical digestion, but no absorption of nutrients occurs in the stomach because the pieces are still too large. The only substance absorbed in the stomach is alcohol, which can enter the bloodstream here. The stomach is made up of three layers of smooth muscle which help to mix up the food. The parietal cells that line the inside of the stomach release hydrochloric acid which helps to dissolve the food and kill off the bacteria present. These cells also release another digestive enzyme, pepsinogen, which produces protein breakdown. The stomach takes around one to four hours to empty completely, depending upon the size of the

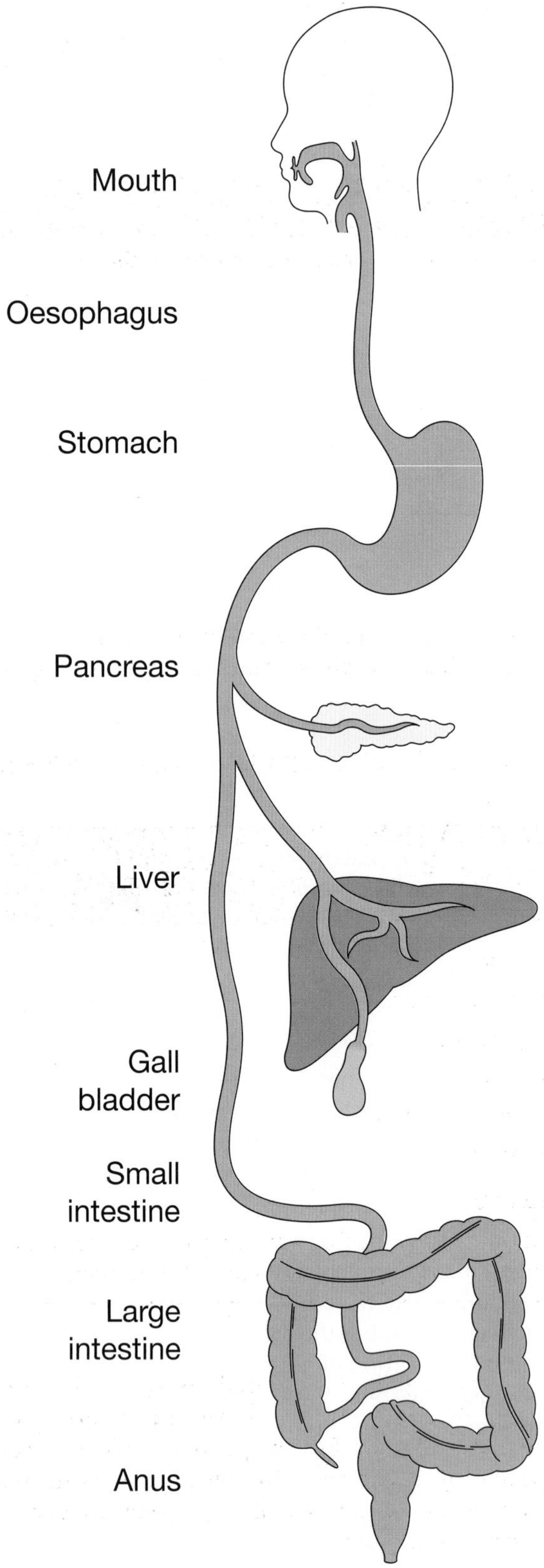

Fig 11.12 Structure of the digestive system

meal. Carbohydrates leave the stomach most quickly, followed by proteins and then fats.

Small intestine

Around 90 per cent of digestion occurs in the upper two-thirds of the small intestine with help from the pancreas, liver and gall bladder. The small intestine is between five and six metres long and consists of three areas:

- the duodenum, the first 25 cm
- the jejunum, the next 2 m
- the ileum, around 3 to 4 m long.

The partly digested foods (called chime) move through the small intestine partly by gravity and mainly through the peristaltic action of the smooth muscle present in the intestine walls. The peristaltic action is also aided by the action of the villi and microvilli, which pushes the food along. These structures line the walls of the intestine and absorption of nutrients occurs between the villi. Any waste is passed into the large intestine.

Pancreas

The pancreas is an important organ in digestion because it secretes around 1.5 litres of a juice that contains three digestive enzymes. These are amylase to digest carbohydrates, lipase to digest fats and trypsin to digest protein.

Liver

The liver is bypassed by the food but it does secrete bile, which helps to emulsify and digest fats. Bile is synthesised in the liver and is stored in the gall bladder, which sits just below the liver.

Large intestine

The large intestine, or colon, performs the following functions:

- storage of waste before elimination
- absorption of any remaining water
- production of vitamins B and K
- breakdown of any toxins that might damage the colon.

The colon contains many millions of bacteria that work to keep the colon healthy through detoxifying the waste and producing vitamins. They are intestinal micro-flora and there are as many of these present in the colon as there are cells in the body. These can be supplemented by yoghurt drinks that promote and increase the number of friendly bacteria.

Anus

The anus is the end of the gastrointestinal tract and is the opening to allow the elimination of waste products of digestion.

Key learning points 5

- The aim of the digestive system is to produce the mechanical and chemical breakdown of the nutrients into their smallest units.
  - Carbohydrates are broken down into glucose.
  - Proteins are broken down into amino acids.
  - Fats are broken down into fatty acids.
- The main structures of the digestive tract are:
  - mouth
  - oesophagus
  - stomach
  - small intestine (duodenum, jejunum, ileum)
  - large intestine
  - anus.
- Other organs are vital in releasing digestive juices to aid in the chemical breakdown of foods.
  - The pancreas releases amylase to digest carbohydrates, lipase to digest fats and trypsin to digest proteins.
  - The liver produces bile to digest fats.

Student activity 11.2 — 30 minutes — P2

Digestion

In order for our body to use the foods that we have eaten, they need to be digested. The digestive system consists of many different parts.

Task 1

By hand, draw a diagram of the digestive system and include in your drawing:

- mouth
- oesophagus
- stomach
- small intestine
- pancreas
- liver
- large intestine
- anus.

Task 2

Write a paragraph that describes the structure and function for each part of the digestive system.

11.4 Energy Intake and Expenditure in Sports Performance

P3 M1

Energy intake and expenditure can be measured in either calories or joules. One calorie is defined as the amount of energy, or heat, needed to raise the temperature of one litre of water by 1°C. A calorie should be referred to as a kilocalorie (kcal). Whereas in Britain we use calories, the international unit for energy is a joule or, more specifically, a kilojoule. To convert a kcalorie into a kjoule you need to use the following calculation: 1 kcal = 4.2 kjoules.

Energy value of food

To discover how much energy foods contain, a scientist in a laboratory would use a bomb calorimeter which is used to burn foods completely and see how much energy is liberated. We know that different nutrients provide different amounts of energy:

1 g of carbohydrate = 4 kcals
1 g of protein = 4 kcals
1 g of fat = 9 kcals

Energy produced by the body

The amount of energy produced by the body can be measured through direct and indirect calorimetry. Direct calorimetry involves having an athlete working in an airtight chamber or human calorimeter. There are coils in the ceiling that contain water circulating at a specific temperature. The athlete has a mouthpiece leading outside the chamber to enable them to breathe. As they work, the circulating water heats up, dependent on the amount of heat and energy the athlete gives off during their activity.

Indirect calorimetry is done by working out how much oxygen an athlete consumes. This works because all reactions in the body that produce energy need oxygen to be present.

Measuring body stores of energy

Our body stores any excess food that we consume as fat. This fat can be stored in and around our body organs and also just underneath the skin (subcutaneous fat). A store of too much body fat is not good for us and can lead to a variety of other health problems, including CHD, diabetes and cancer. In order to help determine whether a person has too much body fat there are different measuring techniques that can be used.

Skinfold analyses

The skinfold assessment test is done using skinfold callipers. It is done using the Durnin and Wormsley sites, as described below. It is carried out as follows:

1. Take the measurements on the left-hand side of the body.
2. Mark up the client accurately.
3. Pinch the skin 1 cm above the marked site.
4. Pull the fat away from the muscle.
5. Place the callipers halfway between the top and bottom of the skinfold.
6. Allow the callipers to settle for one or two seconds.
7. Take the reading and wait 15 seconds before repeating for accuracy.
8. Add up the total of the four measurements.
9. Calculate body fat percentage using the table on the opposite page.

Bioelectrical impedance

The bioelectrical impedance technique involves placing electrodes on one hand and one foot and then passing a very small electrical current through the body. The theory is that muscle will conduct the electricity while fat will resist the path of the electricity. Therefore, the more electricity that comes out of the body, the more muscle a person has; the less electricity that comes out, the more fat a person has.

This technique has benefits over skinfold measurement because it is easier to do and does not mean that the client has to remove or adjust any clothing. However, it has been shown to be not such an accurate measure of body fat percentage.

Hydro densitometry

Hydro densitometry or underwater weighing is a technique that is based on the Archimedes principle. It involves a person being weighed on land and then when fully submerged in water. Muscle and bone are denser than water while fat is less dense. A person with more bone and muscle will weigh more in water, have a higher body density and therefore less fat. Once the weight on land and weight in water are taken, a formula is used to work out percentage body fat.

This technique involves the use of a large pool of water and significant amounts of equipment. It is impractical for use outside a sport science laboratory.

Energy balance

Basal metabolic rate

Basal metabolic rate (BMR) is the minimal caloric requirement needed to sustain life in a resting individual. This is the amount of energy your body would burn if you slept all day or rested in bed for 24 hours. A variety of factors affects your basal metabolic rate. Some speed it up so you burn more kilocalories per day just to stay alive, whereas other factors slow down your metabolic rate so that you need to eat fewer kilocalories just to stay alive.

- Age: as you get older you start to lose more muscle tissue and replace it with fat tissue. The more muscle tissue a person has, the greater their BMR, and vice versa. Hence, as you get older this increased fat mass will have the effect of slowing down your BMR.
- Body size: taller, heavier people have higher BMRs. There is more of them so they require more energy.
- Growth: children and pregnant women have higher BMRs. In both cases the body is growing and needs more energy.

- Body composition: the more muscle tissue, the higher the BMR, and the more fat tissue, the lower the BMR.
- Fever: fevers can raise the BMR. This is because when a person has a fever, their body temperature is increased, which speeds up the rate of metabolic reactions (to help fight off an infection) and results in an increased BMR.
- Stress: stress hormones can raise the BMR.
- Environmental temperature: both heat and cold raise the BMR. When a person is too hot, their body tries to cool down, which requires energy. When a person is too cold they shiver, which again is a process that requires energy.
- Fasting: when a person is fasting, as in dieting, hormones are released which act to lower the BMR.
- Thyroxin: the thyroid hormone thyroxin is a key BMR regulator – the more thyroxin produced, the higher the BMR.

Student activity 11.3 — 30 minutes — P3

Working out your BMR

Task 1

Use the BMR calculations in the box below to estimate your BMR.

BMR Method 1

There is a very basic calculation that takes into account your body weight and gender. This calculation does not take physical activity or age into consideration.

Males: BMR = kg (body weight) × 24 = kcal/day

Females: BMR = kg (body weight) × 23 = kcal/day

BMR Method 2

This method is called the Harris–Benedict equation. It is a more accurate method of assessing a person's BMR because body size (weight and height) and age both affect your BMR.

Males: BMR = 66 + (13.7 × wt in kg) + (5 × ht in cm) − (6.8 × age in yrs)

Females: BMR = 655 + (9.6 × wt in kg) + (1.8 × ht in cm) − (4.7 × age in yrs)

BMR Method 3

This calculation takes into account a person's activity levels. The more active they are, the more calories they will burn on a daily basis.

Males

0–3 yrs (60.9 × wt) – 54

3–10 yrs (22.7 × wt) + 495

10–18 yrs (17.5 × wt) + 651

18–30 yrs (15.3 × wt) + 679

30–50 yrs (11.6 × wt) + 879

over 60 yrs (13.5 × wt) + 487

Females

0–3 yrs (61.0 × wt) − 51

3–10 yrs (22.5 × wt) + 499

10–18 yrs (10.2 × wt) + 746

18–30 yrs (14.7 × wt) + 496

30–60 yrs (8.7 × wt) + 829

over 60 yrs (10.5 × wt) + 596

To include exercise – multiply BMR by the appropriate activity factor:

Level type of activity factor

A	Very light cooking, driving, ironing, painting, sewing, standing	1.3 men, 1.3 women
B	Light walking at 3 mph, electrical trades, sailing, golf, childcare, house-cleaning	1.6 men, 1.3 women
C	Moderate walking 3.5–4.0 mph, weeding, cycling, skiing, tennis, dance	1.7 men, 1.6 women
D	Heavy manual digging, basketball, climbing, football, soccer	2.1 men, 1.9 women
E	Exceptional training for professional athletic competition	2.4 men, 2.2 women

Task 2

Which method do you think gives the most accurate estimate of your BMR and why?

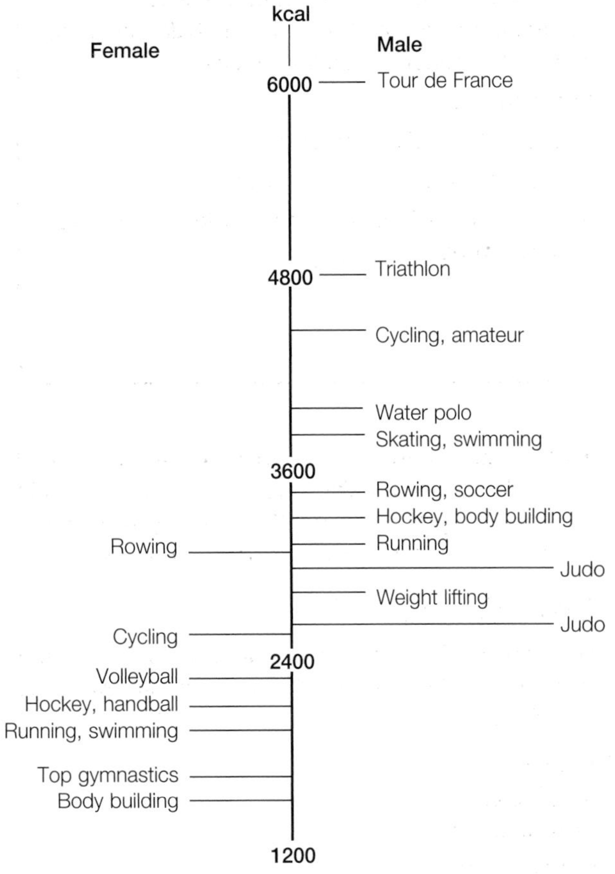

Fig 11.13 Daily energy expenditure (Source: van Erp-Baart *et al.*, 1989)

Figure 11.13 shows how differing athletes expend different amounts of energy. Here you can clearly see that a male cyclist on the Tour de France is expending by far and away more kcals than many other athletes. The reason behind this is that athletes on the Tour de France are exercising at high intensities for prolonged periods of time. Athletes who are body-building are at the bottom of this list as they exercise at very high intensity but for relatively short periods of time.

Key learning points 5

- Fat contains the most amount of energy per g compared with protein and carbohydrate.
- Direct calorimetry involves measuring the heat production of an athlete directly; indirect calorimetry involves working out how much oxygen a person consumes.
- Body fat stores can be measured by skin folds, bioelectric impedance and hydro densitometry.
- Basal metabolic rate can be affected by age, body size, body composition, fever, stress, environment, fasting and thyroxine.

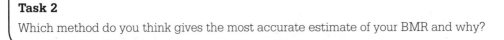

Q Quick quiz 4

Answer the following questions:

1 What is the definition of a calorie?
2 What is the international unit for energy?
3 Which macronutrient contains the most kcalories per gram?
4 Describe the process of direct calorimetry.
5 Name and describe factors that can affect a person's BMR.
6 Name three different methods of measuring a person's body fat.
7 Where is body fat stored?
8 What are the problems associated with having too much body fat?
9 Name five different types of sports where excess body fat does not affect performance.

Student activity 11.4 60–90 mins P3 P4 M1 M2 D1

Energy intake and expenditure

In order to train and compete, most athletes need to make sure they are taking in sufficient amounts of energy, but not too much energy that they store excess as body fat.

Task 1

Prepare a written report that:

- describes and explains energy intake
- describes and explains energy expenditure.

Task 2

Describe and explain the importance of energy balance in relation to an athlete's sporting performance.

Task 3

Analyse the effects of energy balance on an athlete's sporting performance – for this task you may like to consider three different athletes who take part in different sports and how energy balance affects each of their sporting performances.

For example:

- Usain Bolt – 100 m sprinter
- Steve Backley – javelin thrower
- Stefka Kostadinova – female high jump world record holder.

11.5 Hydration and its Effect on Sports Performance

P5

It is possible to survive for six or seven weeks without food because the body stores energy in the form of fat, protein and a small amount of carbohydrate. However, you could survive for only two or three days without drinking water. Every day we lose roughly two litres of water through breathing, sweating and urine production. This is increased if we train or compete as water is sweated out to control the heat produced as a waste product of energy production. Therefore, we need to drink at least two litres of water a day – and more if we train or drink caffeinated or alcoholic drinks. The advice is that we should continually sip water throughout the day or take two or three mouthfuls of water every 15 minutes.

Dehydration

Dehydration is a condition that occurs when fluid loss exceeds fluid intake. The signs and symptoms of dehydration are:

- thirst
- dizziness
- headaches
- dry mouth
- poor concentration
- sticky oral mucus

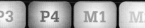

- flushed red skin
- rapid heart rate.

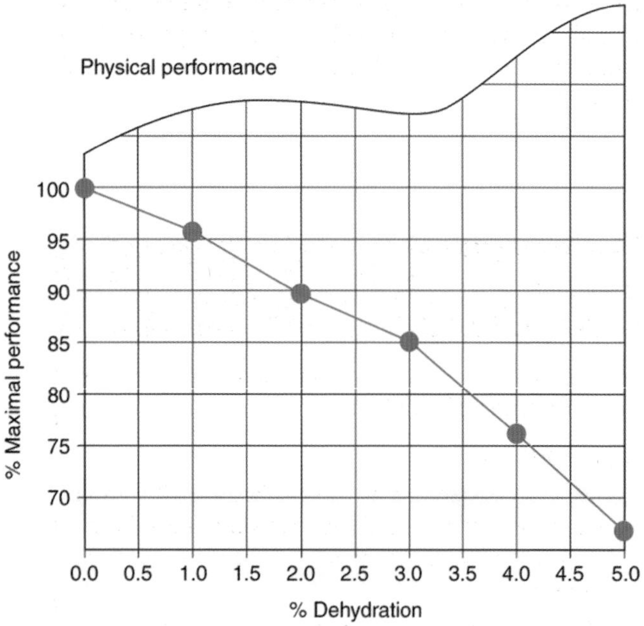

Fig 11.14 Dehydration index

Dehydration causes a significant loss of performance. This is because dehydration, also called hypo hydration, causes a loss of blood plasma affecting blood flow and the ability to sweat. Thus temperature starts to increase steadily. When we sweat it is predominantly blood plasma that is lost and thus cardiac output (the amount of the blood leaving the heart per minute) is reduced. Therefore, dehydration affects the circulation of the blood and the body's ability to control temperature.

Hyper hydration

Hyper hydration is when an athlete drinks extra water before exercising. This is done when they are exercising in a hot environment to prevent the negative effects of dehydration and to minimise the rise in body temperature. The advice is to increase fluid intake over the preceding 24 hours and then drink around 500 ml of water 20 minutes before the event starts. This does not replace the need to continually top up water levels during the competition.

Fluid intake

It is advised that an athlete continually takes on enough fluid to cover the 'cost' of their training or competition. This may involve them consuming around 2.5 to 3 litres of water a day. It should be taken on continually and then some extra taken on 20 minutes before the event. During the event they should top up their water levels when they have a chance. Finally, they should drink water steadily for around one to two hours after their performance, depending upon the demands of the event.

Choices of fluid intake

Water is a good choice, particularly bottled water served at room temperature. Chilled drinks, although refreshing, need to be warmed up in the stomach before they can leave the stomach to be absorbed in the small intestine. This slows down the speed of their absorption.

Sports drinks have a benefit over water in that they provide energy as well as fluid replacement.

Sports drinks are now a common sight at all sports grounds and there are three types of sport drink.

- Isotonic: these drinks have a similar concentration of dissolved solids as blood and as a result are absorbed very quickly. They contain 6 mg of carbohydrate per 100 ml of water and thus provide a good source of fuel as well as being good for hydration. These drinks are useful before, during and after performance, and are the most commonly used.
- Hypotonic: these drinks have a lower concentration of dissolved solids than blood and are absorbed even more quickly than isotonic drinks. With only 2 g of carbohydrate per 100 ml of water they are a relatively poor source of energy. They are used to hydrate after performance.
- Hypertonic: these drinks have a higher concentration of dissolved solids than blood and are absorbed relatively slowly. They contain 10 g of carbohydrate per 100 ml of water and are a very good source of energy but relatively poor for

Student activity 11.5 — 15 minutes — P5

Sports drinks

Task

Name as many different sports drinks as you can. Look through magazines, on the internet or in sports shops to help you. Note down the prices of these drinks and any claimed benefits of consuming them.

hydration. They are mostly used in endurance events of over an hour and a half.

These drinks also contain the correct amounts of the electrolytes, which ensure optimum speed of absorption. On the negative side, they often contain additives such as sweeteners and colourings which have a negative effect on health. They are also relatively expensive when compared with water.

An easy and cheaper alternative is to make your own sports drinks by taking 500 ml of unsweetened fruit juice, 500 ml of water and a pinch of salt to aid absorption. You will have made yourself an isotonic sports drink which is cheaper and without the additives.

Student activity 11.6 — 60 minutes — P5

Designing a sports drink

The aim of this practical is to make a sports drink. You need to decide which athletes you are making the drink for, and when it should be consumed (i.e. if you want to make an isotonic, hypertonic or hypotonic drink).

For this experiment, if you are using equipment taken from the science lab, it must have been thoroughly sterilised. You will need:

- measuring cylinders
- beakers
- weighing scales
- glucose
- sweeteners
- flavourings – your choice
- colourings – your choice
- tasting cups
- drinking water
- salt.

Method

Isotonic drink

- If you are designing an isotonic drink, you need to ensure that the carbohydrate content of your drink is between 6 and 8 per cent. To do this, for every 100 ml of water, you need to add between 6 and 8 g of glucose.
- You can then add other flavourings to your drink to make it taste better. These flavourings should not contain any carbohydrates, so use things that contain sweeteners, such as reduced-sugar squash.

Hypertonic drink

- If you are designing a hypertonic drink, it should contain at least 9 per cent carbohydrates. This means for every 100 ml of water, you need to add at least 9 g of glucose.
- You can then add other flavourings which can contain carbohydrates.

Hypotonic drink

- If you are designing a hypotonic drink, it should contain 5 per cent or fewer carbohydrates. To do this, to every 100 ml of water add 5 g of glucose or less.
- You can then add other flavourings, but these should not contain any carbohydrates, so you could use things that contain sweeteners.

Experiment with different flavours and quantities of flavour. Ensure that, each time, you write out exactly how much of each ingredient you use. When you have made a drink that you think tastes acceptable, place it in a beaker.

Results

Go around the class and sample other people's sports drinks. Do this by pouring their drink from the beaker into your own tasting cup. Ensure that you rinse out your cup after each tasting. Draw up a table for your findings.

Conclusion

In your conclusion answer the following questions:

1. Who was your drink designed for?
2. Did your drink taste acceptable?
3. Would people buy your drink?
4. What could you have done to improve the taste of your drink?
5. Out of the class tasting session, which drinks tasted the best and why?

Key learning points 6

- We need to drink at least 2 litres of water a day to keep hydrated, and 2.5 to 3 litres if we are active. It is best to regularly sip water, taking two or three mouthfuls every 15 minutes.
- There is a range of sports drinks available to provide fuel and rehydration:
  - Isotonic drinks are of the same concentration as blood and provide good fuel and good hydration.
  - Hypotonic drinks are less concentrated than blood and provide good hydration but will be a poor source of fuel.
  - Hypertonic drinks are more concentrated than blood and provide a good source of fuel but will be poor for hydration.

Quick quiz 5

Hypo hydration	2 litres	Dizziness
Hyper hydration	Hypotonic	Isotonic
Hypertonic	2.5–3 litres	Blood plasma

Select a word or words from the table to match the correct statement below:

1 This is how much water we lose per day through breathing, sweating and urine production.
2 This is a symptom of dehydration.
3 This is another name for dehydration.
4 This occurs when a person drinks excessive water.
5 An athlete should aim to drink this quantity of water per day.
6 This type of sports drink has similar concentration of dissolved solids as blood.
7 This type of sports drink has lower levels of dissolved solids than blood.
8 This type of sports drink has higher levels of dissolved solids than blood.
9 Sweat is produced from this.

Student activity 11.7 — 30 minutes — P5

Hydration and its effects on sports performance

As you now know, hydration levels are very important as dehydration can have a significant impact upon an athlete's performance.

Task 1

Design a leaflet that could be given to athletes that describes hydration and its importance in relation to sports performance.

11.6 Planning a Diet for a Selected Sports Activity

P6 P7 M3 M4 D2

A balanced diet consists of the following quantities:

- 50–60 per cent of kcals from carbohydrates
- 10–20 per cent of kcals from proteins
- 30 per cent of kcals from fats
- a plentiful supply of vitamins and minerals from fruit and vegetables
- 2 litres of water.

For an athlete these percentages are slightly different:

- 65–70 per cent of kcals from carbohydrates
- 10–20 per cent of kcals from proteins
- 30 per cent of kcals from fats.

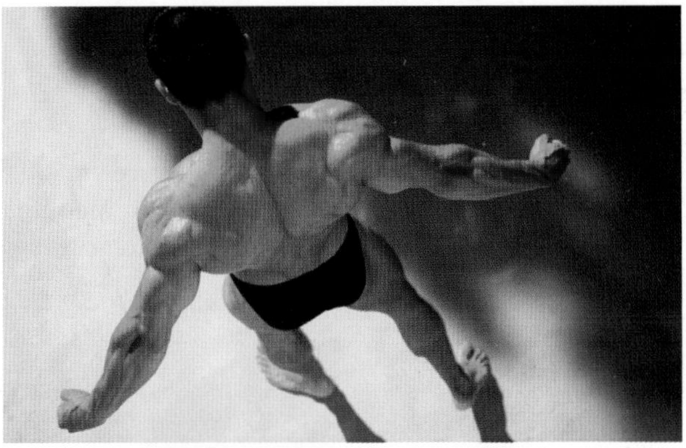

Fig 11.15 A body builder

When choosing foods there are some guidelines that will help you make a good choice:

- eat foods which are naturally occurring rather than processed
- eat foods that look as they occur in nature
- limit processed or take-away foods
- the best foods will not have a label containing ingredients
- avoid additives or E numbers
- eat organic foods where possible as they will contain more vitamins and minerals.

Basically what you eat will become a part of your body or affect the way your body functions, so be very particular about what you choose to eat.

When deciding upon a nutritional strategy for any person, you need to look at the physiological demands placed upon them and the effect these have on their body structures and fuel consumption. You may also have to make a decision about whether to use food alone or to combine food with supplements, protein shakes or multi-vitamins.

Student activity 11.8

60 minutes P6 M3

Components of a balanced diet

A balanced diet that includes carbohydrates, fats, proteins, water, fibre, vitamins and minerals is important for all people, athletes and non-athletes.

Task

Write a report that describes and explains the components of a balanced diet – you will need to include details on:

- carbohydrates
- fats
- proteins
- water
- fibre
- vitamins
- minerals.

Aerobic athletes

The physiological demands on the aerobic athlete are considerable and you will have to consider the following:

- replacing the energy lost during training
- maintaining high energy levels
- repairing any damage done to the body's structures during training
- the need for vitamins and minerals to ensure correct functioning of all the body's systems
- replacement and maintenance of fluid levels.

Anaerobic or power athletes

The physiological demands on the anaerobic athlete differ from the aerobic athlete and they will be:

- repairing the considerable damage occurring to the muscles and other structures of the body during training
- replacing the energy lost during training
- the need for vitamins and minerals to ensure correct functioning of all the body's systems
- replacement and maintenance of fluid levels.

Catabolism and anabolism

Catabolism refers to the breaking down of the structures of the body. Training, especially weight training, is catabolic in nature because it causes damage to the muscles being trained. We know this has occurred because we tend to feel sore and stiff the next day until the body has repaired itself. The process of catabolism releases energy.

Anabolism refers to the building up of the structures of the body. When the body is resting and recovering it will be in an anabolic state. Eating also promotes anabolism. While training is the stimulus to improving our fitness and strength of the body's structures, it is actually when we rest that the body builds up and becomes stronger. The process of anabolism requires energy.

When looking at different athletes' diets we need to give advice on two of the nutrients specifically. They are carbohydrate to replace the energy used and protein to repair the damage that has occurred to the structures. Each performer will still require around 30 per cent of kcals to come from fats, with 10 per cent from saturated fats, 10 per cent from monounsaturated and 10 per cent from polyunsaturated. They will each require at least five to nine portions of fruit and vegetables a day and enough water to replace their fluid loss.

Recommended protein intake

The amount of protein recommended is dependent upon the activity in which the individual is involved. Table 11.7 gives estimated recommended amounts.

Therefore, if you have a sedentary person of 70 kg you would work out their requirements in the following way:

$70 \times 0.8 = 56$ g of protein

Or a body builder at 90 kg:

$90 \times 2.0 = 180$ g of protein

Protein is best utilised if it is taken on in amounts of 30 to 35 g at a time. If any more is taken on it is

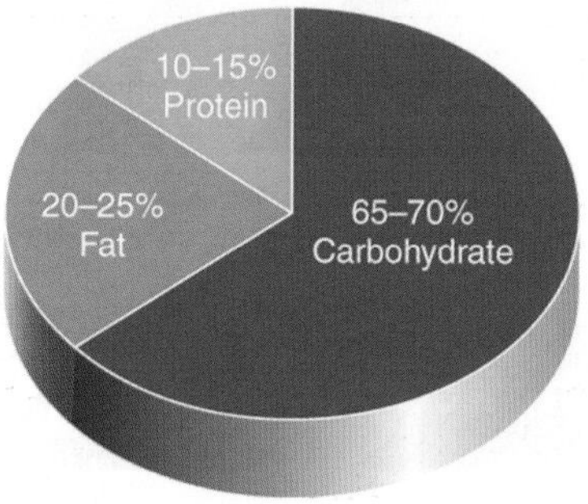

Fig 11.16 Pie chart showing how an athlete's calorie intake should be balanced

Activity	Grams of protein per kg of body weight
Sedentary adult	0.8 g
Recreational exerciser	0.8–1.5 g
Endurance athlete	1.2–1.6 g
Speed/power athlete	1.7–1.8 g
Adult building muscle (hypertrophy)	2 g

Table 11.7 Estimated recommended amounts of protein intake based on activity
(Source: Adapted from Franklin, 2000)

either excreted in the urine or stored as body fat. A chicken breast, tin of tuna or a small steak gives 30 g of protein. The best advice for the body builder would be to consume six portions of 30 g of protein rather than three large protein meals.

Recommended carbohydrate intake

The amount of carbohydrate recommended is based on the activity level of the individual in terms of its length and intensity.

An endurance athlete would need 10 g a day, mainly from complex carbohydrate sources.

The continuum in Figure 11.13 shows an estimated calorie intake and clearly depends upon the size and weight of the individual.

Athlete group	Carbohydrate %	Protein %	Fat %	Kcals per kg of body weight
Triathlete:				
Male	66.2	11.6	21.2	62.0
Female	59.2	11.8	29	57.4
Cyclist:				
Male	54.3	13.5	31.7	46.2
Female	56.5	14.0	29.5	59.1
Swimmer:				
Male	50.3	15.0	34.7	45.5
Female	49.3	14.2	36.5	55.6
Runner:				
Male	48.0	14.0	38.0	42.2
Female	49.0	14.0	36.0	42.9
Basketball:				
Male	49.0	15.0	36.0	32.0
Female	45.3	160	34.7	45.6
Gymnast:				
Male	49.8	15.3	34.9	37.8
Female:	44.0	15.0	39.0	53.3
Dancer:				
Male	50.2	15.4	34.4	34.0
Female	38.4	16.5	45.1	51.7
Rower:				
Male	54.2	13.4	23.7	
Female	55.8	15.3	30.3	
Footballer:				
Male	47	14	39	
Weight lifter:				
Male	40.3	20.0	39.7	46.5
Marathon runner:				
Male	52	15	32	51

Table 11.8 Percentage of macronutrients needed by different types of athletes

Daily intake of carbohydrate, protein and fat

Table 11.8 shows a summary of the studies done into male and female athletes to show the percentage of macronutrients different types of athletes should be consuming in order to maximise their sporting performance.

Protein shakes

Recently there has been a boom in the use of protein shakes as a supplement to training. They are employed by athletes who want to lay down more muscle and need to gain more protein on a daily basis. Protein shakes are usually high in whey protein because it contains high levels of three essential amino acids: leucine, isoleucine and valine. These are important because they are the amino acids that are broken down most during training.

Protein shakes contain plentiful supplies of amino acids and are quick and convenient to use. However, there are several issues to consider:

- The human body has evolved to gain its protein from natural rather than processed sources (meats rather than powders).
- They often contain additives such as sweeteners, sugars and colourings.
- The process of drying the proteins into powder form damages the structure of the amino acids, making them unusable by the body.
- They are often very expensive.

Diet plans

If the amount of energy taken in (via food) equals the amount expended (physical activity and BMR) then a person will remain at the same weight. To lose weight, energy intake must be less than energy expenditure and to gain weight energy intake must exceed expenditure. Therefore, in order to lose weight a person needs to reduce intake (eat less) and increase expenditure (do more physical activity).

To lose one pound in body weight (approximately 0.45 kg) the energy deficit needs to be around 3500 kcals per week. If you expended 250 kcals per day and consumed 250 kcals less you would have a daily deficit of 500 kcal. In seven days you would have a deficit of 3500 kcals and hence you would have lost eleven pounds in body weight.

Weight loss

We have established that in order to lose weight it is necessary to consume fewer calories than your body needs. Athletes may not be overweight, but may need to lose excess weight to compete in a lower weight category. Excess weight in the form of fat usually acts to hinder a person's performance because a heavier body requires more energy for transport. Therefore, athletes may diet to get rid of any unessential fat. The best type of diet to help the person lose weight but still have enough energy to train seems to be a low-fat diet.

Low-fat diets

A low-fat diet recommends low-fat options whenever possible, plus regular consumption of complex carbohydrates like potatoes and brown bread. Low-fat diets are usually quite filling because they involve eating large amounts of complex carbohydrates, which include fibre. Weight loss is steady at about 1.5–2 pounds (0.5–1 kg) per week. Most experts agree that faster weight loss is not sustainable as the weight lost is from the glycogen stores and not from the fat stores of the body.

Here is an example of what you might eat on a low-fat diet.

A typical breakfast:

- glass of freshly squeezed orange
- large bowl of cereal with fat-free milk
- toast with no margarine, and yeast extract (for example Marmite) or jam
- tea/coffee.

A typical lunch:

- large brown bread sandwich with lean meat, and large salad with low-fat dressing
- low-fat yoghurt.

A typical dinner:

- 4 oz lean chicken with potatoes (no butter) and two helpings of vegetables
- chopped fruit topped with low-fat ice cream or low-fat fromage frais.

Typical snacks:

- fruit
- whole-wheat sandwiches
- low-fat yoghurts
- cereal.

Key learning points 7

- A typical athlete's diet should consist of:
  - 65–70 per cent of kcals from carbohydrates
  - 10–20 per cent of kcals from proteins
  - 30 per cent of kcals from fats.
- An aerobic athlete's diet should be designed to provide sufficient energy, repair damage and maintain fluid levels – these are usually high carbohydrate diets.
- An anaerobic athlete's diet should repair muscle damage, replace energy and maintain fluid levels – these are usually high protein diets.
- In order to lose weight a person needs to consume fewer calories than their body needs – this can be achieved through a low-fat diet.

Q Quick quiz 6

Answer the following questions.

1. What percentage of macronutrients should a typical athlete consume?
2. Describe catabolism and how it affects athletes.
3. Describe what anabolism is and how it affects athletes.
4. What is the main function of carbohydrates for athletes?
5. What is the main function of proteins for athletes?
6. Work out your recommended amount of protein per day.
7. Work out your recommended amount of carbohydrates per day.
8. What are the benefits of taking a protein shake?
9. Which athletes may benefit from protein shakes and why?
10. How many kcals are there in a pound of body fat?

Student activity 11.9 — 60–90 mins — P7 M4 D2

Planning a two-week diet plan for a sports performer

Select a sports person of your choice – they could be an aerobic or an anaerobic athlete.

Task 1

(a) Think about what sort of foods your athlete should consume and the percentages of each.

(b) Draw a spider diagram to show the different types of foods your athlete could consume, for example carbohydrates – rice, pasta, baked potato.

Task 2

Produce a two-week plan for your selected athlete of all the meals, snacks and drinks they should eat that meets with their dietary requirements.

Task 3

Write a report that explains and justifies your choice of foods and drinks in your two-week diet plan for your selected sports person.

Useful websites

www.ausport.gov.au/ais

Provides invaluable tips on nutrition for sports participants, including suitable recipes that can be downloaded easily

www.netfit.co.uk/nutrition/nutrition/index.htm

Free useful food facts with the focus on health and fitness.

www.nutrition.org.uk/healthyliving/lifestyle/how-much-physical-activity-do-i-need

Nutrition tips relating to physical activity from the British Nutrition Foundation

References

Burke, L. and Deakin, V. (1994) *Clinical Sports Nutrition*, McGraw-Hill.

Clark, N. (2003) *Sports Nutrition Guidebook*, Human Kinetics.

Eisenman, P., Johnson, S. and Benson, J. (1990) *Coaches' Guide to Nutrition and Weight Control*, Leisure Press.

Franklin, B. (2000) American *College of Sport Medicine's (ACSM) Guidelines for Exercise Testing and Prescription*, 6th edn, Lippincott, Williams and Wilkins.

McArdle, W.D., Katch, F.I. and Katch, V.L. (1999) *Sports and Exercise Nutrition*, Williams & Wilkins.

McArdle, W.D., Katch, F.I. and Katch, V.L. (2001) *Exercise Physiology: Energy, Nutrition and Human Performance*, Williams & Wilkins.

van Erp-Baart, A., Saris, W., Binkhorst, R., Vos, J. and Elvers, J. (1989) nationwide survey on nutritional habits in elite athletes, *International Journal of Sports Medicine*, 10, 53.

12: Current Issues in Sport

12.1 Introduction

The state of current sport and the issues prevalent in sport today can be understood and interpreted only if we examine the society they are played in and how sports have developed. Sport in some way affects the lives of most people in our society, whether it is through playing or watching sport, getting caught up in the excitement of a tournament or supporting the activities of others. Sport in Britain has developed as a result of the development of our society, and the values and features prevalent in sport are also reflected in the values and features of our society. Sport has also been used to address some of the problems in society and to improve the quality of the society in which we live.

By the end of this unit you should:

- know how sport has developed in the UK
- know how media and technology influence modern sport
- know how contemporary issues affect sport
- understand the cultural influences and barriers that affect participation in sports activities.

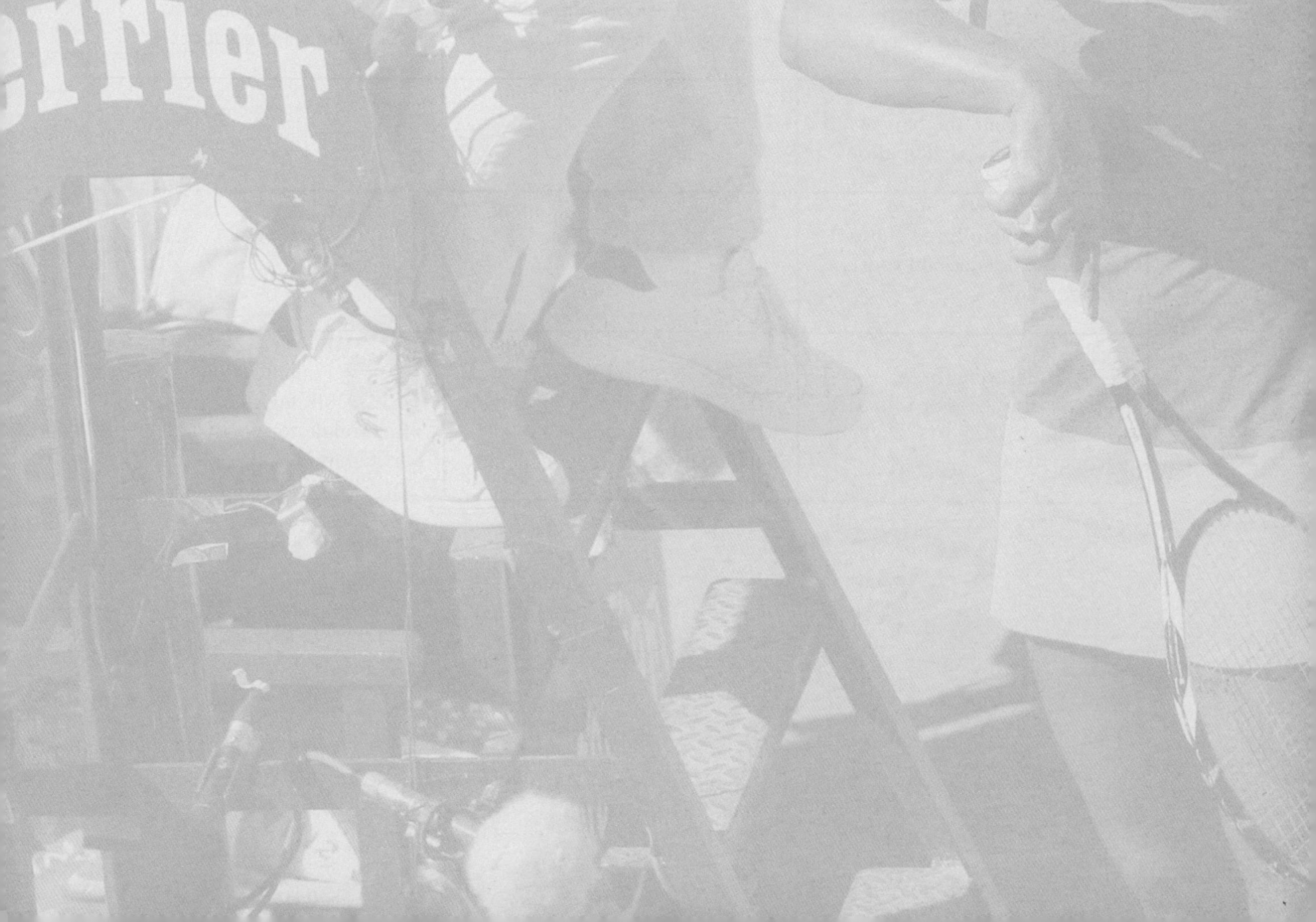

Assessment and grading criteria		
To achieve a PASS grade the evidence must show that the learner is able to:	**To achieve a MERIT grade the evidence must show that, in addition to the pass criteria, the learner is able to:**	**To achieve a DISTINCTION grade the evidence must show that, in addition to the pass and merit criteria, the learner is able to:**
P1 describe the development and organisation of a selected sport in the UK	**M1** explain the development and organisation of a selected sport in the UK	
P2 describe the influence of the media on a selected sport in the UK	**M2** explain the influence of the media on a selected sport in the UK	
P3 describe the effect that technology has on a selected sport	**M3** explain the effect that technology has on a selected sport	
P4 describe the effects of four contemporary issues on a selected sport	**M4** explain the effects of four contemporary issues on a selected sport	**D1** evaluate the effects of four contemporary issues on a selected sport
P5 explain the barriers to sports participation		
P6 explain three cultural influences on sports participation		
P7 describe three strategies or initiatives which relate to sports participation.	**M5** explain three strategies or initiatives which relate to sports participation.	**D2** evaluate three strategies or initiatives which relate to sports participation.

12.2 How Sport has Developed in the UK

P1 M1

Pre-Industrial Sports

There are two distinct periods in Britain: sport before the Industrial Revolution and sport after it. The Industrial Revolution covers a specific period of time from 1780 to 1850. In 1800, only one in five people lived in towns, but by 1851 for the first time over 50 per cent of the population lived in urban environments. By the 1880s, this had risen to 75 per cent of the population.

This was a period of major development in society because the ways people lived and worked were changing. Rather than being a country where people lived predominantly in the countryside and farmed areas of land, Britain became a society of city dwellers who worked for a wage in factories. This had a profound effect on leisure time and the form that sports took. It led to rapid changes in sports, with sports taking on the features we recognise in these activities today. Prior to the Industrial Revolution, Britain was described as being an agricultural society where people lived in the countryside and farmed the land.

The pre-industrial sports that people played were crude forms of sports we would recognise today. For example, folk football was a sport that was played between teams from different villages with the aim being to get the ball, which was an inflated pig's bladder, between the opposition village's church gates. There were no regulations regarding the numbers of players, boundaries of the pitch, time or conduct of the players. The game would go on over the period of a bank holiday weekend and was characterised by violence and unruly behaviour. Pre-industrial sports required large amounts of land and were totally unsuitable for the urban environment that the industrial revolution created.

The Industrial Revolution (1780–1850)

From around the mid-eighteenth century, the English economy underwent a vast transformation. It had been based on agriculture, with particularly busy periods of work for planting and harvesting. Working hours varied and there were long periods of free time available for workers to enjoy leisure activities.

The Industrial Revolution saw the development of factories producing a wide range of consumer goods. Factory owners required their workers to accept longer hours and less free time. Typically, a worker would have a six-day week, working from 7.00 in the morning to 7.00 at night. There may also have been a night shift; this was to maximise the output of factories and reduce the unit costs. Overhead costs were high and could be reduced only if machinery was being worked for as many hours as possible. The second issue was that there was a shortage of people living in the towns and cities where these factories were based, so they had to attract workers from their countryside homes. This was done by offering better wages and the lure of consumer goods to raise standards of living.

The reality was a little different from the promise because these workers traded increased wages for longer working hours and less leisure time. Also, the standards of housing were much worse than in the countryside where they enjoyed plenty of space. The perceived rise in spending and standard of living never occurred because it was more expensive to live in cities. In the cities, families and workers were herded into 'slum' accommodation with little space.

Leisure activities became a problem because violent sports could result in serious injuries, and its associated excessive drinking led to hangovers and absenteeism, and gambling undermined the work ethic. Leisure cost the factory owners money and affected output. Factory owners supported the middle-class efforts to clean up society and impose a new form of morality. Campaigns were mounted against excessive drinking, idleness, sexual promiscuity, gambling, violent sports and the excessive holidays. The aim of the middle classes was to impose a work ethic on the population and make behaviour more polite and respectable.

The agricultural industry also underwent a parallel revolution with the scope and quantity of production increasing. This meant that the population of England became better fed, healthier and had more energy for work.

The economic forces contributed to changes in traditional sports because the employees had to bow to their employers' demands and, moreover, they had little time or energy to play aggressive contact sports. These demands were supplemented by the efforts of religious reformers, who believed violent sports led to moral corruption, and sport on the Sabbath was eventually banned. The Royal Society for the Protection of Animals (RSPCA) put pressure on the authorities to ban sports involving cruelty to animals. The Industrial Revolution led to a growth in the size of towns and cities and a reduction in the amount of space available for recreation. Folk football, which was played across vast swathes of countryside, was completely inappropriate for the urban setting. The result of all these changes was that sports activities slowly disappeared.

Sports, such as fox hunting, for the leisured upper classes and middle classes were still popular and carried on in pre-industrialised forms.

The 1830s and 1840s started to see an upturn in fortune for the workers, because the development of the railways led to an increased mobility. The sports of cricket and horse racing benefited from the easier access to the countryside, allowing the workers to go and watch meetings and matches. The 1840s saw a genuine improvement in real wages (meaning an increased spending power), improving diets and standards of living. There was also money available to spend on entrance fees into sports events.

The 1860s saw the development of nationally agreed rules, known as the codification of sport, and a changing attitude of the middle-class factory owners to their employees' sports activities. Two groups promoted the benefits of sport. First, the industrialists, who saw sport as promoting values which would make their workers more productive, such as teamwork and loyalty. Second, a group called the Muscular Christians took team sports to working-class communities to teach the Bible through sport and promote the value of a healthy mind in a healthy body.

Figures from the time suggest sport was still a minority activity, but spectating was growing, as was professionalism in the sports of football, cricket and horse racing. Social change included the urban population growing from 50.2 per cent in 1851 to 77 per cent in 1900. Working-class wages rose by 70 per cent and a half-day holiday was granted on Saturdays. This meant sport could be played and watched on Saturday afternoons and is the origin of the three o'clock kick-off in football matches.

Rationalisation and Regulation

'Rational recreation' is the term given to the introduction of leisure activities which were seen as being productive and moral. Up until the 1860s and 1870s the workers had relied on their public houses for amusement and entertainment, which were often socially destructive. Rational recreations were brought in by various philanthropic groups, such as the Muscular Christians and other middle-class groups who introduced new alternatives. Thus, societies such as the Mechanics Society, the Boys Brigade and the Young Men's Christian Association developed, and facilities such as libraries, public baths and sports grounds offered more purposeful activities.

This is an example of using sport and leisure as a means of social control, whereby people are persuaded to take part in positive, socially acceptable activities to prevent them from participating in otherwise socially destructive activities such as drinking, gambling and fighting. The middle-class philanthropists wanted to provide better activities for the working class to improve their standard of living, but their ulterior motive was to make sure they were healthier, fitter and more productive workers.

Twentieth-Century Development

Globalisation of Sport

The forms of sport that were established in England in the late nineteenth century quickly spread around the world, particularly through the influence of the British Empire. Officers and soldiers brought the new codified forms of sport to the countries in which they were stationed, and the sports in turn were adopted by the natives. By the end of the nineteenth century, the Olympic movement, under the influence of the French, was finding its feet and starting to involve more and more nations.

The influence of sport by the end of the twentieth century can be seen by the fact that three of the four largest international organisations were sporting organisations:

- The IAAF (International Amateur Athletic Federation) with 184 member countries
- FIFA (Fédération Internationale de Football Association) with 178 members
- The IOC (International Olympic Committee) with 171 members.

The non-sporting organisation was the United Nations, with 180 member countries.

Professionalism

The increasing playing demands of the sports of rugby, football and cricket mean that players have had to devote increasing amounts of time and energy to their sports. By the end of the nineteenth century, these three sports had all embraced professionalism. As the standards of the sports rose, payments had to be made to players to compensate for the wages they would otherwise have earned. Professionalism was initially looked down upon because the upper classes thought that sport should be played purely for the enjoyment derived from the activity. A class distinction arose between the upper-class amateurs and the working-class professionals, which remained until the latter part of the twentieth century. By the end of the twentieth century, professionalism was an accepted part of all sports and necessary to uphold the high standards of play demanded by the sophisticated audiences.

The Development of Sport as a Profitable Industry

As sports have increasingly embraced professionalism, their expenditure has increased. As a result, they have had to increase the amount of money coming into the sport to pay these expenses. Sports and their clubs have increasingly sought sponsorship as a source of income, along with trying to make the sport more attractive and increase the number of spectators coming to matches. As sports have become more popular and widely watched, they have increasingly drawn the attention of the media. This has opened up new sources of revenue to sports and has led to increased profits.

There is also an expanding industry in sport for non-competitive participants, and this has created a variety of opportunities for private companies to invest their money and make profits. It has also resulted in a growing industry with new, exciting employment opportunities.

The Development of Sport in Education

The key element in the expansion of sport in the education system was the 1944 Education Act, which made it policy for local authorities to provide adequate facilities for the teaching of physical education. Sport and physical education became compulsory elements of children's education and are now key features in the National Curriculum. Added to that, there are now many more opportunities to study sport at GCSE, AS and A2 level, National Diploma and degree level.

The Influence of War

The two world wars had a major effect on the development of sport. During World War I, in which the Allies (Britain, France, Russia, Italy and the USA) defeated the central powers (Germany, Austria, Hungary and Turkey), all sports stopped at national and international level as young people were recruited for the war and many were then killed during the fighting. The Olympic Games scheduled for 1916 had to be cancelled.

Between the wars, the upper classes returned to their leisure activities, playing tennis, golf and cricket, and also indulged in overseas holidays and nights of partying. The development of the railways allowed them to visit the seaside in the summer months. The working classes returned to watching football on Saturday afternoons and the first dog-racing meeting was held in 1926 at Belle Vue in Manchester.

During the 1930s, Great Britain experienced a series of financial and economic problems as a result of strikes and industrial unrest. Unemployment rose to three million and the development of Nazism and Fascism led the country to feel insecure, with a negative effect on national morale.

World War II again saw the cessation of sporting activities as all energy went into the war effort and training the young troops for war. The training used by the troops started to appear in schools, forming an integral part of physical education lessons.

The Organisation of Sport in Britain

The government in Britain still plays a key role in influencing the direction sport takes and the opportunities for participation in sport. Rather than directly being involved in sport, the government has developed agencies to influence policy for sport and this is backed up by the provision of funding. In this way, the government can keep sport 'at arm's length' but still maintain some control over it. The current government's major success has been to attract the Olympic Games to London in 2012.

Central Government Control of Sport

Sport in central government is administered through the Department for Culture, Media and Sport (DCMS) under the control of a Secretary of State for Culture, Media and Sport and a Minister for Sport. The DCMS looks after the interests of world-class sports people and also ensures that everyone has an opportunity to take part in sport. The roles of the DCMS in relation to sport are to:

- Widen access to sport for all citizens and offer Sport for All
- Promote the achievement of excellence in national and international competition
- Promote physical education and sport for young people and work with the Department for Children, Schools and Families (DCSF) to promote children's play through education
- Attract major sporting events to Britain, such as the successful bid for the 2012 Olympic Games
- Manage schemes to support the training of athletes, such as TASS (Talented Athletes Scholarship Scheme), which supports athletes in full-time education, and funding of athletes through lottery money.

The DCMS is not the only department representing the interests of people playing sport in Britain. Sport in schools and developing the physical education syllabus is under the control of the DCSF. Sports development departments are under the control of the local authorities within the Department for Communities and Local Government.

- **The CCPR (Central Council for Physical Recreation)**: represents the interests of national governing bodies (NGBs).
- **NGBs (national governing bodies):** all sports clubs are members of the NGB, which runs the leagues, and provides officials and disciplinary measures. For example, the Football Association (FA) is football's NGB.
- **ISFs (International Sports Federations):** in order to be involved in international competition the NGB needs to be affiliated to a relevant ISF.
- **The BOA (British Olympic Association):** selects, funds and manages the team to represent Great Britain and Northern Ireland at the Olympic Games.
- **The IOC (International Olympic Committee):** organises and manages each Olympiad.

Central Council for Physical Recreation

The Central Council for Physical Recreation (CCPR) (www.ccpr.org.uk) was set up against the bleak backdrop of 1930s Britain, which was experiencing economic unrest and high levels of unemployment. The school leaving age was 14 and, with the exception of students in private education, this was when education stopped. There was little opportunity after school to play sport and even in state schools sport was limited.

The CCPR was the first attempt to provide government influence in sport and aimed to promote the benefits of sport. Initially, the CCPR supported the work of the National Fitness Council to provide training for physical education teachers. In 1946, it was offered the use of Bisham Abbey at a low rent to be used as the national Physical Recreation Centre. Lilleshall was acquired in 1947 and Plas y Brenin in 1955; Crystal Palace was built in 1964 and Holme Pierrepoint in 1973. These national sports centres were the central facilities to provide high-quality, residential training facilities and venues for national and international competition.

The CCPR worked to gain the support of the national governing bodies and within six months of its inception 82 NGBs were signed-up members. The CCPR prepared an influential report into sport in Britain, called the Woolfenden Report, which was published in 1960. Among its main recommendations was the formation of a sports council to promote sport in Britain. The Sports Council was formed in 1965 in an advisory capacity and became an executive body in 1972 when it was decided that the CCPR should be taken over by the Sports Council and transfer all its staff and assets. This was not agreed and the CCPR still exists today, representing the members of the NGBs.

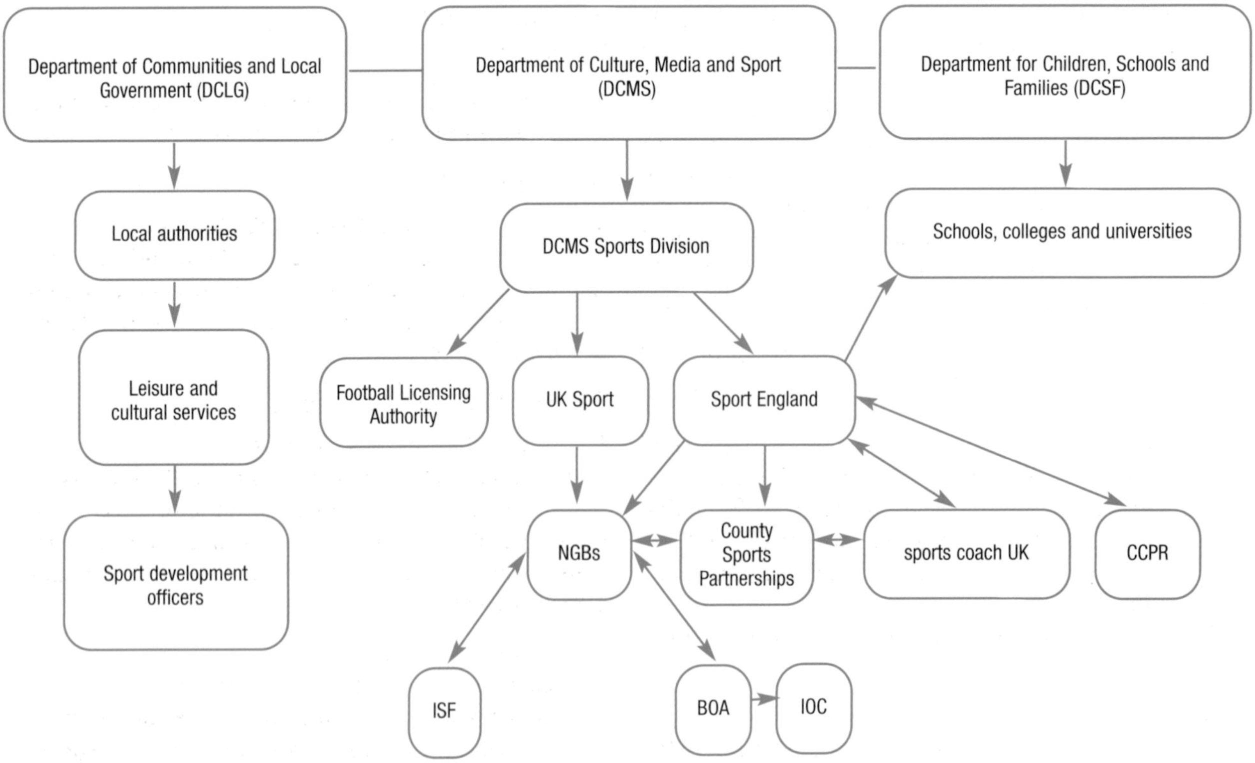

Fig 12.1 Bodies governing sport in England

UK Sport

UK Sport (www.uksport.gov.uk) was established in 1997 through a Royal Charter as the twin roles of the Sports Council were separated. The Sports Council had two remits: first, to promote excellence in sports achievements and, second, to promote participation in sport. These were seen as being radically different and it was decided to let the Sports Council (now Sport England) continue to promote participation in sport but to give the role of developing excellence to a new body with responsibility across the UK.

UK Sport directs the development of sporting excellence within the home countries; it supports athletes to become world-class performers through its World Class Performance Programme. Between 1997 and 2008, UK Sport invested £235 million into supporting athletes in summer Olympic sports. UK Sport's World Class Events Programme supported around 120 events between 1997 and 2009 of World, European or Commonwealth status and has £20 million to invest in events between 2006 and 2012. It used to be responsible for drug control in British sport; however, since December 2009, this responsibility has been taken on by UK Anti-Doping (UKAD).

Sport England

Sport England (www.sportengland.org) was formed from the old Sports Council by Royal Charter in 1997 and is responsible to the Secretary of State for the Department for Culture, Media and Sport. Sport England also operates nine regional offices across England.

It has responsibility for promoting and investing in sport and helping the government to implement its sporting objectives through the distribution of lottery funds. The vision of Sport England is 'to make England an active and successful sporting nation'. The business objectives of Sport England are to allocate its resources to:

- **Grow:** to get one million people taking part in more sport and to get school children taking part in five hours of PE a week
- **Sustain:** to ensure more people are satisfied with their sporting experience and reduce the number of 16–18 year olds dropping out from nine targeted sports (badminton, basketball, football, hockey, gymnastics, netball, rugby league, rugby union and tennis)
- **Excel:** to improve the development of talent in at least 25 sports.

Regional offices

There are nine regional offices, which administer the regional policies of Sport England and deliver local initiatives (see Figure 12.2):

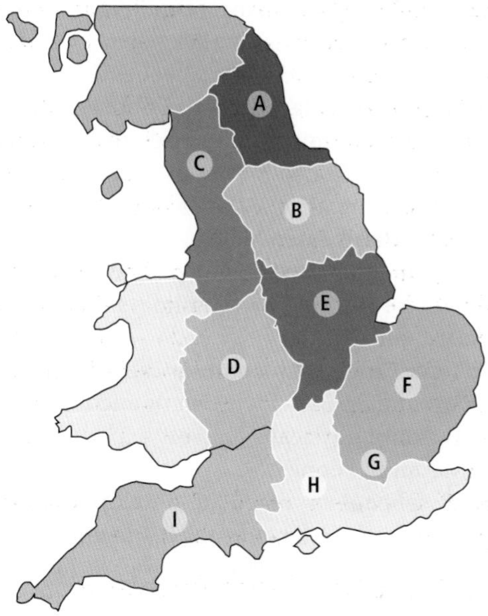

Fig 12.2 Regional offices of Sport England

- North East (A)
- North West (C)
- East Midlands (E)
- London (G)
- Yorkshire (B)
- West Midlands (D)
- East (F)
- South East (H)
- South West (I).

There are also regional offices for the other three countries of the United Kingdom, as outlined below.

Sport Scotland

Sport Scotland (see **Useful Weblinks**) distributes lottery funding to help people in Scotland discover and develop their own sporting experiences, to help increase participation rates and to support the development of excellence.

The Sports Council for Wales

The Sports Council for Wales (www.sports-council-wales.co.uk) has been in action since 1972 and has its head office at the Welsh Institute of Sport in Cardiff. It has several programmes to encourage young people, adults and communities to become more active and achieve excellence:

1. Active Young People
   This includes a variety of schemes:
   (a) Dragon Sport – this involves getting primary schools to sign up for out of school sports activities
   (b) 5 × 60 – this is designed to get secondary

school pupils taking 60 minutes of physical activity five times a week

(c) PE and School Sports Scheme (PESS) □ a scheme managed by the Sports Council of Wales to improve standards of PE lessons in Welsh Schools

(d) Free swimming – this is a scheme funded by the Welsh Assembly Government to offer free swimming sessions to people aged 16 and under during school holidays.

2 Active Adults
Schemes, such as Community Chest, Development Grant and Sportsmatch Cymru encourage adults to be more physically active.

3 Developing People
This scheme is aimed at developing sporting opportunities for disabled people in the community. It is delivered by a network of Development Officers in every local authority in Wales.

4 Delivering Performance
Elite Cymru is a lottery-funded project that provides financial, medical and sport science support to elite and aspiring athletes to allow them to develop their full potential.

Sport Northern Ireland

The aims of Sport Northern Ireland (see **Useful Weblinks**) are to work with partners to:

- Increase and sustain committed participation, especially among young people
- Raise the standards of sporting excellence and promote the good reputation and efficient administration of sport
- Develop the competencies of its staff, who are dedicated to optimising the use of its resources.

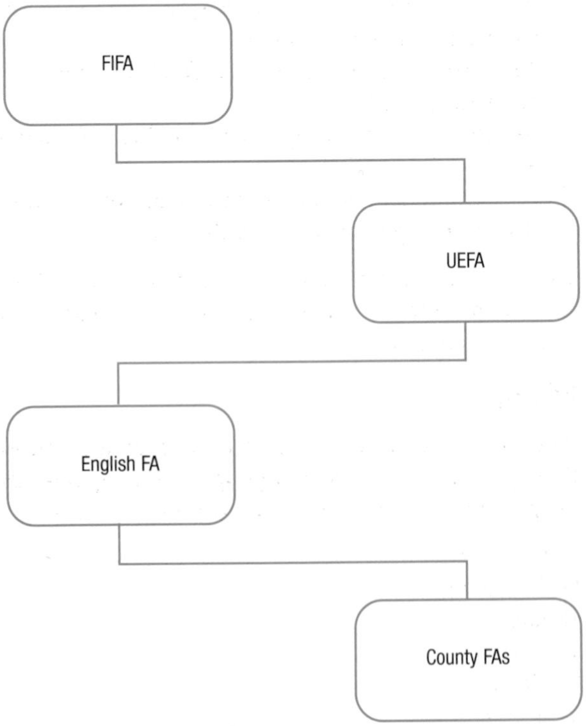

Fig 12.3 The structure of football's governing bodies

National Governing Bodies

To be recognised as a sport there must be a national governing body (NGB) to oversee the activities of the participants involved in that sport. Governing bodies are found at a county, regional, national and international level. If we look at football, for example, we find the structure shown in Figure 12.3.

Football has an international governing body (FIFA), a European governing body (UEFA), a national governing body (English FA) and county governing bodies (e.g. Herts FA), each of which has different responsibilities. You will find similar structures in all sports, although some sports, such as boxing, have more than one body governing the sport. When looking at a governing body, it is useful to look at features such as its membership, funding and policies as this will help to explain what its aims are and what the body is able or not able to do.

The regulation of the sport by a governing body involves setting and implementing the rules for the sport and organising events, such as leagues and tournaments.

- Key Learning Points
- The effects of the Industrial Revolution led to an increase in working hours and a decline in leisure time. Many activities were banned because they became costly in terms of working hours and productivity being lost.
- The workers had a low spending power in reality.
- The urban setting provided an inappropriate environment for playing sports.
- The Department for Culture, Media and Sport is responsible for promoting excellence in sport.
- UK Sport is responsible for promoting excellence in sport.
- National Sports Councils are mainly responsible for increasing participation rates in sport.

Quick quiz 1

Using the following table, match the bodies involved in the administration of sport in Britain and Northern Ireland to a description of what they do.

Administrative body	Description of their responsibilities
Department for Culture, Media and Sport	Manages and organises each Olympic Games
Central Council of Physical Recreation	Selects, funds and manages team to represent GB and NI at the Olympic Games
National Governing Bodies	Represents the interests of NGBs
British Olympic Association	Responsible for administering sport in Central Government
International Olympic Committee	Runs leagues, provides officials and implements disciplinary measures in a sport<TT end>

Student activity 12.1

90 minutes P1 M1

Taking a sport of your choice, research and then describe how the sport has developed and been organised since the mid-nineteenth century. You could look at when the first rules were developed for the sport, when the first competitions took place and how these have developed up to the present day. To achieve M1, you need to explain these developments and show a deeper level of research.

12.3 How the Media and Technology Influence Modern Sport

P2 P3 M2 M3

It is interesting to compare how much we know about different sports and different sports performers. For example, we know a lot about footballers and their private lives; you could probably name the wives/girlfriends of five or six England footballers, even if you don't follow football. But could you name five or six of the current England women's football team? This is despite the England women's team being runners-up at the 2009 European Championships and the England men's failure to reach the finals of the 2008 European Championships. We have world champions as diverse as Beth Tweddle (gymnastics), Amir Khan (boxing), Tom Daley (diving) and Jessica Ennis (athletics), yet we know varying amounts about each of them. This leads to questions such as:

- Why does the media report extensively on football, including off-the-field activities, but very little on gymnastics or trampolining?
- How does this media attention affect the sport and its participants?
- Are there issues of gender equality in media reporting?
- How do the media portray sports performers and why do they portray them in this way?

To answer these questions, we need to look at how sport is presented by the media and who reads and watches sports media.

Media

'The media' refers to the means of communication that reach large numbers of people. The happenings in sport are reported through a variety of media:

- Newspapers
- Television
- Radio
- Internet
- Films
- Books
- Magazines

- Teletext services
- Mobile phones.

Local and National Press

Each area in the UK has its own local newspaper. The local newspaper has a small circulation compared with the national newspaper and its aim is to provide local information only. It will therefore print only local sports stories. It will give reports on the best local teams and will cover national news only if there is a local angle, such as 'Local girl wins national judo championships'. In the same way, national newspapers report world events primarily if there is a UK angle, such as 'England win 2006 Women's World Team Squash Championship'.

It is the editors who make decisions about what news we receive. They decide which news is most important and which news is most relevant. An editor will always have one eye on whether people will be interested in a particular story and if they can relate to it.

Television

Television is the most important aspect of the media in sport. Since the first televised World Cup in football in 1970 to the Sky deal with the Premiership

Channel	Average daily reach		Weekly reach		Average weekly viewing	Share
	Thousands	%	Thousands	%	Hrs/mins per person	%
ALL/ANY TV	32,101	72.9	40,913	92.9	23:37	100.0
BBC 1 (incl. Breakfast News)	20,232	46.0	35,294	80.2	4:33	19.2
BBC 2	10,338	23.5	26,967	61.2	1:31	6.4
TOTAL BBC1/BBC2	22,567	51.3	36,815	83.6	6:04	25.7
ITV (incl. GMTV)	17,131	38.9	32,695	74.3	4:21	18.4
CHANNEL4/S4C	11,037	25.1	28,137	63.9	1:39	7.0
CHANNEL 5	7,502	17.0	22,632	51.4	1:05	4.6
TOTAL/ANY COMMERCIAL TERRESTRIAL TV	22,534	51.2	37,056	84.2	7:05	30.0
Total terrestrial	27,764	63.1	39,195	89.0	13:09	55.7
Sky One	2,757	6.3	9,935	22.6	0:22	1.6
Sky Two	1,239	2.8	5,721	13.0	0.08	0.6
Sky Three	1,391	3.2	6,367	14.5	0.7	0.5
Sky News	1,367	3.1	4,591	10.4	0:07	0.5
Sky Sports 1	2,033	4.6	6,109	13.9	0:34	2.4
Sky Sports 2	1,752	4.0	5,795	13.2	0.18	1.3
Sky Sports 3	598	1.4	2,375	5.4	0:05	0.3
Sky Sports News	1,832	4.2	5,902	13.4	0:09	0.6
Sky Premiership Plus	82	0.2	523	1.2	0.:01	0.1
Sky Sports Extra	264	0.6	1,329	3.0	0:02	0.1
All Sky Sports	4,284	9.7	10,625	24.1	1:08	4.0

Table 12.1 Hours of viewing, share of audience and reach – multi-channel homes: including timeshift (week ending 24 September 2006) (*Source*: Broadcasters' Audience Research Board Ltd, 2006)

to pay £1.7 billion for three years from 2007/8, it has often been about money. TV companies are prepared to pay high prices for the rights to show the best sporting events. The largest events are the FIFA World Cup, the Olympics and the Superbowl. Some 800 million people worldwide watch the Superbowl each year. And the Superbowl viewing figures occupy nine out of the ten most watched sporting events on television in the USA. Only the women's figure skating from the 1994 Winter Olympics can make it into the list, at number 10! With these types of viewing figures, the TV networks are able to hike up their advertising rates and, at their peak in 2000, 30 seconds of airtime during the Superbowl could cost US$2.5 million!

In the UK, 20.4 million viewers tuned in to watch Italy win the 2006 World Cup final. During the match, this figure dropped to as low as 13.6 million. But for the penalty shootout, it rose back to the peak with 17 million watching BBC and 3.4 million watching ITV. In contrast, the Wimbledon men's tennis final, which was shown earlier, had an audience of 7.1 million on the BBC, watching Roger Federer take the title. The average Premiership football game shown on Sky TV in 2006 attracted audiences of 1.25 million. Pay-per-view games in 2006 attracted audiences of 215,000. The average crowd at a Premiership football match in 2006 was 34,000. In 2001, the Office for National Statistics reported that UK children aged between six and sixteen watch three hours of TV per day, compared with two hours elsewhere in Europe.

Table 12.1 shows the viewing figures for one week in September 2006. It shows how terrestrial channels (BBC1 and 2, ITV, Channel 4 and Five) still dominate overall viewing figures, but that channels like Sky Sports 1 have a relatively large share of viewers considering they show only sports programmes.

What is the effect of the media on sport? Table 12.2 lists some of the positive and negative effects.

Sport is presented on television in a 'mediated' form, meaning that television professionals have made decisions about how the sport is presented. It is usually done to make the sports event more attractive to the floating viewer. They know that the devoted sports fans will watch anyway, so they are seeking to attract the attention of viewers who are less committed to the sport, but may enjoy the sense of occasion. As a result, television changes sport to maximise its attractiveness and its number of viewers.

The effects of increasing television coverage of sport are as follows.

- **Money:** increased sums of money come into the sport from television companies who pay for the rights to broadcast the sports. Also, sponsors become more willing to spend more money on sponsoring sport as they know it will receive national attention. Hence, sports' finances receive a boost on two fronts, and this enables them to spend more money on players, players' wages and stadiums. The development of football in the 1990s was based on increased income from television companies and firms offering sponsorship. This extra income enabled the owners of the clubs to spend money on players from overseas, who were superstars of the sport. In turn this makes the sport more attractive to the viewers, who are willing to pay more to watch sport on television and at the grounds. For world events the risks

Positive	Negative
More participation may result from the desire to emulate the superstars	Less participation as people become couch potatoes, watching too much TV
Increased amount of money in the sport which can go to help grassroots	The majority of the money goes to players/clubs – very little goes to grassroots
Allows the players to be full-time professionals and so raises standards	Only certain sports get enough TV money to allow them to be professional
Clubs can provide better facilities/equipment/players	The popular/successful clubs get richer and the poor clubs remain poor
Positive role models can promote good behaviour	Negative role models can promote poor behaviour
Can bring different ethnic groups together – e.g. the multi-ethnic French World Cup squads in 1998 and 2006	Increased media hype may lead to nationalism and 'anti' feelings towards others<TT end>

Table 12.2 Positive and negative effects of the media on sport

can be great as evidenced by some Olympics that did not turn a profit, but the earnings can also be huge. The 2006 World Cup made profits of £741 million, with the cost of staging the event outstripped by sales of tickets, merchandising, sponsorship and media rights.

- **Changes in the rules of the game:** in order to make sports more attractive, the rules can be amended to make the action faster or to penalise negative play. In rugby union, the points for a try have risen from four to five, and bonus points are now given to teams scoring four or more tries or for losing by fewer than five points. One-day cricket has punished bowlers delivering no balls by offering batsmen a free hit on the next delivery from which they cannot be out. In hockey, the offside rule was changed and in netball players no longer have to wait for the umpire's whistle to restart play.
- **Changes in the presentation of the sport:** the introduction of Twenty20 cricket addressed the problem of low attendances by looking at a way to fit cricket into the lives of busy people. In England, a match will typically begin at 5.30pm and be over by 8.30pm, so this caters for people who are at work during the day but are keen to watch a match in the evening. The matches themselves have been organised as part of family entertainment, where the players are introduced by music, and there is additional entertainment such as firework displays, bouncy castles and barbecues on offer. To make the game look more spectacular, the players wear coloured clothing and use a white ball with black stumps. Such has been the popularity of Twenty20 cricket, it has spread quickly to other countries (e.g. Indian Premier League) and there is now a Twenty20 World Cup. It has changed the perception of cricket as being a dull, time-consuming sport and has introduced the sport to different types of spectators who would not attend county cricket. Also, it has brought increased finance into cricket and offered increased incentives to the players.
- **Changes in starting times:** the start times of matches are regularly changed to suit the needs of the television audience. Football games may kick off any time between 11.00am and 10.00pm, depending on where the game is played and when the audience is available. This is great for the television viewers, but comes at a high cost to the spectators at the game, who become much inconvenienced. Televised games on a Sunday are shown at 4.00pm and not 3.00pm after an enforced change one week attracted a much larger audience. The Monday-night games are an attempt to generate the sort of audience loyalty seen in the USA where Monday-night football is watched religiously.
- **Sponsorship:** in the world of corporate sponsorship, how a brand performs off the pitch is just as important as how the players perform on the pitch. FIFA uses Sponsorship Intelligence, a company that researches the impact of events such as the 2006 World Cup. At this event it claims that Coca-Cola 'won the World Cup' in terms of successful promotion. Its research showed that out of the 15 World Cup sponsors, the best remembered was Coca-Cola, something it says might be attributed to that company's support of the World Cup since Mexico 1970.

Other Forms of Media Coverage

Radio is an increasingly popular medium and due to the wealth of radio stations on air, it is possible to devote stations entirely to sports coverage. BBC Radio Five Live is a current affairs and sports station that offers a viable alternative to television through its in-depth coverage.

Books are increasingly becoming an important source of media coverage, and they have the advantage of interpreting events we may not have fully understood at the time. Recently, Wayne Rooney signed a £5 million deal plus royalties to write five books over the next 12 years: a good example of how a player can make money off the field.

Visit any large newsagents and you will see the wide array of **sports magazines** available. The **internet** has also become a rich source of information for people following sports, and there is a vast number of websites dedicated to sport in general and to individual sports. The problem has been that much information has appeared in an unedited, unmediated format and often reflects the views of a minority.

Technology

As coverage of sport has increased and sport has attracted increased investment through television and sponsorship, so the demand for improved performance and exciting outcomes has increased. Technology has been in used in sport for several reasons:

- To improve the equipment and clothing of athletes/teams
- To make the viewing experience more enjoyable
- To help officials reach the correct decisions
- To inform the training programmes of athletes.

We will now examine these individually.

Clothing and Personal Equipment

The application of knowledge gained through biomechanics has led to changes in the design of the following:

- **Golf** the design of the shaft of the club to get the ideal amount of flex that will impart the greatest force on the golf ball (shafts can be graphite or iron)
- **Cricket bats** have to have a wooden face but technology has focused on the treatment of design of bats for maximum power and bat speed
- **Swimsuits** in the 2008 Olympic Games, swimmers started to wear polyurethane swimsuits that work by pushing the water away and helping the swimmers to stay afloat. The result is that there is less resistance on the swimmer from the water.

There have also been changes to the design of football and rugby strips, skis, speedskates, mountain bikes and tennis rackets to help improve performance.

The Viewing Experience

Although we take it for granted now, the viewing experience of watching sport on television has been revolutionised by the use of multiple cameras to give different views of the same events. When there is a controversial moment in cricket, football or rugby, it is often shown from at least four angles. The use of replays and freeze frames has resulted in increased ways to analyse and understand events. Sky Television has introduced computer-animated reconstructions to help their analysts make points to the viewers. These developments have helped to contribute to the enjoyment for the viewer; however, they can also increase pressure on the officials as all of their decisions come under great scrutiny.

Helping Officials Make the Correct Decisions

The use of the third umpire and the referral system in cricket has had a considerable effect on helping the umpires reach the right decision. Technology such as 'Hawk-Eye', 'snicko' and the 'hot spot' have helped umpires to come to the right decision, while the replay camera can be used to judge whether a batsman has been run out. Hawk-Eye technology and its associated referral system have been successfully implemented into tennis to judge the accuracy of the line calls from the umpire. In rugby union, a referee can refer a decision on whether a try has been scored to the video referee before awarding the try. Football is currently resistant to the use of technology in judging on decisions, such as whether the ball has crossed the touchline or to adjudicate on incidents where the referee has not had a full view. Preference is given to the human judgement of the referee and their assistant as it is felt that video replays will slow down the action and undermine the authority of the on-field officials.

Informing the training programmes of athletes

The introduction of science into sport has helped to develop a range of scientific techniques to test and analyse the fitness and skill levels of athletes. The ability to accurately carry out VO_2 max, lactate threshold, anaerobic power tests has enabled coaches to evaluate the effectiveness of their training programmes.

Key learning points 1

- Media refers to the means of communication used for reaching large numbers of people.
- Forms of media include television, newspapers and internet services.
- Television has impacted on sport by increasing the amount of money in sport, changing the presentation of sport and influencing when sports are played.
- Technology has influenced sport by contributing to the design of sports clothing and equipment, and by informing about the effectiveness of an athlete's training techniques. It has also influenced how sport is viewed and how it is officiated.

Q Quick quiz 2

1 List four effects that increased television coverage has on a sport.

2 List four effects technology has had on sport.

Student activity 12.2 90 minutes P2 P3 M2 M3

Task 1

Using examples from televised coverage and newspaper (or online) reports, describe how a sports event is changed for presentation by media professionals and why this is done. To achieve M2, you need to explain and provide more detail about the changes.

Task 2

Choose a sport and describe the effect that technology has had on the sport over the last ten years and what these changes are aiming to achieve. To achieve M3, you need to explain these changes in more detail.

12.4 How Contemporary Issues Affect Sport

P4 M4 D1

Deviance

Deviance is a form of behaviour which is considered to violate society's norms and therefore to be unacceptable. In sport, this manifests itself in a number of ways such as drugs, gamesmanship and violence. A sports person can exhibit positive and negative deviance.

Positive deviance equals over-commitment. For example, over-training or playing on through injury and pain and much of the 'no pain, no gain' philosophy supports this behaviour. In many sports, we applaud the images of athletes covered in blood but carrying on for their country.

Negative deviance equals either a desperate or calculated breaking of the rules or playing outside the spirit of a sport. This is the more recognisable side of deviance (e.g. using banned substances to win a race).

Drugs in Sport

The most notorious drug cheat in history was probably Canadian sprinter Ben Johnson, who tested positive at the 1988 Seoul Olympics for an anabolic steroid called stanozolol. Johnson had been beaten by his nearest rival, Carl Lewis, about a month before in an emphatic manner. When the Olympic 100 m final came around, Johnson led from gun to finish and won easily in a new world record time of 9.79 seconds. Two days later, he tested positive for drugs and was stripped of his medal and world record. It was common knowledge that Johnson had been using illicit drugs for years, but he maintains that the drug he was using was not stanozolol and that he had been set up.

But the problem hasn't gone away. Statistically speaking, Athens 2004 was twice as bad as the previous worst Olympic Games for doping offences. By the time the flame was extinguished in the Olympic Stadium, 24 doping violations had been uncovered. That is double the previous highest number of 12 at Los Angeles in 1984.

More recently we have seen sprinter Justin Gatlin, 100 m world record holder, testing positive for elevated levels of testosterone. And in 2003, Dwain Chambers, the former European 100 m champion became the first athlete in the world to be punished for taking tetrahydrogestrinone (THG), a previously undetectable steroid. Chambers' positive test caused his 4 × 100 m team to be stripped of their European gold in 2002 and silver in the World Championships in 2003. When he had served his ban and was reinstated in the 4 × 100 m team for the European Championships in 2006 and the team won gold again, Darren Campbell, who had lost both previous medals because of Dwain Chambers, refused to take part in the lap of honour. Under British Olympic Association rules, Dwain Chambers can never compete at the Olympics for Team GB as it has imposed its own life ban on anyone who fails a drug test.

The World Anti-Doping Agency

The World Anti-Doping Agency (WADA) (www.wada-ama.org) has the following mission statement:

> *'WADA is the international independent organization created in 1999 to promote, coordinate, and monitor the fight against doping in sport in all its forms. Composed and funded equally by the sports movement and governments of the world, WADA coordinated the development and implementation of the World Anti-Doping Code (Code), the document harmonizing anti-doping policies in all sports and all countries.'*

Gamesmanship

We often talk about sports performers playing fairly, but find it hard to define what playing fairly is. Is a player who appeals for every decision playing fairly or trying to influence the referee? Some definitions may help.

Key terms

Gamesmanship: not playing within the unwritten rules of the game and destroying the ethics, spirit, goodwill, fairness, etc.

Letter of the game: written rules of play.

Spirit of the game: playing fairly and abiding by unwritten rules, and expressing the correct attitudes and ethics of the game.

Sportsmanship: playing within both the written and unwritten rules.

As sport has become increasingly pressured with a 'win at all costs' approach taking over from the old ideals of athleticism (playing fairly as an amateur), so we have seen a rise in gamesmanship. Much sport is professional and the rewards for winning are great. There is pressure from fans, managers and, in world competitions, the nation, all desperate for a win. It is becoming less and less likely to find role models who will not compromise their ethical stance.

Sports Initiatives

Sport has often been used as a power for good. It has been argued that sport is good for society and has a positive influence. For example, those who believe it is functional claim it can increase participation, reduce crime and anti-social behaviour, and improve the nation's health. The government certainly subscribes to this view. It spends millions each year to provide sport and leisure opportunities for all and is particularly interested in deprived areas or those with high incidences of crime. There are a number of anti-crime initiatives the government has introduced which use sport as a vehicle for providing an alternative to committing crime. Sport England (which receives money from government funds) has a representative within the Home Office who has been working closely with the Community Cohesion Unit to show how sport can unite communities, especially in deprived areas.

Social Exclusion

To understand social exclusion it helps to look at occupations and income. Type of employment and income can be considered together as one is dependent on the other. This is addressed further in the next section.

Health Initiatives

Sport England also believes it can make an important contribution to improving health and reducing the estimated £8.2 billion cost of inactivity to the NHS. The 'Everyday Sport' physical activity campaign encourages even the most inactive people to incorporate a little more activity into their daily lives, taking small steps that can make a big difference – from taking the stairs instead of the lift or getting off the bus a stop early, to joining a sports club. Other initiatives include 'Sporting Champions', a scheme that takes sports stars into schools and communities to inspire young people about sport.

Racism

If we look at Britain as a whole, we can see that some sports are more popular in some areas and less popular in others. One of the major factors influencing the sports we play is where we are brought up. For example, rugby league is more prevalent in the north of England and rugby union in the south of England and Wales. Scotland has its own sports, such as skiing, curling and its Highland Games, and Ireland has sports such as hurling and Gaelic football.

Britain has developed into a multi-racial society. Many members of the population are from African-Caribbean or various Asian and European backgrounds. Their parents or grand-parents had been initially drawn to Britain by the need for jobs during the 1950s.

Some ethnic groups choose to retain separate cultural identities within British society, but black sports people participate successfully in most sports in Britain. However, racism does still occur in British sport, although it is not usually the overt racism that black footballers suffered in the 1980s and early 1990s.

Key terms

Race: the physical characteristics of a person.

Ethnicity: the cultural adherence of a person or group, characterised by their customs and habits (religious beliefs, diet, clothing, leisure activities and lifestyle).

Racism describes the oppression of a person or group by another person or group on the grounds of physical differences. Racism in British sport occurs in two ways, through racial stereotyping and stacking.

- **Stereotyping:** historically, racial discrimination has excluded black people from achieving in the workplace, so many black people entered sport

as an arena where they could improve their life chances. Thus, many young black people spent more time improving their sporting ability at the cost of their academic abilities. This produced two stereotypes:
– black people are naturally good at sport
– black people are not intelligent.

- **Stacking:** black people tend to be guided into certain sports and certain positions within teams. They tend to predominate in sports such as track-and-field athletics, football, basketball and boxing. These sports tend to be inexpensive, requiring little specialist equipment, and can be practised relatively cheaply. Within these sports, black people tend to dominate in certain positions or events, usually those requiring physical rather than intellectual or decision-making qualities, such as wingers in rugby rather than positions of centrality.

This stacking comes from a stereotype that black people have a natural, genetic ability to be quick and powerful, but lack high intellectual abilities. This stereotype has in the past been perpetuated by teachers and coaches of sports who, when choosing teams, place black people in a position or an event because they believe all black people are fast and powerful.

More recently, black and Asian players have broken down these stereotypes. In football in the 1980s and 1990s, the majority of black players were forwards. That stereotype no longer exists, with players like Rio Ferdinand and Ashley Cole dominating in their defensive positions. However, an Asian football star is yet to emerge in the England football team.

Racism has been tackled on the football terraces under the Football Offences Act 1991, which makes it illegal to take part in racist chanting. An arrest can be made only if there are one or more people chanting and if the chants are causing distress to the person they are aimed at.

The 'Kick it Out' campaign to combat racism in British football has been fairly successful and it is now less of an issue. However, there are constant allegations of racism against black players in British teams when they are involved in international competitions.

This is a very difficult area of sport to debate. Many arguments can be made on each side. However, it is important to remember that social influences are as strong as other factors. Peer pressure, role models, historical success and society's norms all exert big pressures on young people looking for a sport and an identity. Concepts such as 'white flight' – the avoidance of seemingly black-dominated sports such as sprinting – may occur. In the same way, financial implications may simply be at the root of it all. There is no one answer and looking for a simple 'yes' or 'no' is not the way to answer this question.

Sexism

Before starting a discussion of the relationship between sex and sports participation, it is useful to examine the definitions of the terms we will use.

Key terms

Sex: the biological and therefore genetic differences between males and females.

Gender: the learned social and cultural differences between males and females, in terms of their habits, personality and behaviour.

Sexism: sexism means different things to different people. The following definition gives us a framework to work within:

'Sexism is a practice based on the ideology that men are superior to women. The ideology is expressed through a system of prejudice and discrimination that seeks to control and dominate women. It is systematically embodied in the structures and organisations of that society.' (Hargreaves, 1994)

Here is a comparison of men's and women's sport (General Household Survey figures, 1996):

- 71 per cent of men participate in sport, compared with 57 per cent of women
- 42 per cent of men participate in outdoor sports, compared with 24 per cent of women
- Twice as many men as women watch sport
- There are very few female professionals as compared with men
- There are few women in administrative positions in sport; IOC members for GBR are HRH The Princess Royal, Craig Reedie and Phil Craven
- The history and growth of sport is documented mainly in terms of the development of male sport
- Sport on television and in the written media is dominated by male sports.

Here are some possible reasons why women's participation rates are lower than men's.

- Historically, women in partnerships with men have taken on domestic responsibilities and thus any sport is fitted in between responsibilities of childcare, cooking, working, cleaning, washing, and so on. Sport can be time-consuming and costly, especially if childcare is needed.

- Class inequalities accentuate gender inequalities. Middle-class women have much higher participation rates than working-class women, as they typically have more money and access to private transport. The fitness boom has mostly benefited middle-class women.
- The major biological difference between men and women is that women can bear children and this has psychological and social repercussions. Women are allocated to reproductive, mothering and childcare roles, which limit the time and opportunity they have for sports activities. However, women are waiting longer now before having a family and this has improved their situation. Also, gender equality has meant that childcare and nurturing roles are more commonly shared between partners.
- Every society has a set of beliefs and values that dictate what is acceptable behaviour for women (and men) in all spheres of their lives, and sport is included in these values. Many people consider that some sporting activities can induce masculine traits in women, especially in competitive sports. Strong opinions are held as to what sports are acceptable or unacceptable for girls or women. Even strong peer pressure may prevent women from considering certain sports.

The conventional image of sport is based on chauvinistic values and male identity formation. Sport is the arena for the celebration of masculinity. To be successful at sport, you need to show skill, power, muscularity, competitiveness, aggression, assertiveness and courage. To be successful at sport is to be successful as a man, and to be uninterested or not talented is to be less of a man.

However, more recently body image has changed to accept a fitter, stronger female. Successful sportswomen have broken the old stereotypes and fashion has changed to support the image of a toned body as opposed to a flabby unfit one. Of course, there is also the argument that successful female athletes are a threat to the male-dominated world of sport. The reticence of males towards female sport could be simply viewed as a threat to male hegemony.

It could be argued that to be successful at sport a woman must show masculine traits that contrast with the so-called feminine traits of agility, balance, flexibility, coordination and gentleness. Successful sportswomen not only have to be exceptional athletes, they also have to retain their femininity.

Commercialisation of Sport

Commercialisation refers to the practice of applying business principles to sport. The advantages and disadvantages of commercialisation are outlined in Table 12.3.

Advertising

This is the way a company makes itself known to the public. In sport, this can be through using advertising boards around stadiums, placing an advert in the programme, TV commercials using sport stars, etc. Sponsorship, merchandising and endorsement all act as types of advertising.

Sponsorship

An agreement between a company and a team/governing body/stadium/competition. The company agrees to pay a certain amount to have its logo appear on kit or merchandising.

Advantages	Disadvantages
Sponsorship can help an event that would otherwise not happen without the money provided	The event becomes reliant on the sponsors and would not happen if they pulled out
Endorsements can help boost a performer's wages and sales of a product	The product may be unethical; the performer may not actually wish to use the product; the company may drop a performer who behaves badly or underperforms
Merchandising can help a club provide better facilities and buy better players	The fans could feel like they are being cheated, especially when shirts constantly change and prices are too high
Advertising can be a way for a performer to make extra income or back a worthy cause such as a charity	It can appear the performer has 'sold out' or it may seem like they are not taking their sport seriously enough

Table 12.3 The advantages and disadvantages of commercialisation

Merchandising
The sale of goods that are linked to the club, player or competition. Usually this is replica kits, flags, scarves, stickers, etc.

Endorsement
When a player promotes the use of a product. Companies pay well for a sports star to say their product is worth buying.

Commercialised sports do not work in all societies. They are predominantly found in developed societies where people have enough free time to be involved in watching sport, enough disposable income to spend on sport and the means of private transport to travel to the venues.

Education and Sport in Schools

Sport in schools has often been controversial. When working-class schools first started in the 1870s, children were drilled in military fashion so that they could be prepared for war. More recent controversy in the 1980s saw teacher strikes over pay lead to a withdrawal of teacher support for after-school sports fixtures when their pay demands were not met. When the National Curriculum started in the early 1990s, the suggestion was that all school children should receive two hours of PE per week, but in reality many schools provided less. Alongside this in the 1990s was the scandal of many schools selling off their playing fields for redevelopment.

The government response in the mid-1990s was a report called 'Raising the Game', which promised funding and increased status for schools that could persuade their teachers to provide more after-school activities and raise money for new facilities. The result was Sportsmark status for many schools and new specialist sports colleges with PE teachers taking on new roles such as school sports coordinators. The future for schools PE in the UK will no doubt centre on the 2012 London Olympics. The first response to this has been the proposal for school 'Olympics' to be held across the country each year in the run-up to 2012.

Other issues centre on how we do things in the UK. For example, countries like Australia have talent identification programmes in schools, which test students and assess their suitability for different sports. In this way they have encouraged a number of school children to take up events they would previously not have thought of, such as rowing. In the UK, we have been accused of having a laissez-faire approach to identifying talent. Although some might argue that this allows us to value all equally.

Child Protection

Following a number of high-profile child abuse cases involving sports coaches, new legislation has been put in place. All people working with children must be police-checked for any convictions involving children, and child protection training is now mandatory on most coaching courses.

Key learning points 2

- As sport becomes more important, the prevalence of gamesmanship activities increases.
- Racism in sport can be overt in terms of discrimination against certain racial groups and more covert in terms of stereotyping and stacking.
- Sexism is present in sport as female athletes are not provided with the opportunities on offer to male athletes.
- Commercialisation is the application of business principles to sport and includes advertising and sponsorship.

Q Quick quiz 3

Answer true or false to the following statements.

1 Deviance in sport is a label given to breaking the rules of a sport.

2 Gamesmanship is the deliberate breaking of rules of a sport.

3 Racism in sport occurs when different opportunities are offered to people of different racial groups.

4 Males and females have different rates of participation in sport.

5 Commercialisation always has positive effects on a sport.

Student activity 12.3 90 minutes P4 M4 D1

Choose four contemporary issues in sport and use a poster to present the issues in a visual form for the rest of your group to see. To achieve M4, you need to explain each of these issues on your poster. To achieve D1, in addition to your poster, you will need to write about each issue and evaluate its effect on contemporary sport.

12.5 Cultural Influences and Barriers that Affect Participation

P5 P6 P7 M5 D2

Barriers to Sports Participation

As we will see later in this section, there is a clear relationship between gender, ethnicity, age and socio-economic group and sports participation; these could be perceived as barriers to participation. All these under-represented groups have something in common: they all have special requirements. Sport is predominantly marketed at young, white males and this group is well represented in sport. So arrangements have to be made to ensure that sports activities are accessible to all.

There are also other barriers which may have to be overcome:

- Time
- Resources
- Fitness levels
- Ability
- Lifestyle
- Medical conditions.

Time

Time is a major reason cited by people as a barrier. There are 24 hours in a day and we have to choose how to spend them. The management of time involves allocating time for work requirements, family responsibilities, activities for survival, such as eating and washing, sleep and time for relaxation. People need to find activities which fit in with their weekly schedule and put these times into their diary. They can then make arrangements for work and time to fit these activities in.

Resources

Resources include facilities, equipment and clothing. There is an uneven spread of facilities across the UK. Provision is dependent upon location (city or countryside), natural resources (such as water or mountains), the policy of the local authority on spending for sport and the demand from consumers. Equipment and clothing requirements can seriously deter people from sports – for example, the expense of going skiing or playing golf.

Fitness Levels

It is perceived that people who play sport or take exercise are fit and will look down on those who are not. This perception puts people off because they see their current situation as being miles away from where most people are or want to be. It needs to be explained to these people that there are many activities which can be performed at their own pace and as they get fitter they can increase the intensity they work at. Walking would provide adequate exercise for an unfit person and they can then move on to brisk walking, jogging or even running in their own time.

Ability

Not having the required skills and ability is a concern for some people as they do not want to look foolish or show themselves up. It is important that relevant coaching is provided to enable people to acquire the skills needed and to develop their ability. This is done through local sports development initiatives and government-sponsored schemes.

Lifestyle

Lifestyle issues, such as stress, smoking, alcohol and drug consumption, place barriers in front of people. All these activities will detract from attempts to do sport because smoking, alcohol and drug use all negatively affect health and make a person feel less likely to want to exercise. Stress and stressful situations mean a person is focusing on other issues and cannot contemplate playing a sport or taking exercise. These lifestyle issues need to be dealt with before a person can consider playing sport regularly and being successful.

Medical Conditions

These are a serious consideration for a person playing sport because if a person exercises inappropriately with a medical condition it can make the condition worse; in the case of heart disease it may lead to their death. Having said that, there is virtually no medical condition which does not benefit or improve through regular exercise. Before a person plays sport or exercises they will be screened by a qualified person and then appropriate interventions need to be put in place to ensure the person takes part in the activity safely.

While we can see that sport benefits people and fulfils needs in their lives, it is important to point out that not all people have an equal access to sporting opportunities. These may be issues you take for granted, but in reality these differences exist because of the way our society is organised and how it has developed. A range of factors affect participation in sport, including:

- Gender
- Ethnic origin
- Age
- Socio-economic classification.

Gender

Statistics prepared by Sport England clearly show that women have lower participation rates than men (see Table 12.4).

With the odd exception, we can clearly see that men are more active than women. The figures show that, as a group, 65 per cent of men and 53 per cent of women had participated in at least one sporting activity in the four weeks before the interview. The only discrepancies were in sports such as keep fit and yoga, which traditionally attract more females.

Ethnic Origin

Recent statistics have shown a direct relationship between ethnic origin and participation in sport (see Table 12.5).

Table 12.5 and other research shows that:

- White ethnic groups have the highest participation rates

Sport	Men %	Women %
Walking	34.6	33.7
Swimming	12.3	15.2
Keep fit/yoga	7.1	16.5
Weight training	8.6	3.5
Running	7.1	3.1
Golf	8.3	1.3
Soccer	9.8	0.5
Tennis	2.2	1.6
Badminton	2.2	1.5
Fishing	3.1	0.2

Table 12.4 Percentage of men and women aged 16≤ participating in sport in the four weeks before interview (*Source*: Sport England, 2002)

Ethnic group	Participation excluding walking	Participation including walking
White	44.1	59.4
Any minority ethnic group	34.6	45.5
Indian	30.4	46.3
Pakistani/Bangladeshi	21.7	25.9
Black (Caribbean, African, other)	33.2	43.7
Other (Chinese, none of the above)	45.1	56.5

Table 12.5 Percentage of adults aged 16≤ participating in the four weeks before interview, by ethnic origin (*Source*: Sport England, 2002)

- People of Pakistani origin have the lowest participation rates
- Women of Pakistani origin have particularly low rates of participation
- Certain ethnic groups are well represented in some sports but very poorly represented in others.

Britain is now regarded as a multi-racial society and we must work to meet the needs of all groups. Sports development officers are working hard to offer opportunities to people from all ethnic groups and meet their specific needs – e.g. offering women-only swimming sessions for Muslim women.

Age

Age and also an individual's stage in the life cycle are key factors in influencing the level of participation and also the choice of sports. Younger people tend to choose more physical contact sports such as football and rugby, while older age groups will still be active but in more individual sports with less physical contact (see Table 12.6).

The relationship between participation and age is not always clear-cut, as swimming and keep fit have fairly stable levels of participation across the age groups. Fishing and golf increase slightly with age before falling off again, and soccer and running decline is related to age.

Socio-Economic Classification

Socio-economic classification is a system of classifying people based on their occupation and thus potential income (see Table 12.7).

Strategies and Initiatives

Sport England and local authorities are well aware of the problems faced by people from different cultures and the barriers faced by the general population. Since its inception in 1972, the Sports Council (now Sport England) has run a series of campaigns which started with 'Sport for All' and included 'Ever thought of sport?' and '50≶ and all to play for'. These campaigns were aimed at specific groups with low participation rates, such as women and older people.

Recent strategies have included:

- Game Plan
- Every Child Matters
- Sporting Equals
- Talented Athlete Support Scheme (TASS)
- Plan for Sport 2001
- Active Sports
- Sportsmark.

Game Plan

Game Plan was published in December 2002 to present the government's vision for sport up to 2020 and the strategy to deliver this vision. It includes strategies for developing excellence in performance and promoting mass participation.

Every Child Matters

Every Child Matters is a national policy which is to be achieved through local initiatives. The aim is for school provision to improve the children's attainment and life chances involving the actions of pupils, parents, teachers and governors. Sport and leisure

Sport	16–19	20–24	25–29	30–44	45–59	60–69	70≶
sWalking	40.7	47.1	42.3	50.5	52.0	46.1	26.8
Swimming	46.2	46.3	47.6	48.2	33.3	19.8	8.1
Keep fit/yoga	29.8	33.2	33.3	27.9	19.8	10.7	6.2
Snooker	42.5	41.3	30.3	19.4	10.7	6.2	3.5
Weight training	18.6	19.8	20.4	12.3	5.6	1.4	0.5
Running	19.7	18.1	18.0	13.9	4.6	1.0	0.2
Golf	14.6	17.4	17.1	14.5	10.9	8.1	4.0
Soccer	33.5	26.1	20.2	10.9	2.1	0.3	0.1
Tennis	24.0	14.7	10.1	8.7	4.8	2.1	0.5
Fishing	8.1	5.2	5.2	6.1	6.3	4.9	1.6
At least one activity	90.1	88.3	88.3	85.1	77.2	64.4	39.4

Table 12.6 Percentage of adults aged 16≶ participating in the four weeks before interview, by age (*Source*: Sport England, 2002)

Sport	Large employers/ higher managerial	Higher professional	Lower managerial & professional	Intermediate	Small employers	Lower supervisory & technical	Semi-routine	Routine	Long-term unemployed
Walking	47.1	46.2	41.7	32.7	30.0	29.4	28.5	23.5	19.5
Swimming	24.0	19.9	17.7	13.7	11.9	11.2	8.8	7.8	7.4
Snooker	9.9	9.2	9.6	10.2	9.4	9.1	8.5	7.0	5.5
Keep fit/yoga	20.8	18.3	15.3	14.8	11.1	9.4	7.1	6.3	4.6
Weight training	11.4	8.5	7.3	6.9	5.1	4.0	4.0	2.5	2.0
Running	10.1	8.1	6.6	5.2	3.3	3.4	2.2	2.3	3.2
Golf	9.5	8.4	6.1	4.2	4.8	4.7	3.3	3.8	4.2
Soccer	6.1	5.4	5.5	4.2	4.9	3.6	1.8	1.7	0.0
Tennis	3.1	4.0	2.7	1.8	1.7	0.5	0.8	0.5	1.0
Fishing	1.1	1.1	1.2	1.5	2.5	2.3	1.6	1.5	0.80

Table 12.7 Participation in sport, by socio-economic classification (*Source*: Sport England, 2002)

activities are a part of this scheme by using school facilities to deliver courses.

Sporting Equals

Sporting Equals is a strategy to promote racial equality in sport with the specific aims of developing a society where:

- People from minority ethnic groups can influence and participate equally in sport at all levels, as players, officials, coaches, administrators, volunteers and decision-makers, working with partners to develop awareness and understanding of racial equality issues that impact on sport
- Governors and providers of sport recognise and value a fully integrated and inclusive society
- A sporting environment is established where cultural diversity is recognised and celebrated.

Talented Athlete Support Scheme

The Talented Athlete Support Scheme (TASS) aims to provide funds for talented athletes at schools, colleges and universities to gain access to support for the development of their excellence. Money is provided for equipment, travel costs and sport science support, such as nutritional advice, sport psychology and physiological testing, and medical support such as physiotherapy and sports massage.

Plan for Sport 2001

This document was published in 2001 under the title 'A sporting future for all' and was an action plan setting out the vision and how it will be delivered. The action plan covers initiatives to develop sport in education and the community, and the modernisation of sporting organisations.

Active Sports

Active Sports is delivered on a local county basis and outlines the steps local authorities are taking to develop partnerships to deliver increased opportunities to participate in sport. For example, in Oxfordshire there is a network of partners working together to achieve the following aims:

- To increase participation in sport and active recreation
- To improve the levels of performance in sport
- To widen access to sport and active recreation
- To improve health and well-being.

Sportsmark

Sportsmark was introduced in 2004 as a partnership between the Departments for Education and Skills and for Culture, Media and Sport. It is an accreditation scheme for secondary schools to reward their commitment to developing out-of-hours sport provision as well as a well-designed PE curriculum. There are two levels of award: Sportsmark and Sportsmark Gold, at which a school can achieve a distinction award.

Key learning points 3

- Each individual may have barriers to prevent them from participating in sport.
- Time, facilities and cost are common barriers to participation.
- Gender, ethnic origin, age and socio-economic classification can all influence participation rates.

Q Quick quiz 4

Choosing from the list of words below, fill in the blanks to complete the following paragraph regarding the barriers to sports participation:

- Fitness
- Facilities
- Management
- Ability
- Equipment
- Schedule
- Clothing.

Time or the __________ of time is a major barrier to participation; however, if activities are fitted into their weekly ________ it will increase their chances of being active. Resources include the availability of ________ for sport but the expense of ________ and ________ can have a prohibitive effect. Also a person may not feel they have an appropriate _________ level or the ________ to play a sport or they may have a medical condition that they feel could be made worse.

Student activity 12.4 90 minutes P5 P6 P7 M4 D2

Prepare a presentation to be carried out in front of the rest of the group that covers the following information:

- An explanation of four barriers to sports participation
- An explanation of three cultural influences on sports performance
- A description of three strategies or initiatives to increase sports performance.

To achieve M5 and D2, you will need to explain these initiatives in more detail and then evaluate the success of these strategies in improving sports performance.

References

Broadcasters' Audience Research Board (2006) 'Hours of viewing, share of audience and reach-multi-channel homes: including timeshift (w/e 24/09/06)', www.barb.co.uk (accessed 26 January 2010)

Hargreaves, J. (1994) *Sporting Females – Critical Issues in the History of Women's Sport*, Routledge.

Sport England (2002) 'Participation in Sport, 2002', www.sportengland.org/research (accessed 26 January 2010)

Further reading

Cashmore, E. (2010) *Making Sense of Sport*, Routledge.

Craig, P. and Beedie, P. (2008) *Sport Sociology*, Learning Matters.

Hargreaves, J. (1994) *Sporting Females – Critical Issues in the History of Women's Sport*, Routledge.

Polley, M. (1998) *Moving the Goalposts – A History of Sport and Society Since 1945*, Routledge.

Sport England (2001) *A Review of the Economic Importance of Sport*.

Tomlinson, A. (ed.) (2007) *The Sports Studies Reader*, Routledge.

Useful websites

www.bbc.co.uk/sport

Provides regularly updated reports and articles on sports-related topics

www.sportengland.org/support__advice/equality_and_diversity.aspx

Provides information about how participation in sport is being promoted in Britain by Sport England

13: Leadership in Sport

13.1 Introduction

Leadership has been defined as 'the behavioural process of influencing individuals and groups towards set goals'.

In sport and exercise, leadership has many dimensions, including decision-making processes, motivational techniques, giving feedback, establishing interpersonal relationships and directing a group or team effectively. A leader knows where the group is going (its goals and objectives), and provides the direction and resources to help it get there.

By the end of this unit you should:

- know the qualities, characteristics and roles of effective sports leaders
- know the importance of psychological factors in leading sports activities
- be able to plan a sports activity
- be able to lead a sports activity.

Assessment and grading criteria		
To achieve a PASS grade the evidence must show that the learner is able to:	**To achieve a MERIT grade the evidence must show that, in addition to the pass criteria, the learner is able to:**	**To achieve a DISTINCTION grade the evidence must show that, in addition to the pass and merit criteria, the learner is able to:**
P1 describe four qualities, four characteristics and four roles common to effective sports leaders	**M1** explain four qualities, four characteristics and four roles common to effective sports leaders	**D1** analyse four qualities, four characteristics and four roles common to effective sports leaders
P2 describe four psychological factors that are important in the leading of sports activities	**M2** explain four psychological factors that are important in the leading of sports activities	
P3 produce a risk assessment for a selected sports activity		
P4 produce a plan for leading a selected sports activity		
P5 lead a selected sports activity, with tutor support	**M3** independently lead a selected sports activity	
P6 review the performance of participants, within activity, identifying strengths and areas for improvement		
P7 review own performance in the planning and leading of the sports activity, identifying strengths and areas for improvement.	**M4** review the performance of participants and self, explaining strengths and areas for improvement.	**D2** justify suggestions made relating to development of participants.

13.2 The Qualities, Characteristics and Roles of Effective Sports Leaders

P1 M1 D1

Qualities of Effective Sports Leaders

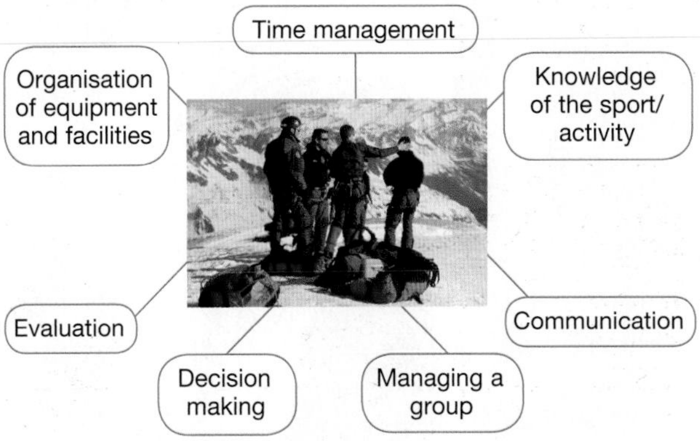

Fig 13.1 Qualities of effective sports leaders

Knowledge of Sports and Rules/Laws

A person leading a sports activity session will need to have a good knowledge of many areas. This process is not an instant one and requires a great deal of practice. First-hand experience and willingness to learn new things will give you a better understanding of delivering sports sessions. A sports leader will need to have a good understanding of the many health and safety factors associated with sports. This should include having a good understanding of emergency procedures and awareness of the facilities being used, as well as having some basic first aid knowledge.

Good fitness levels are linked with good sports performance. Therefore, a sports leader will need to have a good understanding of the different components of fitness and how they can be improved.

A sports leader must also have an in-depth understanding of the sport itself. When delivering a session, it is important to have an understanding of the rules, techniques and tactics required in the sport and how to deliver them. Most sports require the use of different equipment. A leader must first be able to use the equipment properly and safely themselves, and then be able to show others the correct way to use it.

It is also important to have some knowledge of the group of people you are working with. Knowing which people have specific circumstances, such as illness, asthma or prior injuries, is important in case of a potential incident. In sports matches, it is useful to have some knowledge of your opponents so that you can expose their weaknesses.

Knowledge is gained through experience, but can be improved through undertaking a variety of external awards run by national governing bodies.

Communication

This is one of the most important skills for any sports leader to have. The art of good communication is a difficult skill to learn. Communication is successfully sharing information with other people. There are many ways of communicating within a sporting environment, but for communication to be successful you must know that the message sent has been understood.

A sports leader can communicate to a group in many ways, including:

- verbally
- non-verbally
- listening
- demonstrating
- assisting.

Verbal communication

It is important to speak clearly to help the participants understand what it is you are telling them. Try to be concise and avoid any jargon that may confuse them. It is also important to be constructive and positive, as being negative or critical can upset the sports performers and affect motivation.

Non-verbal communication

Sometimes it can be difficult to be heard in a sporting environment, so we may need to use a range of non-verbal communication methods. These can include the use of body language, gestures, hand signals and facial expressions. *Remember, actions speak louder than words!*

Listening

Listening is a vital part of the communication process; however, it is often forgotten. A good sports leader will listen to their group, when appropriate.

Demonstrating

Demonstrating is a method of communication that helps participants learn new skills. It is important when showing people demonstrations that they are kept simple and that they are done correctly, so that the participants do not pick up incorrect techniques.

Assisting

This is the part where the sports leader helps individuals who cannot perform a sports skill correctly. This method will include using a range of the previously mentioned techniques to help them understand what it is they should be doing.

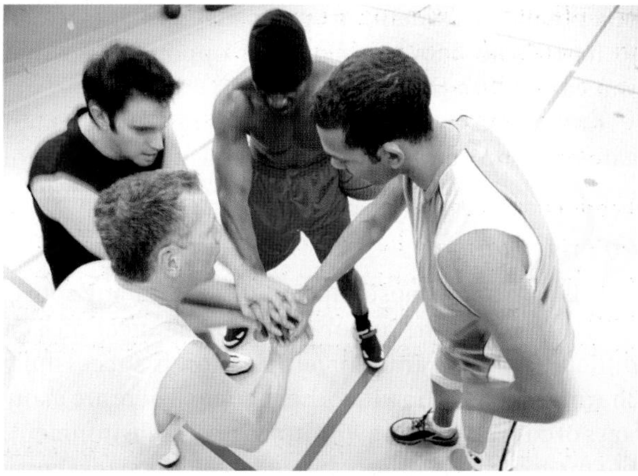

Fig 13.2 A sports leader

Managing a Group

A sports leader may have to work with a large number of people in their group. There can often be conflict within a group of people, and a group leader must ensure that the group is able to work together. Effective management of the group will ensure that you get the best out of them.

Decision-making

A sports leader will have to make many different types of decisions when working with sports performers. What to do, and why, will need to be considered when making decisions. Knowing how to make the right decision will come through relevant experience.

Evaluation

A good sports leader will take time to evaluate their own performance as well as that of their participants. Evaluating your own sessions will help you improve them in the future. Consider what worked well, what could be improved, how you can make your session more enjoyable in the future, what feedback you received from the participants, and so on.

Organisation of Sports Equipment and Facilities

It is important for sports leaders to be organised when arranging their sports sessions. They should consider what facilities are available when planning and organising a session. Once you know what facilities are available, you can start to organise the sports equipment that you will need.

There are many equipment factors that a sports leader will need to consider before their session. These include what equipment is available and whether there is enough equipment for the group. It is important that any equipment that is to be used is in safe working condition, and that it is returned in the same condition in which it was lent out.

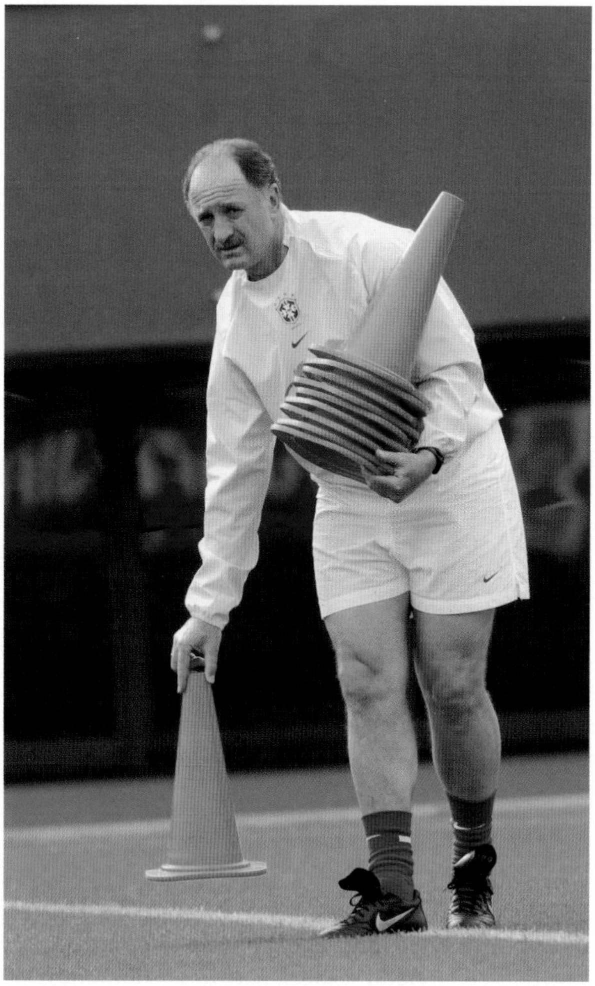

Fig 13.3 A coach setting out equipment

Time Management

Time management is an important skill to develop if you want to be successful. Sports leaders take on many responsibilities, so it is important that they manage their time wisely. Time management is linked to having good organisational skills. It is also important that a sports leader can prioritise items when required.

A sports leader also needs many personal qualities in order to be successful. Such qualities include:

- a good personal appearance
- having ambition
- being positive
- showing empathy
- being motivated
- being confident
- having enthusiasm.

The personal appearance of a sports leader is very important. Sports leaders must remember that they are setting the standard. By dressing in the appropriate attire, you will gain the respect of the group, some of whom may see you as a role model. It is therefore very important to look smart. This can also make you feel more confident when delivering your session. What you wear can also differentiate you from the rest of the group so that you can be spotted easily.

Characteristics of Effective Sports Leaders

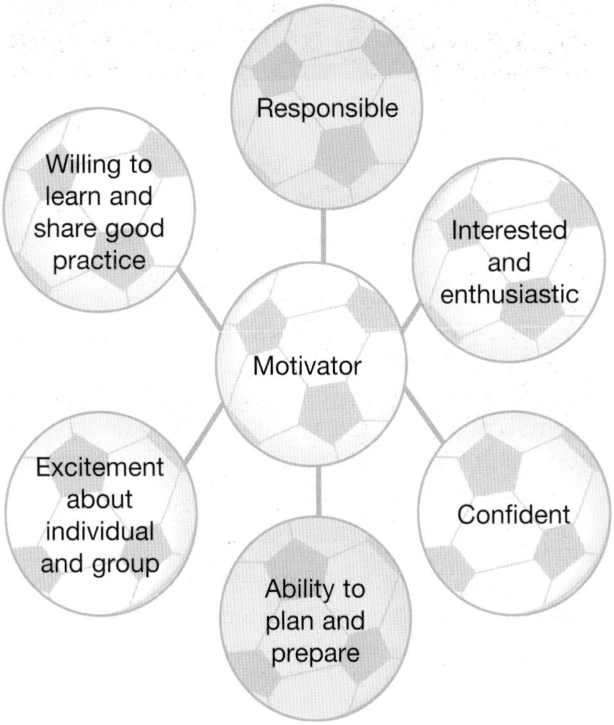

Fig 13.4 Characteristics of effective motivators

Patience

It is very important for leaders to be controlled and responsible in every situation, especially when their patience is tried. People can test the patience of leaders in a variety of ways:

- they may be particularly slow to learn
- they may have annoying or antisocial habits
- they may disrupt the group.

Often leaders encounter problems that are beyond their control. It is essential that leaders develop a strategy for coping with such problems.

Approachable

It is very important that leaders are accessible to a range of different people. People who are in the group that is being led need to feel that they can approach the leader on a range of potential issues, such as:

- difficulty in learning a new technique
- a personal, health-related problem
- conflict between group members
- simply not understanding a task and requiring extra explanation.

Leaders should also consider how they appear to others – not just the group, but others involved in the leadership process, such as parents, teachers, other instructors and possibly authority figures, such as governing bodies of sport or emergency services.

Empowering

Sports leaders must inspire and motivate their groups. In order to motivate others, leaders need to consider what methods they could use to inspire and encourage their participants, such as prizes, fun, targets or general praise.

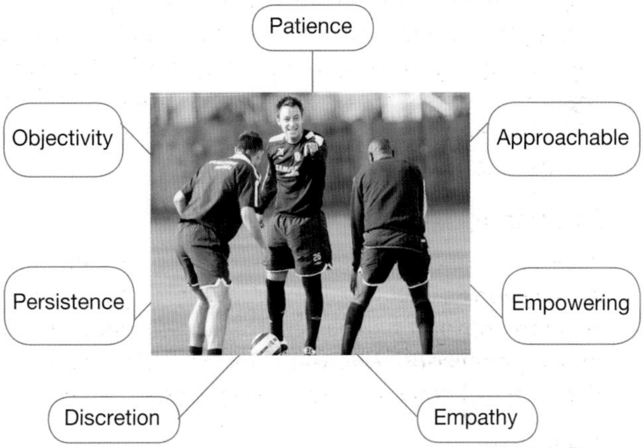

Fig 13.5 Characteristics of effective sports leadership

Empathy

Empathy is the ability to understand the needs of others. Most groups will have people of mixed ability. Some groups will have examples of different cultures, backgrounds and possibly health status.

Leaders must identify the needs of each member of the group and establish effective ways of ensuring that everybody gains from their activity experience.

Some organisations and good leaders gather information before activities in the form of questionnaires or perhaps even an interview.

Discretion

For the purpose of maintaining the rights of an individual, it is absolutely necessary for leaders to develop policies and procedures that are completely confidential. It may be necessary for leaders to gather information about their group, such as personal details, names, addresses and health information.

Many organisations are required by law not to divulge personal information under the Data

Protection Act, which makes it illegal to use personal information inappropriately, whether this is intended or not.

Persistence

In many situations, it is necessary for a leader to be persistent. When participants or groups fail to meet objectives, leaders must re-evaluate the target or intended achievement. In many cases, simply trying a different approach or a variety of approaches can be useful. Consider a group of kayakers who are tired and close to finishing their trip, but in order to do so they must cross a stretch of water that is a busy shipping lane. While all members of the group are capable, some have become tired and are reluctant to cross the stretch of water. In this situation, the leader must find a way of persuading these paddlers to complete what they are capable of, while ensuring that the safety of any member of the group is not compromised.

Objectivity

Being objective is simply about taking a range of factors into account. A leader may be presented with a great deal of information about a range of issues, including:

- the capability of a group
- the weather or environment
- a conflict within the group.

It is very important that the leader carefully considers the facts and takes a 'bigger picture' view of all situations, particularly those concerning safety, when deciding on the most appropriate course of action.

The Roles of Effective Sports Leaders

Effective leaders tend to find new ways of improving existing practices or theories. Some adapt the way in which they practise, others develop specific strategies for differing situations. Other leaders integrate new developments or technologies to improve performance.

Teacher/educator/instructor

The difference between these is hard to discern. Teaching implies a transfer of learning through demonstration, modelling or instruction. Leaders can also teach emotional and social skills. Young performers in particular can be encouraged to increase their social awareness, learn to cope with losing and winning, and develop self-confidence.

Good leaders will be aware that people learn in different ways, and will adapt and use a range of techniques to ensure that learning takes place.

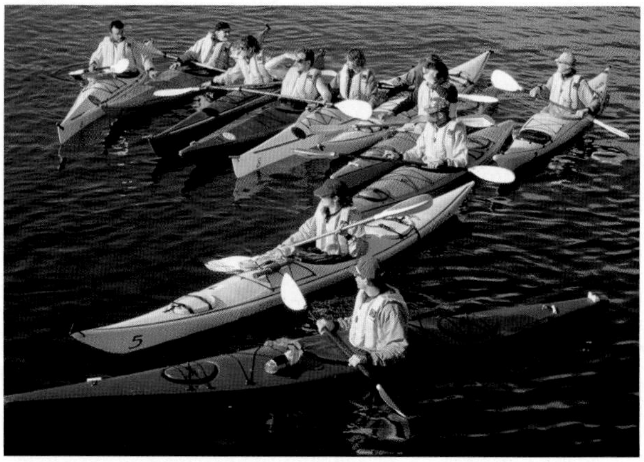

Fig 13.6 Sea kayakers with a leader

Trainer

In some cultures, trainers and leaders are taken to mean the same thing. Since all sport requires some kind of physical exertion, it is important that these physical demands are recognised and that allowance for these demands is incorporated into coaching programmes. A sound knowledge of anatomy, physiology and fitness theory is essential for coaches. In the role of trainer, you might expect to design and implement training programmes for your performers.

Motivator

Motivation can come merely by providing a stable environment in which to learn, creating a positive and safe atmosphere. Performers who constantly find negativity are certain at some point to become despondent and suffer a reduction in self-confidence and improvement.

Evidence suggests that performers who use praise and positive feedback are likely to get more from their performances.

When providing feedback to performers – for example, in the case of skill learning – you could employ the following technique: KISS, KICK, KISS. When communicating with performers, the emphasis with this technique is to start your feedback with a positive comment; there is nearly always something that is positive in any performance. Second, a corrective comment can be presented in as positive a manner as possible. Finally, leave the interaction with a positive comment and possibly an action plan.

For example, consider a tennis player struggling to make a particular shot:

KISS: 'Good positioning prior to the shot and you watched the ball well.'
KICK: 'You should consider how you back-lift the racket; you could prepare your grip earlier.'
KISS: 'If you practise these changes you will almost certainly improve.'

Role Model

In almost every coaching situation, players will look mostly, if not entirely, to the leader as their source of inspiration and knowledge, never more so than when working with children. Children often imitate the behaviour and manner of their coach. For this reason, it is vital that leadership is safe and responsible and that behaviour is considered good practice.

The leader can influence player development in a number of ways.

1 **Social** – sport offers a code of acceptable social behaviour, teamwork, citizenship, cooperation and fair play.
2 **Personal** – players can be encouraged to learn life skills, promote their own self-esteem, manage personal matters like careers or socialising, and develop a value system that includes good manners, politeness and self-discipline.
3 **Psychological** – coaches can create environments that help performers control emotions and develop their own identities, confidence, mental toughness, visualisation and a positive outlook on life.
4 **Health** – taking care to design coaching or training sessions to include sufficient physical exercise, so that good health and healthy habits can be established and maintained.

Leadership Styles

Leaders will vary in the styles and methods that they use with their groups. This includes the way in which they deliver their outcomes and take responsibility for their groups.

The following leadership styles are commonly used in sports leadership:

- The **autocratic** style, which is sometimes known as the command style, is where the person leading the group makes all the decisions and imposes them on the group, who respond by doing what they are told. The leader concentrates more on the outcome than on the group. It is a method that is often used when dealing with large groups or in circumstances where there may be potential hazards.
- The **democratic** method is different to the autocratic style as the leader involves the group and asks for their opinions when making the decisions. This enables the group to take more responsibility for their actions. The leader, however, will have the final say.
- A **liberal** leader will look to use a combination of both autocratic and democratic methods.
- The **laissez-faire** method of leadership allows the group to make all the decisions required. This allows the group much freedom to do what they like. For this method to work, the group needs to be highly motivated, as the leader does not provide any direction.

Key learning points 1

- Communication can be in the following forms:
  - verbal
  - non-verbal
  - listening
  - demonstrating
  - assisting.
- Leaders should have the following qualities:
  - a good personal appearance
  - having ambition
  - being positive
  - showing empathy
  - being motivated
  - being confident
  - having enthusiasm.
- There are several styles of leadership that can be employed in different situations and with different groups. The following leadership styles are commonly used in sports leadership:
  - the autocratic style
  - the democratic style
  - a liberal style
  - the laissez-faire style.

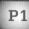

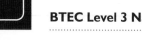

Student activity 13.1 — 60–90 mins — P1 M1 D1

Task 1

Draw a spider diagram that shows the:

- qualities
- characteristics
- roles

that are common to effective sports leaders.

Task 2

Select four qualities, characteristics and roles from your spider diagram and write a report that describes, explain and analyses each one and how they can be used to be an effective sports leader.

Quick quiz 1

1 Give examples of the types of groups that you could lead in the following styles:
   (a) autocratic style
   (b) democratic style
   (c) liberal style
   (d) laissez-faire style.

2 Describe how a leader can influence a player's development.

3 Describe the kiss, kick, kiss technique and when it may be used.

4 Name and give examples of the different methods of communication that a sports leader can use.

13.3 The Importance of Psychological Factors in Leading Sports Activities

P2 M2

Team Dynamics

A group is two or more people interacting with one another so that each person influences and is influenced by the others. Groups have a collective identity and a sense of shared purpose, involving mutual awareness and potential interaction with structured patterns of communication. Here are some examples:

- The crowd at a football match
- A soccer team
- Parents watching their children swim.

Successful groups have a strong collective identity, and members have an opportunity to socialise and share goals and ambitions, as well as ownership of ideas. They also have members who are able to communicate effectively (on the same wavelength), have strong cohesion (see below), value relationships within the group and have a successful leader who ensures that members' contributions to the group are valued.

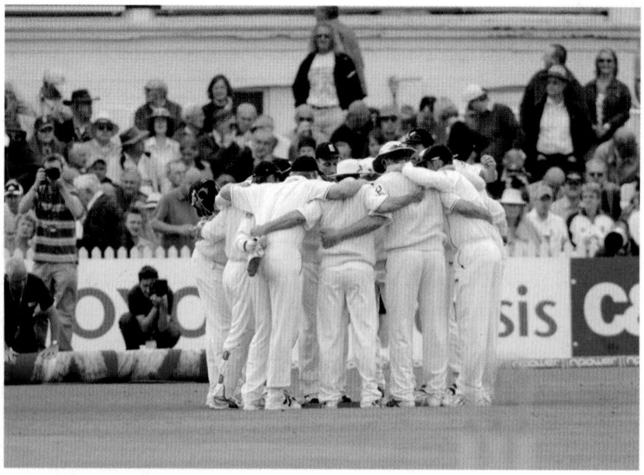

Fig 13.7 The England Cricket Team in a huddle

Team Cohesion

Players and coaches of teams often attribute team success or failure to how well the team works together as a cohesive unit.

Cohesion can be defined as the total field of forces that acts on members to remain in a group. There are two major forces acting on members to remain in a group:

- The first class of forces, attractiveness of a group, refers to the individual's desire for interpersonal interactions with other group members and a desire to be involved in group activities.
- The second class of forces, control, refers to the benefits that a member can derive by being associated with a group.

Several other definitions have also been proposed, all with the common idea that cohesion consists of two basic dimensions: task cohesion and social cohesion.

- **Task cohesion** reflects the degree to which members work together to achieve common goals.
- **Social cohesion** reflects the degree to which members in a team like each other and enjoy each other's company, and is often equated with interpersonal attraction. For example, in an exercise class, a common goal would be to improve fitness, and it has been shown through research that such classes thrive and continue if the social cohesion of the group increases.

Carron (1982) redefined cohesion to include the task and social components, suggesting that cohesion is 'a dynamic process which is reflected in the tendency for a group to stick together and remain united in the pursuit of its goals and objectives'.

The following factors contribute to cohesiveness, which Carron describes as a dynamic rather than a static characteristic:

- Environmental factors
- Personal factors
- Team factors
- Leadership factors.

How can a leader influence group cohesion effectively?
Explain individual roles in a team success
Develop pride within any sub-units that might exist
Set challenging team goals
Encourage team identity
Avoid the formation of social cliques
Avoid excessive turnover of players
Conduct periodic team meetings to resolve conflicts
Know something personal about each member of the group
Stay in touch with the team's attitudes & feelings

Table 13.1 The leader's role in group cohesion

Improving Team Cohesion

One of the key roles of a leader is to keep teams together and to ensure that teams or groups work effectively together. Improving and maintaining cohesion is achieved in a variety of ways, some of which are illustrated in Table 12.1.

Group Formation

A group of sports performers does not necessarily become a team. Realistically, teams evolve, usually through four stages (Tuckman, 1965):

1. **Forming** is a stage where the team members familiarise themselves with other members of the team. They try to determine if they belong in the group and, if so, in what role. Having found their place, the individual forms and tests interpersonal relationships with other members, including leaders. It is at this stage that a sense of team identity is important.
2. **Storming** is characterised by rebellion against the leader, resistance to control by the group and interpersonal conflict, which can even extend to fights as individual members vie for a spot on the team. Most of the in-fighting, however, is social and interpersonal in nature.
3. **Norming** is the stage where hostility is replaced with solidarity and cooperation. The athletes work together for common goals. This is the stage where group cohesion occurs. This usually improves an individual's sense of satisfaction, and sets the foundations for future success. Team roles stabilise and respect develops for the unique role of teammates. Instead of competing for status, members strive for economy of effort and task effectiveness.
4. **Performing** is the final stage where team members rally together to channel their energies towards team success. Structural issues and interpersonal relationships are stabilised. Roles are well defined and the players work with each other towards the primary goal – team success. The coach's job is to maintain this status by providing feedback about individuals' special contributions to the team performance, making sure that nobody is omitted.

Social Loafing

Individual abilities do not make up a group or team performance, and there can be losses in group performance due to faulty processes. Ringelmann (1913, in Carron, 1982) observed that groups of two, three and eight people pulling on a rope did not pull as much as their individual efforts suggested they should.

Later investigations concluded that the faulty processes involved are not due to a decrease in coordination, but rather a loss of motivation.

This **Ringelmann effect** has become known as '**social loafing**' – defined as the reduction of individual effort when working as part of a team or group.

Personality

Personality is how we present our self to the outside world. Each person is unique in this respect and while we compare ourselves to others we are not really like anyone else. However, although we are all different, we can still place people into certain categories which will give us an indication of how they may react in certain situations.

One method of categorising people is to decide if they are an introvert or extrovert. An introvert is a person who is shy, quiet and inward-looking. They are not so good in social situations and like to spend time on their own. Many long-distance runners have been found to have such a personality; this makes sense as they spend a lot of time training on their own. An extrovert is someone who is outgoing, likes talking and mixing with people, and is good in social situations; they do not like to spend too much time on their own and are easily bored. People who take part in team sports are more likely to have an extrovert personality, as such sports usually provide action and excitement.

Motivation

Key term

Motivation: the stimulus for a sportsperson to continue training and competing in their chosen sport.

There are two main types of motivation: intrinsic and extrinsic.

Intrinsic Motivation

Behaviour that is intrinsically motivated has the following features:

- Behaviour is chosen for the pleasure of participating
- Behaviour provides its own satisfaction
- There is no reward outside participating in the activity.

Extrinsic Motivation

Behaviour that is extrinsically motivated has the following features:

- Behaviour where the goal of participation is outside the activity
- Behaviour in the activity is a means to an end rather than for the pleasure of being involved – this can be in the form of rewards, such as a trophy, money or praise
- Success is needed to ensure maximum results.

Stress, Arousal and Anxiety

Arousal and anxiety are terms related to stress. Arousal is seen as being a positive aspect of stress and shows how motivated we are by a situation. The more aroused we are, the more interested and excited we are by a situation. Anxiety can be seen as a negative aspect of stress, and it may accompany high levels of arousal. It is not pleasant to be anxious, and anxiety is characterised by feelings of nervousness and worry. Again, the stress and anxiety responses are unique to each individual. Arousal levels will have an influence on performance; in some cases, as arousal levels increase, performance will also increase (drive theory) – this can be seen mainly in strength-related sports such as weightlifting. However, sports such as snooker or archery that require a lot of concentration and precision can be negatively affected by high levels of arousal.

The inverted U hypothesis suggests that arousal does improve performance, but only up to a point, and once arousal goes beyond this point performance starts to decline. The main point of the theory is that there is an optimum level of arousal before performance starts to diminish, and it is important for leaders to identify this at the right time.

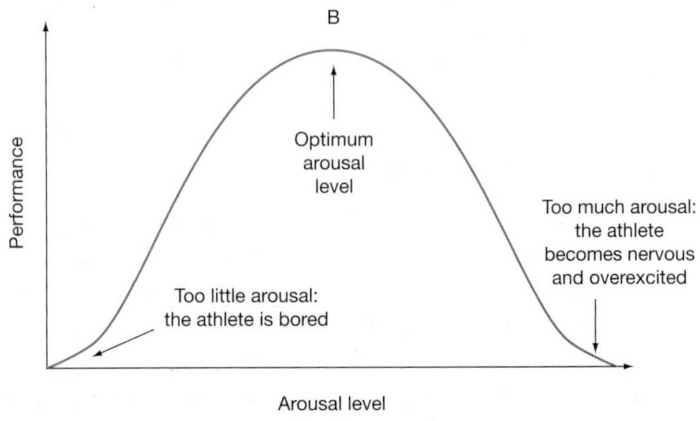

Fig 13.8 The inverted U theory of arousal

Key learning points 2

- A group is two or more people interacting with one another so that each person influences and is influenced by the others.
- Cohesion is 'a dynamic process which is reflected in the tendency for a group to stick together and remain united in the pursuit of its goals and objectives' (Carron, 1987).
- Social loafing is defined as the reduction of individual effort when working as part of a team or group.
- Motivation is the stimulus for a sportsperson to continue training and competing in their chosen sport.

Student activity 13.2 45–60 mins P2 M2

Task 1

Draw a spider diagram that illustrates psychological factors that are important in the leading of sports activities.

Task 2

Select four psychological factors from your spider diagram and then write a report that describes and explains why each one is important in the leading of sports activities.

Q Quick quiz 2

1 Describe team cohesion.
2 Describe the four stages of team evolvement.
3 Describe yourself or a well-known sportsperson and how you/they are intrinsically motivated.
4 Describe yourself or a well-known sportsperson and how you/they are extrinsically motivated.
5 Explain how arousal can affect sports performance in:
   (a) a good way
   (b) a bad way.

13.4. Planning Sports Activities

P3 P4

Risk Assessment

A risk assessment is a technique for preventing any potential accidents, injury or ill health by helping people to consider what could go wrong, either in the workplace or on the sports field. A risk assessment looks at the possible hazards that may occur, the likelihood of them happening and how the hazards could be prevented.

In sporting activities and outdoor pursuits, risk assessments are important and need to be undertaken by a range of people. For example, the manager of a sports centre, a basketball coach and a mountain walker would all need to ensure that they had undertaken a risk assessment prior to starting their activity.

Risk assessments should be logged, kept and reviewed regularly to see if they are up to date, and to ensure that none of the details have changed. Britain's Health and Safety Commission (HSC) and the Health and Safety Executive (HSE) are responsible for health and safety regulation in the workplaces of Britain. All major organisations in sport will have a health and safety policy.

Undertaking a Risk Assessment

We have established that a risk assessment is about identifying hazards and assessing the risks associated with them, but how do we undertake a risk assessment? This is something we do informally in everyday life. For example, a racing car driver, wishing

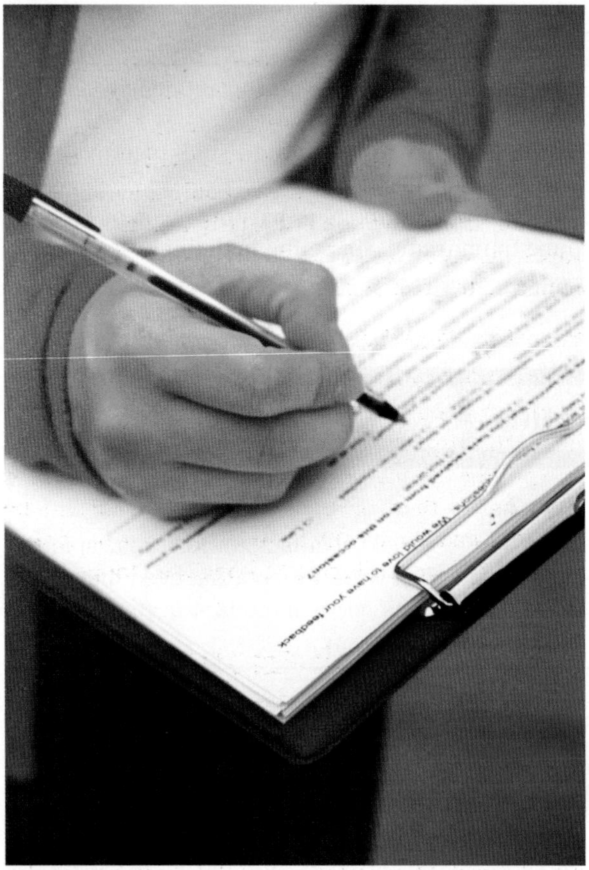

Fig 13.9 A sports leader undertaking a risk assessment

to overtake, will make decisions based on factors such as the speed at which they are travelling, the layout of the track and the weather conditions, so that they can overtake safely. By looking at these factors, the driver is assessing the hazards, so as to minimise the risk of an accident.

Key terms

Hazard: something that has the potential to cause injury or compromise safety.

Risk: the likelihood of something unpleasant happening.

Risk assessment: a list of possible hazards that states the likelihood of them happening, and ways of controlling them.

After you have highlighted a potential hazard, the easiest way to assess any potential problems that may arise is to use the following formula: Likelihood χ Severity.

Likelihood – is it likely to happen:

1 Unlikely.
2 Quite likely.
3 Very likely.

Severity – how badly someone could be injured:

1 No injury/minor incident.
2 Injury requiring medical assistance.
3 Major injury or fatality.

For example, Table 13.2 attempts to assess the risk posed by broken glass on a park football pitch.

By multiplying the likelihood against the severity, you will be able to draw up a chart that looks at the potential problems, and make a decision about whether you want to take the risk or not (see Table 13.3).

In the example in Table 13.2, the likelihood multiplied by the severity is $2 \times 2 = 4$.

Likelihood of happening	Severity
2 Quite likely	2 Injury requiring medical assistance

Table 13.2 Broken glass on a park football pitch

Likelihood × Severity	Is the risk worth taking?	What measures should be considered/ taken prior to activity?
1	Yes, with caution	
2	Yes, possibly with caution	
3	Yes, possibly with extreme caution	
4	Possibly, with extreme caution	
5 or above	No	

Table 13.3 Is the risk worth taking?

Control Measures

Control measures help to reduce the likelihood of an accident happening. This could include having safety goggles, for example, where a person is at risk of getting something in their eye. Having eyewash solution close by could also help somebody if they were to get something in their eye. Cleaners often put up warning signs when they are mopping floors. This is a control measure to alert people that the floor may be wet, and helps reduce the risk of injury by bringing attention to the hazard. Control measures are also known as precautions.

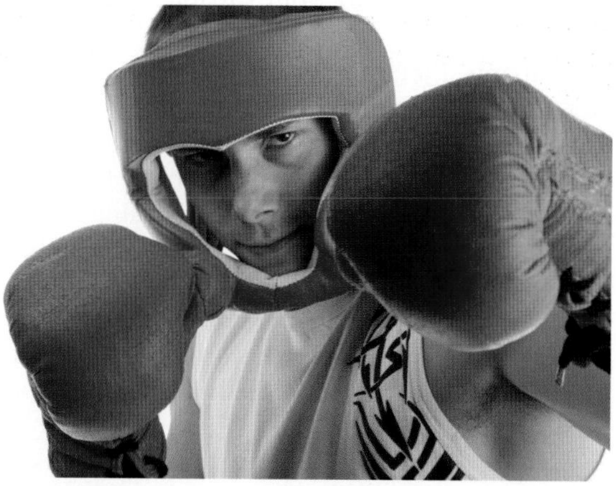

Fig 13.10 An amateur boxer wearing a head guard

Safety Equipment

Specialist equipment is also sometimes used in sport to help minimise the risk of injury. This can include protective clothing, accessories and equipment.

Cyclists wear helmets in case they fall off. A cricket batsman would wear protective equipment such as a box and helmet to prevent injury from the ball. Safety ropes are often used in climbing and abseiling to minimise the risk of potential danger.

Reporting Procedures

Health and safety is the responsibility of everyone. In the workplace everyone should be responsible; however, in sports activities it is often the responsibility of the instructor, coach or leader. If an accident happens or there is a near miss, it needs to be reported and documented, so that it can be looked at, dealt with accordingly and hopefully stopped from happening again.

Reviewing a Risk Assessment

It is important that, once a risk assessment has been undertaken, it is reviewed and updated regularly. As equipment gets older it is more likely to go wrong and, therefore, become more hazardous. Undertaking an activity at a new venue or in a different environment also needs to be looked at, even if it is an activity you are familiar with.

Student activity 13.3 — 60 mins — P3

Task 1

Choose one of your favourite sporting activities and make a list of:

- All the risks and hazards associated with your selected sport
- All the hazards associated with your selected sport
- All the safety equipment you need in order to reduce the risk of injury in your selected sport.

Task 2

Copy and complete the risk assessment form for your selected sports activity.

Example of a risk assessment form

Location of risk assessment:

Risk assessor's name:

Date:

Hazard	People at risk	Likelihood	Severity	Level of risk	Control measures

Fig 13.11 Risk assessment form

Activities

Leadership is more than simply being the person at the front of the room or area telling the others what to do. A variety of activities can be applied to each situation.

Warm-ups

Warm-ups are essential for all activities, and should be fun and relevant to the session and the participants. An example of a warm-up useful with younger children is small-sided games. The concept of small-sided games is that the game has more impact on individuals; it helps people learn and recognise rules and fair play; and it encourages the young to adapt their own games.

These games are typically versions of traditional sports such as basketball, netball or football. The games can be modified by restricting the playing area, changing the equipment (e.g. smaller balls in basketball), changing roles and positions (such as in the game of high five in netball) or adapting scoring to reward fair play.

Activities Suitable for Older People

In an increasingly ageing population, there is a growing need for physical activities for older people. Older people still have a desire and a need to take part in physical activity. While some consideration should be made regarding physical capability, the principles for leadership are the same as for any group.

Activities Suitable for Disabled People

Every effort should be made to include disabled people in mainstream sports, and to promote a general awareness and positive attitude towards disabled people in sport.

Planning Sports Activities

Planning a session means that you will need to look at every detail of the activity and consider every possible eventuality. The time spent planning may be time-consuming, but it will help ensure that you get the best out of your sessions. *Remember, proper planning prevents poor performance!*

There are many things to take into account when planning your activity session; however, the first thing to consider should be what you want to get out of the activity session. It is important to set aims and objectives.

There is an acronym for setting goals that is believed to motivate people in achieving their aims and objectives. These are known as SMARTER targets:

- **S**pecific – your aim must be specific.
- **M**easurable – how can you measure it?
- **A**chievable – it must be possible to achieve the goal.
- **R**ealistic – be realistic with your aims; are they achievable?
- **T**ime-constrained – set yourself a time period to do it in.
- **E**xciting – this will help motivate you to achieve your aims.
- **R**ecorded – record your aims; this will help you stick to them.

This method should be used when setting potential aims and objectives for your session.

Following this, you will need to consider the participants that the session is being planned for. How many participants will there be? Knowing the age and ability of the group is also important, as you can use this information in planning the types of activities that you wish to include. Leading an activity for a group of beginners is completely different to organising a session for more advanced performers. Also, when planning your sports activity session, you might consider what the group has done prior to your session or what they have planned for the following sessions.

Another consideration you may have to take into account is if you have a mixed-sex group.

Lastly, it is important to know, prior to running a session, of any medical or special needs that any of the participants may have. A good way for a leader to know the medical backgrounds of their participants is to get them to complete a PAR-Q prior to taking part in exercise. A PAR-Q is a Physical Activity Readiness Questionnaire, which looks at an individual's medical history and highlights any major factors that could stop them from participating.

If the person answered YES to one or more questions, they should be instructed to talk with their doctor before beginning an exercise programme or taking part in fitness tests.

Planning the Resources

Planning and organising what equipment you will require for your activity should be done prior to the session. Time spent during the activity putting goals up or pumping up balls, and so on, eats into participants' time, so planning this in advance will help the session run more smoothly. You should also consider what facilities you will have to use for your session. These may well need to be booked in advance of the session and this is the responsibility of the activity leader. When planning your session you will need to ensure that you have enough material and activities to last the time allocated; it is a good idea to have a few more activities planned than you think you will

Physical Activity Readiness Questionnaire (PAR-Q)

1 Has a doctor ever said you have a heart condition and recommended only medically supervised physical activity?

2 Do you have chest pain brought on by physical activity?

3 Have you developed chest pain in the past month?

4 Do you tend to lose consciousness or fall over as a result of dizziness?

5 Do you have a bone or joint problem that could be aggravated by the proposed physical activity?

6 Has a doctor ever recommended medication for your blood pressure or a heart condition?

7 Are you aware through your own experience, or a doctor's advice, of any other physical reason against your exercising without medical supervision?

8 Have you had any operations?

9 Have you suffered any injuries?

10 Do you or have you suffered from back pain?

11 Are you pregnant?

12 Have you recently given birth?

If the person answered YES to one or more questions they should be instructed to talk with their doctor before beginning an exercise programme or taking part in fitness tests.

Fig 13.12 Physical Activity Readiness Questionnaire (PAR-Q)

need, then you will never run out of things to do during the session!

The key points for planning an activity session are as follows:

- What space/facilities do you need?
- How many people are there participating in the session?
- How much equipment do you need?
- How long will the session last?

Many sports leaders will use a session planner to highlight the information above and the aims and content of the session.

- A risk assessment is a technique for preventing any potential accidents, injury or ill health by helping people to consider what could go wrong either in the workplace or on the sports field.
- Warm-ups are essential for all activities, and should be fun and relevant to the session and the participants.

- Proper planning prevents poor performance!
- A PAR-Q is a Physical Activity Readiness Questionnaire, which gives details of an individual's medical history and highlights any major factors that could stop them from participating.

Session planner

Date:	Venue:
Time:	Duration:
Group:	No. of participants:
Equipment required:	Aims of session:
Safety checks required:	
TIME	CONTENT
	Warm-up:
	Fitness work:
	Main technical skills work:
	Game play/tactical work:
	Cool-down
Injuries/issues arising	
Evaluation of session	

Fig 13.13 Session planner

Student activity 13.4 — 30 minutes — P4

Task 1

Select a sports activity of your choice and work out who is going to take part in the activity and their ability levels.

Task 2

Complete a session plan for your sports activity, making sure you consider the following points:

- Age of participants
- Ability of participants
- Aims of session
- Equipment required
- Warm-up
- Fitness work (if applicable)
- Technical skills work
- Tactical work
- Cool-down.

13.5 Leading Sports Activities Effectively

P5 M3

Leading a Sports Activity Session

When delivering your session, you will need to do many things to ensure that your participants understand what it is you are trying to cover.

First, you will need to explain and demonstrate the skills that you require them to undertake. Demonstrations should be kept simple and it is important that they are done correctly. This will help to ensure that the group understands what it is you are trying to teach them. Some participants will need additional support when teaching them new skills, so it is important that you move around your group and look at the different individuals' needs.

It is also important to look to progress the session. This will help motivate the participants and help prevent them from getting bored. Spending too much time on one activity can cause participants to switch off and start to do other things as they get bored. Progression also gives encouragement to performers, as they can see their own achievement.

Sometimes you may need to adapt the session, as things are not going to plan, or changes may become necessary due to factors that are out of your control.

What Components Should Go into your Sports Activity Session?

The first thing to consider is what the activity session is that you wish to carry out. Sessions could include:

- A fitness session such as a circuit
- A practical coaching session
- A sports event such as a competition or race
- A competitive match.

A typical sports coaching session will progress through the following stages:

1. **Warm-up**: this will typically involve pulse-raising activities, mobility and flexibility work, and some sports-specific skills that help prepare the performer for what they are about to do. It is important to consider what skill-related components of fitness will be used during the activity and how to integrate them into the warm-up. For example, volleyball players require both power and hand-eye coordination in their sport, so both should be included in their warm-up.
2. **Fitness work**: if time allows, participants should undertake some fitness and training methods that are relevant to their sport. Rugby players, for example, might incorporate aerobic conditioning and muscular endurance training into their sessions.
3. **Technical skills practice**: this is where you normally cover the main aims of your session. This will include your drill and routines that you have prepared. Remember to demonstrate the skills and give people the opportunity to practise them, while assisting those individuals who struggle.
4. **Tactical work**: once you have developed the skills, you should look at how and when you use them to gain an advantage over your opponents.
5. **Game play**: it is important to put the skills learnt into a game context.
6. **Cool-down**: this is used to help reduce the build-up of lactic acid and reduce the risk of DOMS (delayed onset of muscle soreness).

It is important that you record evidence of your sports activity session. You should use the feedback to help you evaluate the session. Evaluation is as important as the planning process, and it can help you with future sessions, as you will know what has worked well, any problems that arose and what should be changed.

Student activity 13.5 15–30 mins P5 M3

Demonstrate effective leadership skills while leading a selected sports activity.

Reviewing a Sports Activity Session

It is important to consider that leadership does not end at the end of a session when everyone has cooled down or even gone home. Leadership is a continuous process and the best leaders reflect on what happened and, more importantly, how to improve. A well-considered evaluation should aid the improvement of subsequent sessions.

The process is something like this:

- **Collect, analyse and review** information about the session from feedback and self-reflection, and from others
- **Session effectiveness** – identify the effectiveness of the session in achieving objectives
- **Review key aspects** (e.g. the drills or practices)
- **Identify development needs** and take steps to action them.

When evaluating a session, a leader should consider the following:

1. **Performance against pre-set goals** – effective leaders will be familiar with the goals for the session, both long-term and short-term. There should be an opportunity to decide to what extent, if at all, the session objectives were met, and to what extent this contributed to the achievement of all the goals.
2. **Participants' progress** – a review will enable leaders to monitor a performer's progress over a period of time and help plan for future sessions. Typical review questions could be:
   (a) How well did the performers learn the skills or techniques introduced to them?
   (b) What performance developments were evident for each participant?
   (c) Are the performers ready to progress to the next session?
3. **Leadership ability** – this is the part where the leader can review their own performance.
   (a) What went well?
   (b) What went less well?
   (c) How did the performers respond?
   (d) Were the performers bored or restless?
   (e) Did the leader behave acceptably?
4. **Future targets** – this is all about planning for future goals and objectives based on achievements and progress made by the participants.

Tools to Help the Review Process

- **Videos** – an excellent way of improving your effectiveness. Videos can be used to judge leadership actions, interaction with your performers, facial expressions and gestures, as well as what you say.
- **Critical analysis and self-reflection** – self-reflection allows you to explore your perceptions, decisions and subsequent actions to work out ways in which performers can improve technical, tactical or physical ability.
- **A mentor** – a mentor leader can help provide you with a role model figure who can help you with practical solutions, work as a sounding board and generally provide you with a range of support.
- **Leadership diaries** – these can act as a permanent source of information to record your own thoughts and feelings, and serve as a true account of what happened and when. Diaries or logs can certainly help with self-reflection and form the basis of action plans for improvement.

Using a Diary or Log

These can come in all shapes and sizes. Most people will have used a diary at some point and this will make them easy to use. Diaries can be useful tools in assisting self-reflection, planning and monitoring progress.

The major benefits of diaries are that they provide a written record over time of progress. It is also easy to record emotions, feelings, and so on.

Critical Analysis and Self-reflection

Everyone has experienced a certain amount of self-reflection. As a leader, it is possible to think back over a competition, but in everyday life, you might think about a driving test or an argument.

This can be a useful process if you review what happened and what you did and then suggest to yourself what you might have done better. This could lead you to determine what you might do in the future.

The process of reflection has several stages (as illustrated in Figure 13.14).

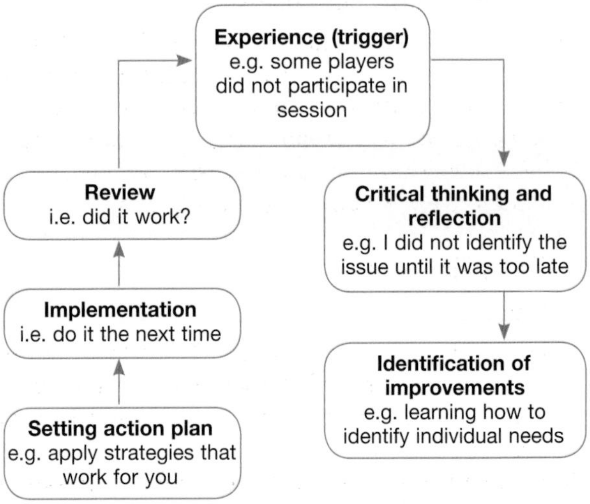

Fig 13.14 Example of the self-reflection process

Using Video

Simply having your performance filmed will provide you with an objective record of what happened, with the advantage of being able to analyse in slow motion or real time. You will see yourself as you see others and there is no need to try to remember everything, as in the case of a diary.

Videos can also be used to form a point of reference. Watching an elite official in action can be beneficial and help to demonstrate the techniques required to improve.

Peer Observation

Information from people in the same situation as you can be some of the most valuable information received. Often, as a new leader, it is easier for peers to relate to the kind of situations that you might be in, and offer you the benefit of their own experiences and ways in which they have dealt with challenging situations. It is very easy for an experienced leader to state the easiest way to deal with a difficult situation, but it should be borne in mind that what works for them is most likely based on the relationships that they have established through years of experience and that an appropriate course of action for you could be completely different from the one that they might take.

Qualifications

In improving as a leader, it is necessary at some stage to become qualified. Qualifications such as the Duke of Edinburgh's Award Scheme and the Community and Higher Sports Leadership Awards are useful, both in terms of your personal development and in introducing you to peers, who will want to update you with all the relevant issues and scenarios relating to leadership.

Message Boards/Chat Rooms

Message boards or chat rooms on internet sites are now a good means of communication between officials. It should be pointed out that while this medium may be very useful, it is open to abuse and it is worth being cautious about all contact unless it is supported by a recognised governing body.

Development

Feedback

- **Formative** – this sort of feedback assists the leader in the improvement of their own performance, and provides corrective advice and guidance for improvement.
- **Summative** – this sort of feedback passes a judgement on performance and can be used as an assessment tool, such as in the assessment of a leaders' course or qualification, or in the formal assessment of leadership performance, measured against a specification authorised by the governing body, such as the British Sports Trust.

Having completed an activity, it is important to gain some feedback on how to improve performance. Feedback can come from a number of sources:

- Yourself
- Your peers
- An assessor
- A supervisor
- An observer.

Whatever the nature and style of your leadership, and whatever the nature of your activity, no two leaders are identical. Information about strengths and weaknesses provides us with a template for improvement. A leader should learn something new from every session.

Examples of development feedback could be:

- Poor or ineffective stroke demonstration
- Unsafe activity
- Ineffective/unsafe knots used (climbing)
- Ineffective communication with the group
- Lack of confidence and experience.

All of the above can be improved. Leaders must review and develop their own self-assessment techniques, paying particular attention to what needs to be improved and in what order.

Target Setting

When you have identified areas for development, it is good practice to apply the SMART principle:

- **S**pecific (e.g. test the effectiveness of your teaching – in this case, to a group of beginners)
- **M**easurable (e.g. test the effectiveness of your teaching – see if you can learn the skill well enough to produce an effective demonstration)
- **A**chievable (e.g. know that you are capable of executing the skill well enough to demonstrate to a group of beginners)
- **R**ealistic (is it possible?)
- **T**ime-constrained (e.g. review the situation in one month).

Evaluating a Session

Once a session is completed, it is important to review and record the practice, to improve the quality of your leadership and the quality of the experience for the learner.

Key learning points 3

- A typical sports activity session will usually contain:
  - warm-up
  - fitness work
  - technical skills practice
  - tactical work
  - game play
  - cool-down.
- Sports sessions take many forms, for example:
  - a fitness session such as a circuit
  - a practical coaching session
  - a sports event such as a competition or race
  - a competitive match.
- Feedback may be formative – assists the leader in the improvement of their own performance; or summative – passes a judgement on performance.
- Self-reflection allows you to explore your perceptions, decisions and subsequent actions, to work out ways in which performers can improve technical, tactical or physical ability.

Student activity 13.6

60–90 mins P6 P7 M4 D2

Task 1

Carry out a review of the performance of participants while they are taking part in the sports activity. Make a list of the participants' strengths and areas for improvement and then write a report that explains and justifies these.

Task 2

Design a feedback form that you could give to the participants in your activity session so that they can provide constructive feedback on how they thought your sports activity session went.

Task 3

Examine the feedback from the participants and speak to your supervisor or teacher to gain their opinion of your planning and leadership. Carry out a self-assessment of how you think you planned and led the activity session. In a written report, carry out a review of your planning and leading a sports activity. Identify and explain your strengths in the planning and leading of the activity.

Task 3

Identify and explain any areas for improvement and justify some SMARTER targets for how you can make these improvements.

Q Quick quiz 3

1 Give examples of the activities and exercises you would include in a:
   (a) warm-up
   (b) fitness work
   (c) technical skills practice
   (d) tactical work
   (e) game play
   (f) cool-down
   for a sports activity session.
2 Describe what formative feedback is.
3 Describe the processes involved in self-reflection.
4 List and explain three tools that can be used to help the review process.

References

Carron, A.V. (1982) Cohesiveness in sport group: interpretations and consideration. *Journal of Sport Psychology*, 4, 123–38.

Crisfield, P. (2001) *Analysing your Coaching*, Coachwise.

Higher Sports Leader Award Resource Pack (2005) *Developing Leadership Through Community Sport*, British Sports Trust.

Miles, A. (2004) *Coaching Practice*, Coachwise.

Stafford-Brown, J., Rea, S., Janaway, L. and Manley, C. (2006) *BTEC First Sport*, Hodder Arnold.

Tuckman, B.W. (1965) Developmental sequence in small groups. *Psychological Bulletin*, 63, 384–99.

Useful websites

www.nspcc.org.uk/inform/cpsu/resources/bullying/bullying_wda60599.html

Free access to online resource outlining how to challenge bullying in sports clubs; includes links to icebreaker exercises and other resources

www.safesport.co.uk

Provides a wealth of articles that give advice on how to engage in sport safely

www.guardian.co.uk/sport/2005/apr/03/rugbyunion.features

Online article from *The Observer* that examines what qualities make a great leader in sport

http://psychology.about.com/library/quiz/bl-leadershipquiz.htm

Fun online quiz that suggests what your leadership style is and how it can be utilised effectively

14: Exercise, Health and Lifestyle

14.1 Introduction

A person's lifestyle can have a huge impact on their long-term health. Lifestyle plays a key role in the prevention of a large number of diseases, including coronary heart disease, cancer and obesity. This unit will give you the knowledge and skills to assess the lifestyle of an individual, provide advice on lifestyle improvement and plan a health-related physical activity programme.

By the end of this unit you should:

- know the importance of lifestyle factors in the maintenance of health and well-being
- be able to assess the lifestyle of a selected individual
- be able to provide advice on lifestyle improvement
- be able to plan a health-related physical activity programme for a selected individual.

Assessment and grading criteria		
To achieve a PASS grade the evidence must show that the learner is able to:	**To achieve a MERIT grade the evidence must show that, in addition to the pass criteria, the learner is able to:**	**To achieve a DISTINCTION grade the evidence must show that, in addition to the pass and merit criteria, the learner is able to:**
P1 describe lifestyle factors that have an effect on health	**M1** explain the effects of identified lifestyle factors on health	
P2 design and use a lifestyle questionnaire to describe the strengths and areas for improvement in the lifestyle of a selected individual	**M2** explain the strengths and areas for improvement in the lifestyle of a selected individual	**D1** evaluate the lifestyle of a selected individual and prioritise areas for change
P3 provide lifestyle improvement strategies for a selected individual	**M3** explain recommendations made regarding lifestyle improvement strategies.	**D2** analyse a range of lifestyle improvement strategies.
P4 plan a six-week health-related physical activity programme for a selected individual.		

14.2 Lifestyle Factors

P1 M1

Physical Activity

Our lifestyle has become much more sedentary over the years. We now have methods of transport that require little physical exertion. Cars and buses have replaced walking and cycling. Recent studies have shown that 30 per cent of children go to school by car, and fewer than 50 per cent walk. This country has less time dedicated to PE lessons than any other country in the European Union. There are now relatively few manual occupations, and the majority of people's careers are spent in an office-based environment. Everyday tasks such as laundry, cleaning and cooking require little effort, as they are all aided by labour-saving devices. It is now even possible to go shopping by sitting in front of a computer and logging on to the internet.

For entertainment, the average person spends less time participating in active leisure pursuits and prefers to sit in front of the TV. The average adult watches over 26 hours of television each week, which is a virtually totally sedentary activity. Children also spend much less time pursuing activity-based play and choose computer games, videos or the TV to occupy their free time. All these factors have led to many people taking part in very low levels of physical activity.

Physical activity can increase a person's basal metabolic rate by around 10 per cent. This elevated basal metabolic rate can last for up to 48 hours after the completion of the activity. By taking part in physical activity kilocalories will be expended. The number of kilocalories used depends on the type and intensity of the activity. The more muscles that are used in the activity and the harder you work, the more kilocalories will be used up to perform the activity. For example, swimming the front crawl uses both the arms and the legs and will therefore use more calories to perform than walking, which mainly uses the leg muscles.

The body weight of the person will also have an impact on the number of kilocalories burnt while taking part in a physical activity. The heavier the person, the more kilocalories are required to move the heavier weight. So a heavier person will burn more calories than a lighter person when performing the same activity at the same intensity.

Key term

Physical activity: the state of being active.

National Recommended Guidelines

In order to gain the health benefits of physical activity, adults should aim to participate in physical activity for 30 minutes at least five times a week. Our national recommended guidelines for children state that they should participate in moderate-intensity exercise for 60 minutes per day, but the European Health Study 2006 found that they should be exercising for 90 minutes per day to gain the health benefits of physical activity.

Health Benefits of Physical Activity

Taking part in regular exercise has consistently been shown to have many benefits to a person's physical and mental health. Many types of disease can be alleviated or prevented by taking part in regular exercise.

Coronary heart disease and physical activity

Coronary heart disease (CHD) is the leading cause of death in the Western world. One-third of all deaths associated with CHD are due to not taking part in physical activity. Coronary heart disease is a narrowing of the coronary arteries, which are the blood vessels that pass over the surface of the heart and supply it with blood. CHD is usually a result of a build-up of fatty material and plaques within the coronary blood vessels. This is known as atherosclerosis.

Key terms

Coronary blood vessels: blood vessels that supply blood to the heart.

Atherosclerosis: build-up of fatty material in the coronary blood vessels, which makes their diameter smaller.

When a person with CHD takes part in a physically demanding task, the coronary arteries may not be able to supply the heart muscle with enough blood to keep up with the demand for oxygen. This will be felt as a pain in the chest (angina). If a coronary artery becomes completely blocked, the area of the heart muscle served by the artery will die, resulting in a heart attack.

Taking part in regular exercise appears to reduce the risk of heart disease directly and indirectly. Research has shown that exercise:

- Increases levels of HDL cholesterol
- Decreases the amount of triglycerides in the bloodstream.

Key terms

HDL cholesterol: the 'good' cholesterol that acts to clean the artery walls, which in turn reduces atherosclerosis.

Triglycerides: another type of fat; high levels in the bloodstream have been linked with increased risk of heart disease.

Hypertension: high blood pressure.

Hypertension and physical activity
A person is deemed to have hypertension if their blood pressure consistently reads at 140/90 or higher. Hypertension is a very common complaint, and around 15 to 25 per cent of adults in most Western countries have high blood pressure. If a person with hypertension does not reduce their blood pressure they are more at risk of suffering a stroke or a heart attack.

Psychological Benefits of Physical Activity

A number of studies have attempted to explore the effects of exercise on depression and found that exercise increases self-esteem, improves mood, reduces anxiety levels, increases the ability to handle stress and generally makes people happier than those who do not exercise. It is thought that one cause of depression may be a decreased production of certain chemicals in the brain, specifically adrenaline, dopamine and serotonin. Exercise has been shown to increase the levels of these substances, which may have the effect of improving a person's mood after taking part in exercise. For the last decade or so, exercise has been prescribed as a method of combating depression.

Smoking

You are probably aware that smoking is bad for you. It actually kills around 14,000 people in the UK each year, and 300 people die in the UK every day as a result of smoking. These deaths occur through a range of diseases caused by smoking and include a variety of cancers, cardiovascular disease and an array of chronic lung diseases.

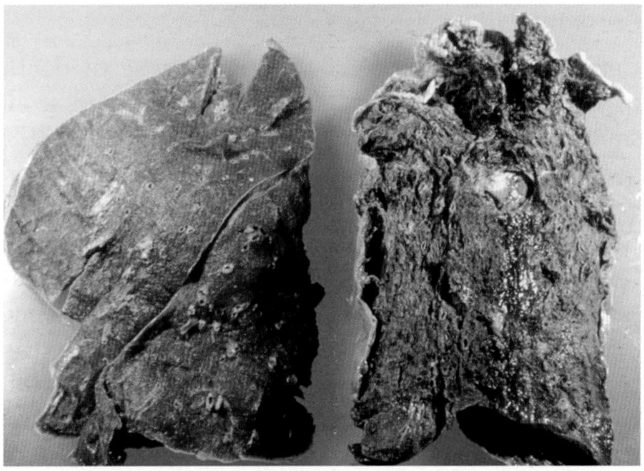

Fig 14.1 A normal lung (left) beside the lung of a smoker (right)

The products in a cigarette that appear to do the most damage include tar, nicotine and carbon monoxide.

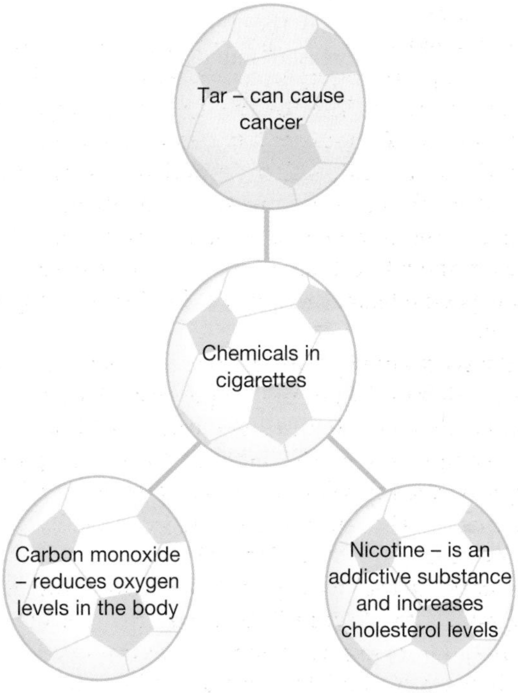

Fig 14.2 Chemicals in cigarettes

Smokers are making themselves much more likely to suffer from a range of cancers; 90 per cent of people suffering from lung cancer have the disease because they smoke or have smoked. You are also four times more likely to contract mouth cancer if you are a smoker. Other forms of cancer that have been linked to smoking include cancers of the bladder, oesophagus, kidneys and pancreas, and cervical cancer.

Cardiovascular Disease

Cardiovascular disease is the main cause of death in smokers. The excess cholesterol produced from smoking narrows the blood vessels.

When the blood vessels become narrower, blood clots are more likely to form, which can then block the coronary blood vessels. A blockage in these vessels can lead to a heart attack. It is estimated that 30 per cent of these heart attacks are due to smoking.

Alternatively, the blood clot may travel to the brain, which can lead to a stroke; or it could travel to the kidneys, which could result in kidney failure; or the block may occur in the legs, which can lead to gangrene, for which the main treatment is amputation.

Chronic Lung Disease

The following diseases are more prevalent in smokers:

- Emphysema – a disease that causes breathlessness due to damaged alveoli
- Bronchitis – makes the person cough excessively because of increased mucus production in the lungs.

> **Key term**
>
> **Alveoli:** air sacs in the lungs in which gaseous exchange takes place.

Smoking is responsible for 80 per cent of these conditions, which basically block air flow to and from the lungs, making breathing more difficult. These diseases tend to start between the ages of 35 and 45.

Other Smoking-Related Health Risks

Smoking can also damage health in a variety of other ways. A person who smokes may suffer from some of the following:

- High blood pressure
- Impotence
- Fertility problems
- Eye problems
- Discoloured teeth and gums
- Mouth ulcers
- Skin more prone to wrinkles.

Alcohol

Alcohol is a legal drug that may be consumed by people aged 18 or over – although by the age of 16, over 80 per cent of young people in the UK have tried alcohol. In fact, in the UK, people aged between 16 and 24 are the heaviest drinking group of the population. Studies reveal that one in two men and one in four women drink more than the recommended daily benchmarks, and over a quarter of males and females drink more than double the recommended daily amount.

The recommended daily benchmarks for alcohol consumption are based on adult drinking; there are no recommendations for children and young people as they should be refraining from alcohol consumption by law.

Recommended Daily Intake

The Health Education Authority recommends that women should drink no more than two units of alcohol per day and males should drink no more than three units per day. Both males and females should have at least two alcohol-free days per week.

It takes around an hour for the adult body to get rid of one unit of alcohol, and this may well be slower in young people.

Effects of Alcohol on the Body

Alcohol affects the brain so that it compromises our judgement and suppresses our inhibitions. It decreases our physical coordination and sense of balance, and makes our vision blurred and speech slurred. Excessive drinking can lead to alcohol poisoning, which can cause unconsciousness, coma and even death. Excessive alcohol consumption can often make a person vomit, and vomiting while unconscious can lead to death by suffocation, as the vomit can block the air flow to and from the lungs. The effects of alcohol have also been implicated in a large proportion of fatal road accidents, assaults and incidents of domestic violence.

Diseases Associated with Excess Alcohol Consumption

Alcohol consumption in excess of the recommended daily guidelines will often cause physical damage to the body and increase the likelihood of getting diseases such as cancer, cirrhosis, high blood pressure, strokes and depression.

Cirrhosis

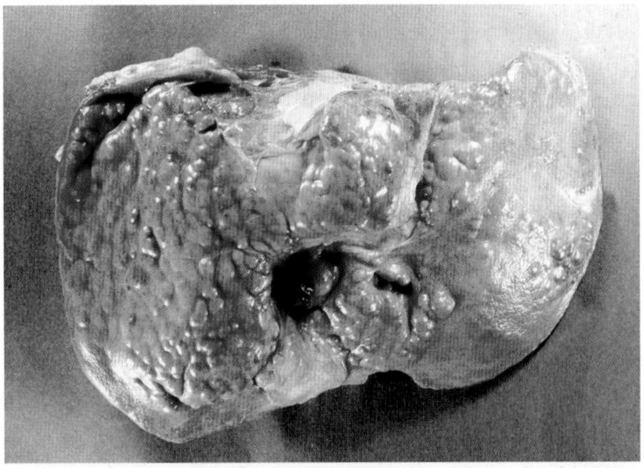

Fig 14.3 A liver affected by cirrhosis

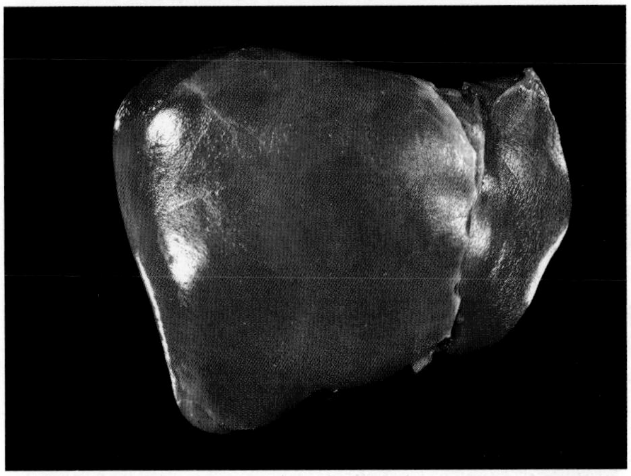

Fig 14.4 A healthy liver

Excessive alcohol consumption can result in cirrhosis of the liver. The liver is the largest organ in the body. It is responsible for getting rid of poisons from the blood, helps our immune system in fighting infection, makes proteins that help our blood to clot and produces bile, which helps with the breakdown of fats. The disease damages the liver and produces scar tissue. The scar tissue replaces the normal tissue and prevents it from working as it should. Cirrhosis is the twelfth leading cause of death by disease and causes 26,000 deaths per year.

Cancer
Around 6 per cent of deaths from cancer in the UK are caused by alcohol (*Oxford Textbook of Medicine*, 2003). A range of cancers have been linked with excess alcohol consumption; these include:

- Cancer of the mouth
- Cancer of the larynx
- Cancer of the oesophagus
- Liver cancer
- Breast cancer
- Bowel cancer.

Depression
Alcohol consumption has been linked with anxiety and depression. One in three young people who have committed suicide drank alcohol before they died, and more than two out of three people who attempt suicide have drunk excessively.

Stress

When we perceive ourselves to be in a situation that is dangerous, our stress response is activated. This has been developed as a means of ensuring our survival by making us respond to danger. For example, if you are walking home at night along a dark street and you hear noises behind you, your body will instigate physiological changes, called the 'fight-or-flight' response, as your body is preparing to turn and fight the danger or run away as fast as it can.

Adrenaline and cortisol are the main hormones released when we are stressed, which have the effect of:

- Increasing the heart rate
- Increasing the breathing rate
- Decreasing the rate of digestion.

It is not healthy for the body to be in a constant state of stress because of the excess production of adrenaline and cortisol. This results in excess cholesterol production that raises blood cholesterol levels and is a risk factor for CHD.

Stress and Cardiovascular Disease

If the excess hormones and chemicals released during stressful periods are not 'used up' through physical exertion, the increased heart rate and high blood pressure place excess strain on our blood vessels. This can lead to vascular damage. Damaged blood vessels are thicker than healthy blood vessels and have a reduced ability to stretch. This can have the effect of reducing the supply of blood and oxygen to the heart.

Stress and the Immune System

Stress can decrease our body's ability to fight infection, which makes us more susceptible to suffering from illnesses. This explains why we catch more colds when we are stressed.

Stress and Depression

Stress is also associated with mental health problems, and in particular with anxiety and depression. Here the relationship is fairly clear. The negative thinking that is associated with stress also contributes to these.

Diet

Our diets have changed significantly over the years. Today we have the largest range of foods available to us, but we are choosing to eat foods that are high in saturated fats and simple carbohydrates. Fast-food restaurants are flourishing because they are used so regularly by our society. Today, the nation's diet tends to be lacking in a number of important nutrients, including fibre, calcium, vitamins and iron. This is because a high proportion of the population relies on snacks and fast foods as their main source of nutritional intake. As a result, the Western diet is generally high in fat and sugars, resulting in a huge increase in obesity.

Estimates in 1990 suggested that 1 in 20 children aged 9 to 11 could be classified as clinically obese. If a person is obese they are much more likely to suffer from coronary heart disease, which is currently the biggest killer in Britain. As we are continuing to rely on foods that do not give us the right balance of vital nutrients, a number of people are suffering from poor nutrition. This not only impairs physical and mental functioning, but can also increase the risk of suffering from a range of diseases, including anaemia, diabetes and osteoporosis. A number of nutrition experts have also linked poor nutrition to emotional and behavioural problems that are seen to occur much more frequently among children today; these include hyperactivity and attention deficit disorders.

A healthy diet contains lots of fruit and vegetables. It is based on starchy foods, such as wholegrain bread, pasta and rice, and is low in fat (especially saturated fat), salt and sugar. Current recommendations for a healthy diet are shown in Table 14.1.

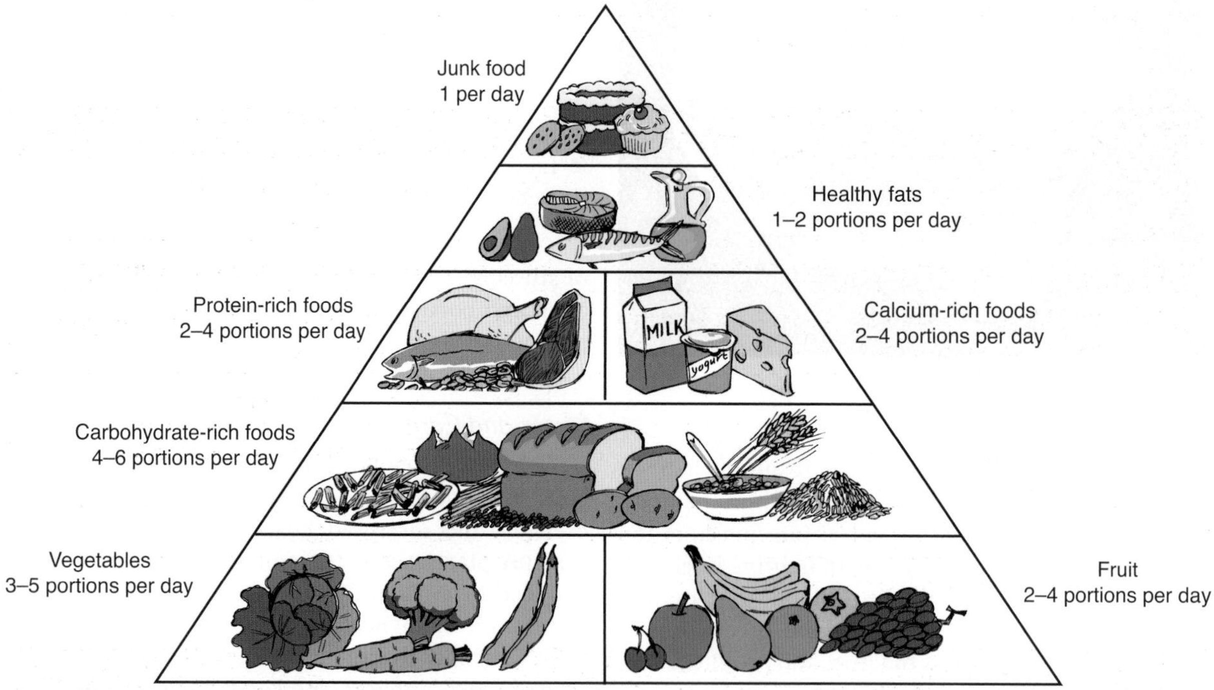

Fig 14.5 The nutrition pyramid

Food	Amount we should eat	Function	Example of food sources
Carbohydrates	50–60%	Provide energy for sports performance	
Sugars		Provide short bursts of energy	Jam, sweets, fruit, fizzy drinks, sports drinks
Starch		Provide energy for longer periods	Pasta, rice, bread, potatoes, breakfast cereals
Fat	25–30%	Provides energy for low-intensity exercise, e.g. walking	
Saturated fats		Insulate the body against the cold	Mainly animal sources: cream, lard, cheese, meat
Unsaturated fats		Help to protect internal organs	Mainly plant sources: nuts, soya, tofu
Protein	10–15%	For growth and repair	Meat, eggs, nuts, fish, poultry

Table 14.1 Recommendations for a healthy diet

Vitamin	Food sources	Function
A	Carrots, liver, dark green vegetables, mackerel	Maintains good vision, skin and hair
B group	Cereals, liver, yeast, eggs, beef, beans	Helps to break down food to produce energy
C	Most fresh fruits and vegetables, especially citrus fruits	Fights infection; maintains healthy skin and gums; helps with wound healing
D	Oily fish, eggs	Helps to build bones and teeth
E	Nuts, whole grains, dark green leafy vegetables	Antioxidant that prevents damage to cells
K	Leafy green vegetables, peas, milk, egg yolks	Helps to form blood clots

Table 14.2 Sources and functions of vitamins

Mineral	Food sources	Function
Iron	Liver, lean meats, eggs, dried fruits	Blood production
Calcium	Milk, fish bones, green leafy vegetables	Helps to build strong bones and teeth; helps to form blood clots
Sodium	Salt, seafood, processed foods, celery	Maintains fluid balance in cells; helps in muscle contraction
Potassium	Bananas	Works with sodium to maintain fluid balance, aids muscle contraction, maintains blood pressure
Zinc	Meats, fish	Tissue growth and repair

Table 14.3 Sources and functions of minerals

Key learning points 1

- People are much more sedentary today and many are not meeting national recommended guidelines.
- Children should be physically active for at least 60 to 90 minutes per day.
- Adults should be physically active for at least 30 minutes five times per week.
- People who take part in physical activity are less likely to suffer from CHD, hypertension, diabetes, obesity and depression.
- Smoking has been shown to cause cancer, chronic lung disease and cardiovascular disease in some people.
- Adult males should have no more than three units of alcohol per day and adult females should have no more than two. Males and females should both have at least two alcohol-free days per week.
- Excess alcohol consumption has been shown to cause cirrhosis, cancer and depression in some people.
- Stress can cause cardiovascular disease, decrease the immune system's response to infection and cause depression in some people.
- Today, many people are eating fast food and not taking in the right quantities of macronutrients, vitamins and minerals.
- A healthy diet contains lots of fruit and vegetables, is based on starchy foods such as wholegrain bread, pasta and rice, and is low in fat (especially saturated fat), salt and sugar.

Q Quick quiz 1

Match each description in the table below to the condition it describes, choosing from the following:

- Excess alcohol consumption
- CHD
- Hypertension
- Emphysema
- Cirrhosis.

Description	Condition
A disease that causes breathlessness due to damaged alveoli	
Damage and scarring to the liver	
A blood pressure reading of 140/90 or higher	
The build-up of fats in the coronary blood vessels	
This can lead to poisoning, unconsciousness and coma	

14.3 Assessing the Lifestyle of an Individual

P2 M2 D1

When assessing the lifestyle of an individual, you will need to gather as much information on them as possible. This can be done effectively through a comprehensive questionnaire. It will be part of an initial consultation and must cover the following as a minimum requirement:

- Medical history
- Activity history
- Lifestyle factors
- Nutritional status
- Any other factors that will affect the person's health.

Lifestyle Questionnaire

Section 1: Personal Details

Name ______________________________

Address ______________________________

____

____

____

Home telephone ______________

Mobile telephone ______________

Email ______________________________

Occupation ______________________________

Date of birth ______________________________

Section 2: Physical Activity Levels

1 Does your occupation require you to take part in physical activity? If so, what?

____

____

2 What are your medium-term goals over the next three months?

____

____

____

____

3 What are your short-term goals over the next four weeks?

____

____

____

____

Section 3: Current Training Status

1 What are your main training requirements?

(a) Muscular strength.

(b) Muscular endurance.

(c) Speed.

(d) Flexibility.

(e) Aerobic fitness.

(f) Power.

(g) Weight loss or gain.

(h) Skill-related fitness.

(i) Other (please state)

____

2 How would you describe your current fitness status?

____

____

3 How many times a week will you train?

____

4 How long do you have for each training session?

____

Section 4: Your Nutritional Status

1 On a scale of 1 to 10 (1 being very low quality and 10 being very high quality), how would you rate the quality of your diet?

____

2 Do you follow any particular diet?
  (a) Vegetarian.
  (b) Vegan.
  (c) Vegetarian plus fish.
  (d) Gluten-free.
  (e) Dairy-free.

3 How often do you eat? Note down a typical day's intake.

____

____

____

____

____

4 Do you take any supplements? If so, which ones?

____

____

Section 5: Your Lifestyle

1 How many units of alcohol do you drink in a typical week?__________

2 Do you smoke?________ If yes, how many a day?______________

3 Do you experience stress on a daily basis?____________

4 If yes, what causes you stress (if you know)?

____

____

5 What techniques do you use to deal with your stress?

____

Section 6: Your Physical Health

1 Do you experience any of the following?
  (a) Back pain or injury.
  (b) Knee pain or injury.
  (c) Ankle pain or injury.
  (d) Swollen joints.
  (e) Shoulder pain or injury.
  (f) Hip or pelvic pain or injury.
  (g) Nerve damage.
  (h) Head injuries.

2 If yes, please give details.

3 Are any of these injuries made worse by exercise?

4 If yes, what movements in particular cause pain?

5 Are you currently receiving any treatment for any injuries? If so, what?

Section 7: Medical History

1 Do you have, or have you had, any of the following medical conditions?

(a) Asthma.
(b) Bronchitis.
(c) Heart problems.
(d) Chest pains.
(e) Diabetes.
(f) High blood pressure.
(g) Epilepsy.
(h) Other

2 Are you taking any medication? (If yes, state what, how much and why.)

Name

Signature Date

One-to-one Consultation

It is always a good idea to follow up a lifestyle questionnaire with a consultation with the individual. The person running the consultation must know when to ask questions and prompt the client, and when to listen and take notes. The main rule of thumb is that the client should be doing most of the talking in a consultation; the consultant's role is to ensure that questions are answered accurately and fully. The client should be made aware that their lifestyle questionnaire and the follow-up consultation are confidential, and the questionnaire should be stored in a secure place.

Communication Skills

When conducting a consultation, you will need to use skills such as questioning and listening. One of the aims of the consultation is to develop rapport with your client, which means that they will start to trust you and accept the advice that you give to them.

Questioning

The consultation is a chance to gain information from your client so that you can use that information to help them improve their lifestyle; however, the quality of the information you gain will depend on the quality of the questions that you ask. There are different types of questions, such as:

- Closed questions
- Open questions
- Indirect questions.

Closed questions can be answered with a simple yes

or no, or by a short phrase. They are used to obtain facts or to clarify a certain point, for example:

- Where do you live?
- What is your occupation?
- Have you tried changing your diet?

Open questions will require a longer and more thoughtful response, as they are used to invite the client into a discussion or to explore an issue, for example:

- What activities do you enjoy doing?
- How are you getting on with your training?

Indirect questions are a softer introduction to a question and they may feel less intrusive, so are good for gaining sensitive information, for example:

- Do you mind me asking what you are trying to achieve?
- I was wondering whether you had thought about giving up smoking?

When you are choosing questions, you need to think about the information you are aiming to gather, as this will influence whether you ask a closed, open or indirect question. You should also think about the wording you use in your question and make sure that the client will understand it, rather than using wording that you think makes you look intelligent!

Listening
Listening is the second part of good communication and is vital in establishing rapport. If you are a good listener, people will like talking to you and you will gather all the information that you need. The following are guidelines on how to listen to people:

- Clear your mind of thoughts, as it is not easy to listen to listen and think at the same time.
- Avoid jumping to conclusions or prejudging a person by how the person looks or talks.
- Establish eye contact, but keep your eyes soft so the client does not feel you are staring at them.
- Once the client has answered your questions, summarise the main points of what they have said and even take notes.
- Give the client your full attention and avoid fidgeting.

As you are consulting, you also need to consider non-verbal communication, which is body language and facial expressions. It is best to keep your body language open, which means that you should not cross your arms or legs, as they look like a barrier, and you should sit in a posture that makes it look like you are interested – for example, leaning forward slightly, but not in a threatening way. You should keep your expression relaxed and maintain eye contact when you are listening. Taken together, working on your questioning and listening skills and your non-verbal communication will help improve your consultation skills.

Key learning point 2

- A lifestyle questionnaire should address levels of activity, alcohol consumption, smoking, stress levels and diet. A one-to-one consultation should follow up a lifestyle questionnaire.

Q Quick quiz 2

Which of the following statements are true and which are false?

1. There should be an equal amount of talking between the trainer and the client during a consultation.
2. Once rapport has been created, the client will accept the advice that you offer.
3. Indirect questions can be used to put a client at ease.
4. 'How do you feel your training is going?' is a closed question.
5. When you are listening, it is important to summarise what the client is telling you.

14.4 Lifestyle Improvement

P3 M3 P2

Physical Activity

When designing a physical activity programme, it is important to make the programme as personal as possible. It must meet the needs of the individual it is written for or it will result in the person being unhappy or unsuccessful. The key to this is gathering as much information as possible on the individual, by asking questions such as:

- What activities do you like to take part in?
- What have you done in the past that you enjoyed?
- Do you like to exercise alone or with other people?

You should take into account the facilities in the person's area. Do they live near a gym or leisure centre? One of the biggest factors to put people off going to a gym is if it is quite some distance away and takes them a while to get there. If the gym is close to where they live or work, this makes it a much more viable option. They could go to the gym in their lunch break or on the way to or from work.

Increasing Daily Activity

It is actually unnecessary to join a gym or go to a swimming pool to increase physical activity levels. There are lots of ways to attain the benefits of physical activity by just adapting everyday life. If a person takes the bus or train to work, they could get off one or two stops earlier and walk the remaining distance. If a person drives to work, they could park further away from their workplace and walk the remaining distance. If cycling to work is a viable option, it is not only good for you but is also cheaper and better for the environment. Many new cycle paths are being constructed to encourage people to cycle. Choosing options such as walking up a flight of stairs instead of taking a lift or escalator also help to increase a person's activity levels.

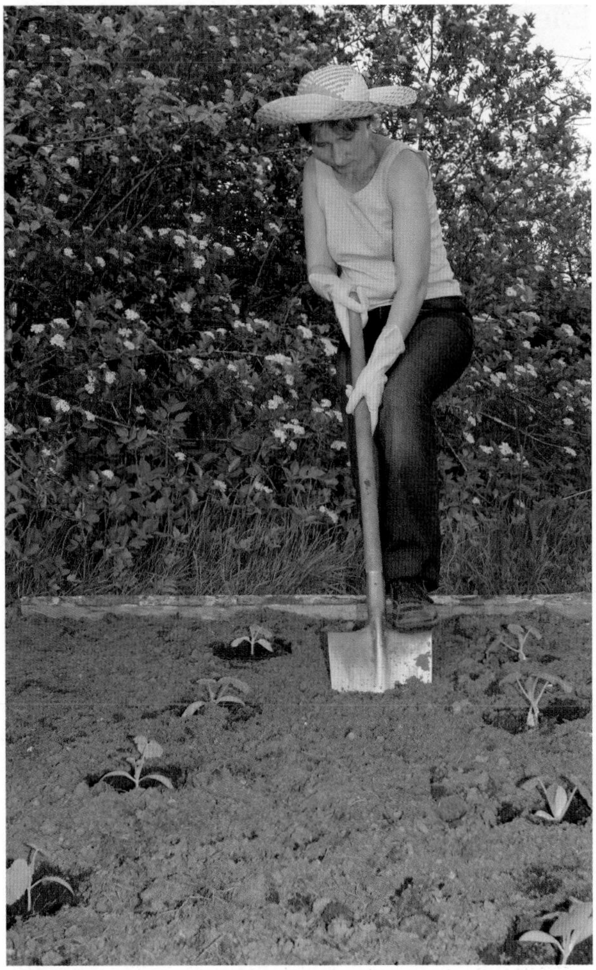

Fig 14.6 Gardening can increase heart rate and help tone muscles

Housework and gardening are productive ways of increasing daily activity levels. Vacuum cleaning and dusting the home, or digging the garden or mowing the lawn will increase heart rate and help tone muscles.

Reducing Alcohol Consumption

If a person is dependent on alcohol they must seek help to prevent the damage it does to their body and mind and to those around them.

In order to determine if a person is drinking more than the government recommended amounts of alcohol, it is a good idea to keep a 'drinking diary'. This involves noting what, how much and when that person drinks alcohol. If the person is just over the limit, simple changes could help them cut down. If they usually drink strong lager, they could opt for one that contains less alcohol. Or if they usually drink wine, they could have a spritzer instead, as this will make their drink last longer and help them to drink less. If they regularly meet up with friends in pubs, they could try to find alternative venues, such as a juice bar or coffee shop.

A GP can provide confidential advice and support. In order to help prevent the withdrawal symptoms of drinking, they may be prescribed antidepressants (e.g. Valium). Two drug treatments are also available to help a person stop drinking. A drug called Disulfiram makes the person feel very ill if they drink even a small amount of alcohol. Another drug called Acamprosate helps to reduce a person's craving for alcohol, but it does have many unpleasant side-effects. A person may attend organisations such as Alcohol Concern and Alcoholics Anonymous to help them stop drinking alcohol.

Stopping Smoking

Smokers have both a physical and a psychological addiction to smoking. The combination of these two factors makes cigarettes one of the most addictive drugs used today. Determining whether you are more physiologically than psychologically addicted to smoking will help to decide the best course of action in trying to stop smoking.

First of all, a person needs to think about why they smoke and identify the things they do that always make them want to light up. Once these triggers have been identified, the person can attempt to remove themselves from them. The next step is to decrease the person's dependence on nicotine. Either they can slowly decrease the amount of cigarettes they smoke over a set period or they could use a nicotine replacement therapy, such as a nicotine patch and/or nicotine gum. This process helps the person break the cigarette habit and also slowly reduces the amount of nicotine being taken into the body.

The NHS has set up a smoking helpline and runs clinics to help advise people on how to give up smoking. Each year there is a national no-smoking day, which has also been effective in making people think about giving up smoking and giving them a clear target day to attempt to stop.

Reducing Stress through Stress Management Techniques

The main methods of stress management are:

- Progressive muscular relaxation
- Mind-to-muscle relaxation
- Meditation/centring.

Progressive Muscular Relaxation

Progressive muscular relaxation (PMR) involves a person tensing and relaxing the muscle groups individually and sequentially to relax their whole body and mind. It is also called 'muscle-to-mind' relaxation, as muscles are tensed and relaxed to induce complete relaxation. Each muscle is tensed and relaxed to teach the person the difference between a tense muscle and a relaxed muscle. After a muscle is tensed, the relaxation effect is deepened, which also has an effect on the involuntary muscles.

The technique is practised using a series of taped instructions, or with the psychologist giving the instructions. It usually starts at the hands by making a tight fist and then relaxing. The tensing and relaxing carries on up the arms into the shoulders, face and neck, then down to the stomach and through the hips and legs.

These sessions last between 20 and 30 minutes, and need to be practised about five times a day to gain the maximum effect. Each time they are practised they have an increased effect and a person can relax more quickly and more deeply. The aim is that when the person needs to use the relaxation technique quickly, they can induce relaxation using a trigger, such as tensing the hand or the shoulders.

Mind-to-muscle Relaxation

Mind-to-muscle relaxation is also called imagery and involves the use of a mental room or a mental place. This is a place where a person can quickly picture themselves to produce feelings of relaxation when they need to relax.

Again, it involves the person using a taped script, or a psychologist giving instructions. Usually the psychologist asks a person to build a mental picture of a room. This is a room where they can feel relaxed and where there is somewhere to sit or lie down. It should be decorated in a pleasing manner. Alternatively, the person may imagine a relaxing place, such as somewhere they went on their holidays, or a beach or quiet place where they feel calm and relaxed. They are taught to imagine this place in detail and to feel the sensations associated with being there. They do this about five times, so that eventually they can go there when they need to and are able to relax more quickly and more deeply. As the person relaxes their mind, they feel the sensations transferring to their muscle groups and they can achieve overall body relaxation. It tends to work best for individuals who have good imagery skills. Other people may feel that PMR is more effective for them.

Meditation/Centring

Meditation/centring techniques involve the person focusing on one thing, such as their breathing (centring) or a mantra (meditation). By focusing their attention they become more and more relaxed. Again, these feelings of relaxation can eventually be produced when needed.

Diet

Food Preparation

The way food is prepared has a huge impact on its nutritional value. We should eat a fair amount of potatoes, but if you fry the potatoes to make chips, the food then belongs in the fats and oils food group, as it now has such a high concentration of fat.

You can prepare foods in certain ways to make them much healthier.

Breads and grains

- Use lots of wholemeal pasta and a small portion of sauce to prepare pasta dishes.
- Make sandwiches out of thick slices of wholemeal bread.
- Mash sweet potatoes and regular potatoes in larger than usual quantities for a shepherd's pie topping.

Fruits and vegetables

- Eat dried fruit, fresh fruit or vegetable sticks (e.g. carrot sticks) as snacks.
- A selection of vegetables or salads can accompany each main meal.
- Make fruit-based puddings, such as poached pears or apple and blackberry crumble.
- Add dried or fresh fruit to breakfast cereals.
- Include more vegetables in casserole dishes.

Meat, fish and vegetarian alternatives

- Use lean meat and remove skin and fat where possible.
- Grill meats wherever possible.
- Include pulses in meat dishes to reduce the fat

content and increase the fibre content, such as kidney beans in a chilli.
- Try to eat two portions of oily fish per week.

Milk and dairy foods
- Choose semi-skimmed or skimmed milk and low-fat or reduced-fat cheeses.
- Replace cream with fromage frais or yoghurt.
- Use strong-tasting cheese in cooking so that you require smaller amounts.

Foods containing fat and foods containing sugar
- Do not fry foods containing fat as it will just add more fat to them. Instead, grill or dry-bake them (without oil) in the oven.
- Use small amounts of plant-based cooking oils (e.g. olive oil or rapeseed) when frying foods.
- Make salad dressings with a balsamic vinegar base instead of oil.
- Sweeten puddings with dried or fresh fruits instead of sugar.
- Drink fresh water instead of fizzy drinks.

Timing of Food Intake

There is a saying that you should 'Eat breakfast like a king, lunch like a prince and dinner like a pauper.' This basically means that you should have your main meal at breakfast time, have a good-sized lunch and then eat your smallest meal at dinner time. The reasoning behind this saying is to have enough energy for the day and then to digest the food properly before going to bed. Heavy meals eaten before bedtime, such as a curry, take a long time to digest, which may disturb sleep. Any excess calories eaten during this meal will most probably be turned into body fat, as very few people actually take any form of exercise after a late heavy meal.

Key learning points 3

- Physical activity levels can be increased by adapting an individual's daily activities.
- A drinking diary can make a person aware of how much alcohol they are consuming.
- Nicotine replacement therapy and NHS support can help people stop smoking.
- Relaxation techniques, such as PMR and mind-to-muscle relaxation, can help reduce stress.
- The way foods are prepared and the timing of their intake can have an impact on an individual's health.

Q Quick quiz 3

Fill in the blank spaces to complete the following sentences.

In order to help a person improve their lifestyle it is important to increase their ______ ______. It would be beneficial to ______ or ______ to work rather than take the car. When at home, gardening and housework can be used to raise the ______ ______. It would improve health if alcohol consumption was reduced by keeping a ______ ______, or, if a person smokes, by using ______ ______ ______. Stress can cause people to smoke or drink more alcohol, but it can be reduced by using ______ techniques or using ______ to take them to a mental place or room. Also, diet can be improved by eating less ______ and more ______ and ______.

14.5 Planning a Health-related Physical Activity Programme

P4

Collecting Information

When a trainer sits down to design a physical activity programme, they need to consider a range of factors to ensure that the programme is appropriate and that it will benefit the person rather than harm them. They will need to consider the following factors:

- PAR-Q responses – have any contraindications to exercise been identified?
- Medical history – does the client have any conditions which may affect the training programme and choice of exercises?
- Current and previous exercise history – this will give an idea about the current fitness level of the client.
- Barriers to exercise – does the client have constraints such as time, cost, family responsibilities or work commitments?
- Motives and goals – what is the client aiming to achieve and what is their time-scale?

- Occupation – what hours does the client work, and is their work manual or office-based?
- Activity levels – what amount of movement does the client do on a daily basis?
- Leisure-time activities – are these active or inactive?
- Diet – what, how much and when does the client eat?
- Stress levels – how does the client deal with stress, either through work or in their home life?
- Alcohol intake – how much does the client consume and how often?
- Smoking – is the client a smoker or ex-smoker, and how much do they smoke?
- Time available – the client needs to fit the training into their schedule and the trainer needs to be realistic when planning the programme.

Goal Setting

Short-term goals are set over a brief period of time, usually from one day to one month. A short-term goal may relate to what you want to achieve in one training session or where you want to be by the end of the month.

Long-term goals run from three months to a period of several years. You may even set some lifetime goals, which run until you retire from your sport. In sport, we set long-term goals to cover a season or a sporting year. The period between one and three months would be called medium-term goals.

Usually, short-term goals are set to help achieve the long-term goals. It is important to set both short- and long-term goals, but particularly short-term goals, because they will give a person more motivation to act immediately.

When goals are set, you need to use the SMART principle to make them workable. SMART stands for:

- **S**pecific
- **M**easurable
- **A**chievable
- **R**ealistic
- **T**ime-constrained.

Specific
The goal must be specific to what you want to achieve. It is not enough to say, 'I want to get fitter'. You need to say, 'I want to improve strength/speed/stamina.'

Measurable
Goals must be stated in a way that is measurable, so a goal needs to state figures, for example, 'I want to cut down my alcohol intake to five units per week.'

Achievable
It must be possible to actually achieve the goal.

Realistic
We need to be realistic in our setting of goals and look at what factors may stop us achieving them.

Time-constrained
There must be a time-scale or deadline for the goal. This allows you to review your success. It is best to set a date by which you wish to achieve the goal.

Strategies to Achieve Goals

Some commonly used and effective strategies are as follows:

- **Using a decision balance sheet**: an individual writes down all the gains they will make by exercising and all the things they may lose through taking up exercise. Hopefully, the gains will outweigh the losses and this list will help to motivate them at difficult times.
- **Prompts**: an individual puts up posters or reminders around the house that will keep giving them reminders to exercise. This could also be done with little coloured dots on mirrors or other places where they look regularly.
- **Rewards for attendance/completing goals**: the individual is provided with an extrinsic reward for completing the goal or attending the gym regularly. This may be something to pamper themselves, such as a massage, and should not be something that conflicts with the goal – such as a slap-up meal!
- **Social support approaches**: you can help people to exercise regularly by developing a social support group of like-minded people with similar fitness goals, so that they can arrange to meet at the gym at certain times. This makes it more difficult for people to miss their exercise session. Also, try to gain the backing of the people they live with, to support them rather than teasing or criticising them.

Principles of Training

In order to develop a safe and effective training programme, you will need to consider the principles of training. These principles are a set of guidelines to help you understand the requirements of programme design. They are:

- Frequency
- Intensity
- Time
- Type
- Overload
- Reversibility
- Specificity.

- **Frequency:** this is how often the person will train per week.
- **Intensity**: this is how hard the person will work. It is usually expressed as a percentage of maximum intensity.
- **Time**: this indicates how long the person will train for in each session.
- **Type**: this shows the type of training the person will perform and needs to be individual to each person.
- **Overload**: this shows that to make an improvement, a muscle or system must work slightly harder than it is used to. This may be as simple as getting a sedentary person to walk for ten minutes or getting an athlete to squat more weight than have done previously.
- **Reversibility**: this principle states that if a fitness gain is not used regularly, the body will reverse it and go back to its previous fitness level. It is commonly known as 'use it or lose it'.
- **Specificity**: this principle states that any fitness gain will be specific to the muscles or system to which the overload is applied. Put simply, this says that different types of training will produce different results. To make a programme specific, you need to look at the needs of the person and then train them accordingly. For example, a person who was overweight would need to take part in lots of low-intensity cardiovascular training in order to burn fat.

Appropriate Activities

When you are devising your training programme you need to be sure that you are including activities that are appropriate to your client. If your client is obese, a training programme that includes jogging would probably not be appropriate. This kind of exercise is a high-impact exercise which places a lot of stress on the joints. If a person is obese, they will be stressing their joints to a greater degree, which means they would be much more likely to injure or damage their joints. Therefore, walking or swimming would be much more appropriate, as these activities place much less stress on the joints.

You should also try to include activities that you know your client enjoys. That way, they will be much more likely to continue their exercise programme.

Exercise Intensity

The intensity of exercise can be monitored by expressing it as a percentage of maximum heart rate. Your maximum heart rate is the maximum number of times your heart could beat. To find this out, you would have to work to your maximum intensity, which for most people would clearly be unsafe. Therefore, we estimate the maximum heart rate by using the following formula:

Maximum heart rate = 220 − age

So, for a 17-year-old, their maximum heart rate would be 220 − 17 = 203 beats per minute (b.p.m.).

To work out the heart rate training zone, we take percentages of heart rate maximum. If we work between 60 and 90 per cent, we would be working in the aerobic training zone, where the exercise we are performing is effective in improving aerobic fitness without being dangerous. However, it is still a wide range for a heart rate to be within, so we change the zone depending on the fitness level of the participant.

Rate of perceived exertion (RPE) is another measure used to monitor exercise. RPE is scale that can be used by the participant to rate how hard they feel they are working between two extremes. Rather than monitoring heart rate, the participant is introduced to the scale and then asked during the aerobic session where they feel they are. Below is Borg's modified RPE scale.

1 Extremely light.
2 Very light.
3 Moderate.
4
5 Somewhat hard.
6
7 Hard.
8 Very hard.
9 Extremely hard.
10 Maximal exertion.

To achieve aerobic fitness gains, the participant needs to be working at around 6 to 7 on the modified scale.

Key learning points 4

- Ensure you collect all relevant information from your client to assess their lifestyle and determine any contraindications.
- Ensure you set short-term and long-term goals.
- Apply the principles of training to your training programme.
- Ensure your training programme incorporates appropriate activities.
- Ensure your client exercises at the appropriate intensity.
- Effective zones for different groups as a percentage of maximum heart rate (MHR) are: beginners – 60 to 70 per cent of MHR; intermediate – 70 to 80 per cent of MHR; advanced – 80 to 90 per cent of MHR.

Student activity 14.1

3 hours

Read through the following case study and then complete the tasks that follow.

Eddie is a full-time student who is studying a demanding course at university; he attends lectures from 9 a.m. to 5 p.m. every day. He also loves playing sport and plays football and cricket for the university; he also enjoys golf. Although he enjoys playing sport, he does not enjoy the training and feels that it gets in the way of his social life. He enjoys socialising and spends most evenings in the pub, even sometimes the night before a match. He worked out his alcohol consumption as 35 units per week, but he thinks it could be higher, and he has been smoking on what he sees as being a 'social basis', consisting of three to four cigarettes a day.

Eddie does not really have a weight issue and he is able to get good food from the canteen. He knows he needs to eat fruit and vegetables, so he makes sure that he eats as much fresh food as he can and only occasionally eats takeaways. However, he hardly ever eats breakfast as he prefers to spend the time in bed.

In terms of his current activity, Eddie plays football at the weekend and he does have a bike, but he chooses to get the university bus each day and occasionally goes training with the football team, which is mainly circuit training.

Task 1

P1 M1

Choose three lifestyle factors from the case study and describe the effect each one has on Eddie's health and well-being. To achieve a merit you need to explain the effects that each of the three lifestyle factors may have on Eddie's health and well-being.

Task 2

P2 M2 D1

1 Design a lifestyle questionnaire that could be used describe the strengths and weaknesses of Eddie's lifestyle.

2 Use a role-playing exercise with a fellow student; you should play the role of the consultant and your fellow student should play the role of Eddie. In this role play, use the questionnaire to gain as much information about Eddie as you can.

To achieve **P2** you need to describe the strengths and areas for improvement of Eddie's lifestyle. To achieve **M2** you need to explain these strengths and areas for improvement. To achieve **D1** you need to evaluate Eddie's lifestyle and make a list of priorities for changing and improving it.

Task 3

P3 M3 D2

Now that you have analysed the areas that Eddie has to improve, you need to decide the strategies you are going to use to help him to do this (**P3**). To achieve **M3** you need to explain why you have made these recommendations to improve Eddie's lifestyle. To achieve **D2** you need to analyse the effectiveness of these chosen methods.

Task 4

P4

Now that you have looked at Eddie's lifestyle you need to focus on his physical activity and produce a six-week physical activity plan to help improve his health. Be sure to incorporate his current activity into the plan. You can use the following template to help him.

	Week 1	Week 2	Week 3	Week 4	Week 5	Week 6
Monday						
Tuesday						
Wednesday						
Thursday						
Friday						
Saturday						
Sunday						

Useful websites

www.bhf.org.uk

Tips on how to keep your heart healthy

www.getbodysmart.com

Free tutorials and quizzes from an American site that looks at human anatomy and physiology, helping you to see the structure of the different body systems.

www.innerbody.com

Free and informative diagrams of the different body systems, including respiratory, cardiovascular, skeletal and muscular

www.topendsports.com

Provides online articles for athletes, covering a wide range of health, exercise & lifestyle issues

Further reading

Baechle, T. and Earle, R. (2008) *Essentials of Strength Training and Conditioning*, Human Kinetics.

Dalgleish, J. and Dollery, S. (2001) *The Health and Fitness Handbook*, Longman.

Sharkey, B.J. and Gaskill, S.E. (2006). *Fitness and Health*, Human Kinetics.

17: Psychology for sports performance

17.1 Introduction

Success in sport is derived from a series of variable factors. The athlete must be prepared physically, have the correct nutritional strategy, and ensure that they are appropriately recovered and in a positive mental state. Sport psychology deals with ensuring that the performer has this correct mental state and is able to control this state during training and training periods.

By the end of this unit you should:

- know the effect of personality and motivation on sports performance
- know the relationship between stress, anxiety, arousal and sports performance
- know the role of group dynamics in team sports
- be able to plan a psychological skills training programme to enhance sports performance.

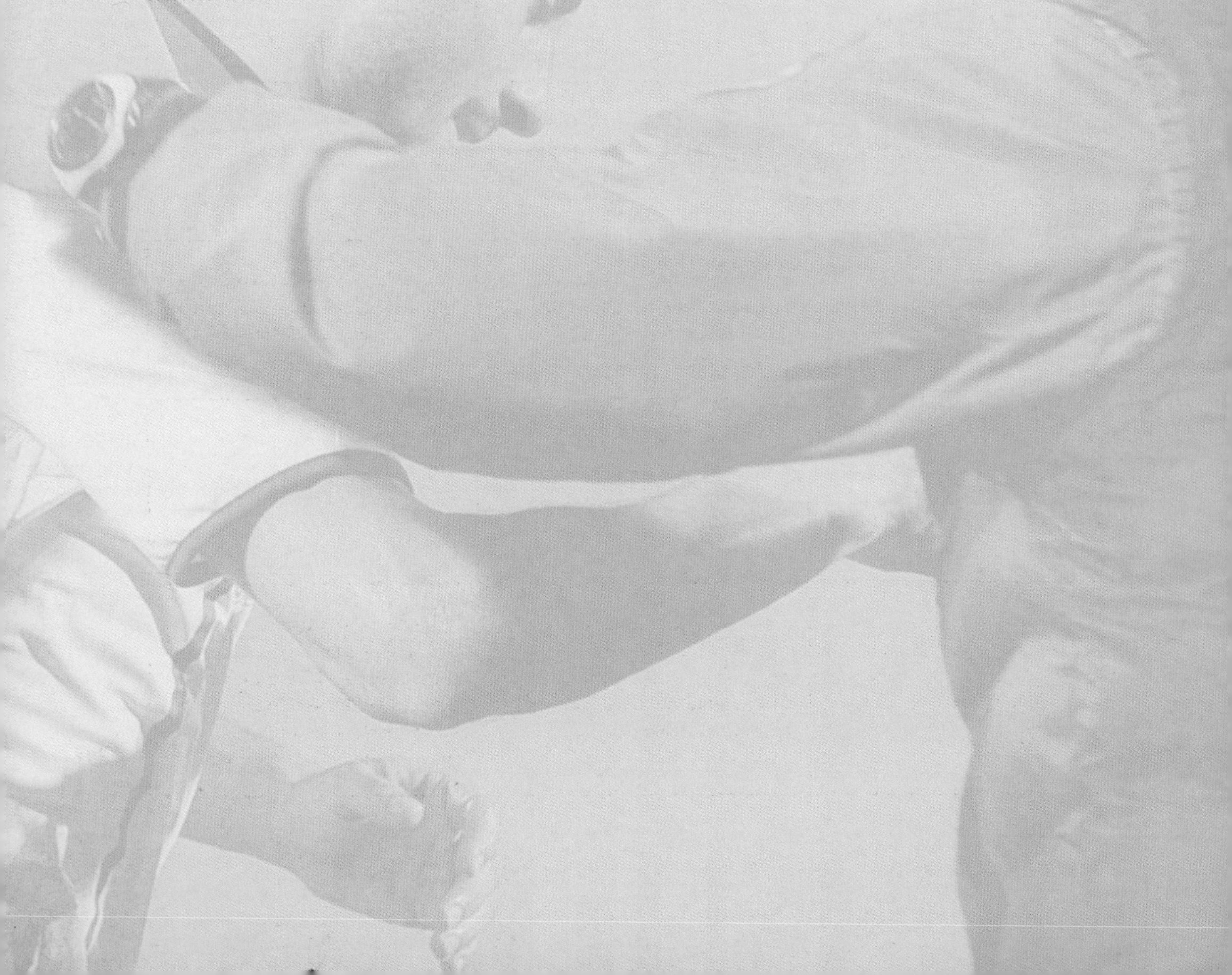

Assessment and grading criteria		
To achieve a PASS grade the evidence must show that the learner is able to:	**To achieve a MERIT grade the evidence must show that, in addition to the pass criteria, the learner is able to:**	**To achieve a DISTINCTION grade the evidence must show that, in addition to the pass and merit criteria, the learner is able to:**
P1 define personality and how it affects sports performance	**M1** explain the effects of personality and motivation on sports performance	**D1** evaluate the effects of personality and motivation on sports performance
P2 describe motivation and how it affects sports performance		
P3 describe stress and anxiety, their causes, symptoms and effect on sports performance		
P4 describe three theories of arousal and the effect on sports performance	**M2** explain three theories of arousal and the effect on sports performance	
P5 identify four factors which influence group dynamics and performance in team sports	**M3** explain four factors which influence group dynamics and performance in team sports	**D2** analyse four factors which influence group dynamics and performance in team sports
P6 assess the current psychological skills of a selected sports performer, identifying strengths and areas for improvement (IE2)		
P7 plan a six-week psychological skills training programme to enhance performance for a selected sports performer.	**M4** explain the design of the six-week psychological skills training programme for a selected sports performer.	**D3** justify the design of the six-week psychological skills training programme for a selected sports performer, making suggestions for improvement.

17.2 The Effects of Personality and Motivation on Sports Performance

41499

P1 P2 M1 D1

The key concept that underpins all studies in sport psychology is personality. It is clear that each person has the same brain structure and that their senses will all work in the same way to provide the brain with information. However, each person appears to be different in the decisions they make and how they behave in specific situations. Personality looks at these individual differences and how they affect performance.

There is a range of definitions of personality, each with its merits and drawbacks. It has been suggested that we all have traits and behaviour that we share with other people, but we also have some particular to ourselves. However, this idea does lack depth of information, as does Cattell's (1965) attempt to define personality: 'that which tells what a man will do when placed in a given situation.'

This suggests that if we know an individual's personality, we can predict their behaviour. However, human beings tend to be less than predictable and can act out of character, depending on the situation. Their behaviour may also be affected by their mood, fatigue or emotions.

Eysenck (1964) sought to address the limitations of previous definitions: 'The more or less stable and enduring organisation of an individual's character, temperament, intellect and physique which determines their unique adjustment to the environment.' Eysenck's statement that personality is more or less stable allows the human element to enter the equation and explain the unpredictable. He also makes the important point that personality is 'unique'. We may have behaviour in common with other people, but, ultimately, every person has a set of characteristics unique to themselves.

In summary, most personality theories state the following: personality is the set of individual characteristics that make a person unique and will determine their relatively consistent patterns of behaviour.

By giving labels to a person's character and behaviour, you have started to assess personality. By observing sportspeople, we are using a behavioural approach – assessing what they are like by assessing their responses to various situations. In reality, our observations may be unreliable because we see sportspeople in only one environment, and although we see them interviewed as well, we do not know what they are truly like. A cognitive psychologist believes we need to understand an individual's thoughts and emotions, as well as watching their behaviour. This we cannot do without the use of a questionnaire or an interview.

Personality Theories

Jarvis (2006) identifies four factors that will determine how an individual responds in a specific situation:

1. Our genetic make-up – the innate aspect of our personality that we inherit from our parents.
2. Our past experiences – these are important because if we have acted in a certain way in the past and it had a successful outcome, it is likely that we will act in the same way in the future; or if we have had a negative experience in the past, the same experience in the future will be seen as being threatening or stressful.
3. The nature of the situation in which we find ourselves – this will cause us to adapt our behaviour in a way that suits the situation.
4. Free will – a difficult concept in psychology, which suggests we have control over our thinking and thus our behaviour; it can be difficult to separate whether a person has chosen to behave in that way or is programmed by their genetics or past experiences.

Martens' Schematic View of Personality

Martens views personality as having three different depths or layers:

- Level 1 – the psychological core is the deepest component of personality and is at its centre. It includes an individual's beliefs, attitudes, values and feelings of self-worth. It is 'the real you' and, as a result, it is relatively permanent and seen by few people.
- Level 2 – typical responses are how we usually respond to situations and adapt to our environment. It is seen as the relatively consistent way we behave. Our typical responses are good indicators of our psychological core, but they can be affected by the social environment. A person who is very outgoing and sociable with his rugby-playing friends may become more reserved at a party with people he does not know.
- Level 3 – role-related behaviour is the shallowest level of our personality, and this level shows how we change our behaviour to adapt to the situation we are in. For example, throughout the day, we may play the roles of sportsperson, student, employee, friend, son/daughter, coach, and so on. In order to survive, we need to adapt our personalities, as it

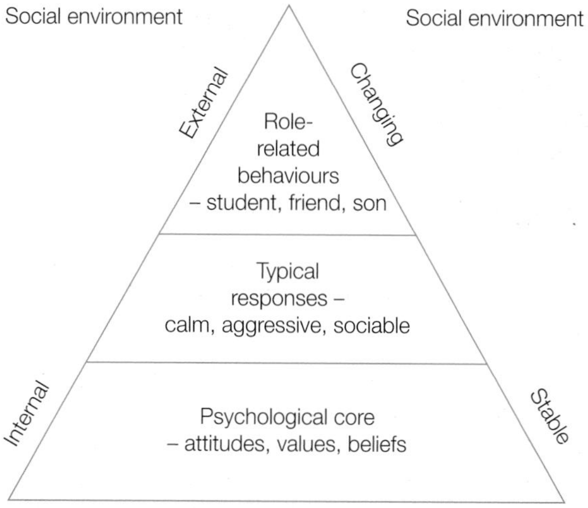

Fig 17.1 Martens' personality levels

would not be appropriate to behave on the sports field in the same manner as when studying in class. We need to modify our personalities to suit the situation.

Trait Theory

The trait approach to personality relates to the first factor of personality. Jarvis (2006) identifies that personality is based in genetics. This is called the nature approach and says that we inherit personality at birth. This has some validity. For example, we can observe how different babies have different personalities from a young age. A trait is defined as 'a relatively stable way of behaving', suggesting that if a person shows a trait of shyness in one situation, they will be shy across a range of situations. Across a population, the traits people have are the same, but they show them to a greater or lesser extent, and this dictates their personality. This theory was very popular in the 1960s, but it is continually criticised for not considering that the situation may influence an individual's behaviour.

Situational Approach

The situational approach, or social learning theory, takes the view that personality is determined by the environment and the experiences a person has as they grow up. Other theories (e.g. trait theory) take the nature or biological approach to personality in that they see it as being largely genetic or inherited. The social learning theory sees personality as the result of nurture or past experiences.

Cox (2007) outlines the two mechanisms of learning: modelling and social reinforcement:

- Modelling: as we grow up, we observe and imitate the behaviour of significant others in our lives. At first, this is our parents and siblings, then our friends, teachers, sports stars and anyone we regard as a role model.
- Social reinforcement: this means that when behaviour is rewarded positively, it is more likely that it will be repeated. Conversely, behaviour negatively rewarded is less likely to be repeated. At an early age, our parents teach us right and wrong by positively or negatively rewarding behaviour.

In sport, there is a system of negative reinforcement to discourage negative behaviour on the sports field. Thus, rugby players are sent to the sin bin, cricketers are fined part of their match fee, and footballers are shown yellow and red cards. In particular, this theory shows why people behave differently in different situations. For example, an athlete may be confident and outgoing in a sporting setting, but shy and quiet in an educational setting. The athlete may have chosen positive role models in the sporting environment and had their successful performances rewarded. In the educational setting, they may have modelled less appropriate behaviour and had their behaviour rewarded negatively.

Interactional Approach

The trait theory of personality is criticised for not taking into account the situation that determines behaviour. The situational approach is criticised because research shows that while situation influences some people's behaviour, other people will not be influenced in the same way. The interactional approach considers the person's psychological traits and the situation they are in as equal predictors of behaviour.

$$\text{behaviour} = f\,(\text{personality, environment})$$

Thus, we can understand an individual's behaviour by assessing their personality traits and the specific situation they find themselves in. Bowers (1973) says the interaction between a person and their situation could give twice as much information as traits or the situational approach alone.

An interactional psychologist would use a trait–state approach to assess an individual's personality traits and then assess how these traits affect their behaviour in a situation (state). For example, an athlete who exhibits high anxiety levels as a personality trait would have an exaggerated response to a specific situation.

Neither personality traits nor situations alone are enough to predict an individual's behaviour. We must consider both to get a real picture.

Type A and Type B Personalities

Friedman (1996) developed a questionnaire to diagnose people who were prone to stress and

Type A behaviour:

- Highly competitive and strong desire to succeed
- Achievement orientated
- Eat fast, walk fast, talk fast and have a strong sense of urgency
- Aggressive, restless and impatient
- Find it difficult to delegate and need to be in control
- Experience high levels of stress.

Type B behaviour:

- Less competitive
- More relaxed
- Delegate work easily
- Take time to complete their tasks
- Calm, laid-back and patient
- Experience low levels of stress.

Name of researcher/s	Questionnaire used and groups studied	Research findings
Schurr, Ashley and Joy (1977)	16PF: 1500 American students – athletes versus non-athletes	Athletes were more: • Independent • Objective • Relaxed. Athletes who played team sports were: • More outgoing and warm-hearted (A) • Less intelligent (B) • More group-dependent (Q2) • Less emotionally stable (C). Athletes who played individual sports were: More group-dependent (Q2) Less anxious (Q4) Less intelligent (B).
Francis *et al.* (1998)	EPQ: 133 female hockey players versus non-athlete students	Hockey players were: • More extroverted • Higher in psychoticism.
Ogilvie (1968)	16PF: athletes versus non-athletes	Athletic performance is related to: • Emotional stability • Tough-mindedness • Conscientiousness • Self-discipline • Self-assurance • Trust • Extroversion • Low tension.
Breivik (1996)	16PF: 38 elite Norwegian climbers	Research showed: • High levels of stability • Extroversion • Adventure seeking.
Williams (1980)	Female athletes versus female non-athletes	Athletes were: • More independent • More aggressive and dominant • More emotionally stable.

Table 17.1 **Trait theory research (from Weinberg and Gould, 2007)**

stress-related illnesses. However, it has some application to sport and exercise.

Type Bs will exhibit the opposite types of behaviour to type As. In sport, we see both personality types being equally successful. However, with people exercising recreationally, we see higher levels of retention on their exercise programmes. Type As would benefit from exercise, as it promotes type B-related behaviour. Type A behaviour is seen as causing a rise in a person's blood pressure and increasing the risk of coronary heart disease (CHD).

Personality and Sports Performance

The majority of research using trait theory was carried out in the 1970s and 1980s. Table 17.1 summarises this research.

Motivation

If a sports psychologist were asked why athletes of similar talents achieve different levels of performance, they would consider several factors, such as personality and ability to cope with stress. However, if one subject could be said to influence everything in sports psychology, it would be motivation – the reasons why we do what we do and behave and respond in the manner particular to us.

Psychologists would say that there is a reason for everything we do in life, and that some of these motives are conscious and some are unconscious. As a result, it can be difficult to assess our own motivating factors, let alone anyone else's.

Motivation is important to coaches and managers as they seek to get the best performances out of their athletes. Arsene Wenger and Alex Ferguson are two football managers who are seen as being great motivators of people.

Motivation can be a difficult subject to pin down and deal with because it is not steady and constant and depends on many factors. Most people will experience fluctuations in motivation. Some days they are fully prepared for the competition mentally, and on other days they just cannot seem to get themselves in the right frame of mind. This applies to everything we may do in a day, as sometimes it takes all our powers of motivation just to get out of bed!

Key terms

Motivation:

- 'Motive – a desire to fulfil a need' (Cox, 2007)
- 'The internal mechanisms which arouse and direct behaviour' (Sage, 1974)
- 'The direction and intensity of one's effort' (Sage, 1977).

When examining motivation, five terms come up again and again:

- Fulfilling a need – all motivation arises as we seek to fulfil our needs. These may be basic biological needs, such as finding food and shelter, or more sophisticated needs, such as self-esteem or the need to belong and be loved.
- Internal state – a state is 'how we feel at any point in time', and this will be subject to change. As we see and feel things, they will trigger an internal state that will need actions to fulfil any needs.
- Direction – the direction of effort refers to the actions we take to move towards what we feel motivated by and feel we need.
- Intensity – the intensity of effort refers to how much effort the person puts into achieving their goal or into a certain situation.
- Energise behaviour – this shows how the power of the brain and the thoughts we have can give us the energy we need to produce the behaviour that is required to be successful in a certain situation.

Intrinsic and Extrinsic Motivation

To expand on Sage's definition, we can see motivation as coming from internal mechanisms or sources inside the body. We can call these intrinsic factors, or rewards coming from the activity itself. These include motives such as fun, pleasure, enjoyment, feelings of self-worth, excitement and self-mastery. They are the reasons why we do a sport and keep doing it.

> Those who are intrinsically motivated engage in an activity for the pleasure and satisfaction they experience while learning, exploring or trying to understand something new.
> (Weinberg and Gould, 2007)

The external stimuli, also called extrinsic rewards, come from sources outside the activity. This would include the recognition and praise we get from other people, such as our coach, friends and family. It could also be the approval we get from the crowd who support us. Extrinsic motivating factors would also include trophies, medals, prizes, records and any money derived from success.

> Those who are extrinsically motivated engage in the activity because of the valued outcome rather than the interest in the activity solely for itself.
> (Weinberg and Gould, 2007)

Theories of Motivation

Achievement motivation

> I do not play to win; I play to fight against the idea of losing. (Eric Cantona, Manchester United, 1997)

Achievement motivation is seen as a personality factor and describes our persistence in striving for success, irrespective of the bad experiences and obstacles that are put in our way. It can be seen as our level of 'competitiveness' or desire for success. Achievement motivation is not that simple, however, as the quote from Eric Cantona shows. Some people are driven to success and have no fear of failure, while others are driven to succeed because they have a deep-rooted fear of failure. This paradox was addressed by McClelland *et al.* (1953) in their theory of the need for achievement.

In certain sporting situations, we may have conflicting feelings: on the one hand, we want to take part and achieve success; on the other hand, we are motivated to avoid the situation by our need to avoid failure. The relative strength of these emotions influences our achievement motivation:

Achievement motivation = need to achieve (nACH) − need to avoid failure (naF)

If our nACH outweighs our naF, we are said to be high in achievement motivation; if our naF outweighs our nACH, we are said to be low in achievement motivation. This will influence our behaviour in sport and the types of challenges we seek.

A sportsperson with a high need to achieve will choose competitive situations and opponents close to their skill level who will challenge them. A person with a high fear of failure will choose opponents of much higher skill or much lower skill because these people are less threatening to them; they will also tend to avoid situations involving personal challenges.

The situation will also affect achievement motivation. If the probability of success is high, it tends to weaken the need to achieve because the reward for success is low; if the probability of success is low and failure is likely, it tends to weaken the need to avoid failure.

Weiner's attribution theory

The reasons we give for an outcome are called attributions. We are attributing that outcome to a certain factor. We all make attributions about our own performances, as well as those of other people. It is important for us to make attributions because:

- they affect our motivation levels
- we need to understand the outcome so that we can learn from our experiences
- they will affect our future expectations of success and failure.

Attributions fall into four categories:

1. **Ability or skill** – a performer's capability in performing skills.
2. **Effort** – the amount of physical or mental effort put into a task.
3. **Task difficulty** – the problems posed by the task, such as the strength of the opposition or the difficulty of a move.
4. **Luck** – factors attributed to chance, such as the effect of the weather, the referee or the run of the ball.

As shown in Table 17.2, these four categories can be classified as internal (inside an individual), external (outside the individual), stable (not subject to change) or unstable (continually changing).

	Internal	External
Stable	Ability	Task difficulty
Unstable	Effort	Luck

Table 17.2 Categories of attributions

Research findings

Research shows that winners tend to give internal attributions and take responsibility for their successes. They will usually say, 'I won because I tried hard', or 'I am more talented'. Losers, meanwhile, tend to give external attributions and distance themselves from their failures. For example, they will say, 'The task was too difficult', or 'The referee was against me'. These attributions can be seen as ego-enhancing and ego-protective, respectively. Winners give internal attributions to make themselves feel even better; losers give external attributions so they do not feel so bad.

Attributions and self-confidence

If we make a more stable attribution – that is, to ability or task difficulty – it is more realistic and gives a clearer indication of future expectations and confidence. However, attribution to unstable factors can act to protect the ego and reduce loss of self-confidence.

This is important because confidence levels will influence motivation – the more confidence we have, the more motivation we will have for a task.

The Motivational Climate

Creating a motivational climate means influencing the factors that affect motivation in a positive way, to help increase the motivation levels of the participants in that environment. Three of the most influential factors are:

1. The behaviour of the leader.

2 The environment itself.
3 The influence of other people in the environment.

Behaviour of the leader

The leader's behaviour can seriously affect the behaviour of other people because the leader will set an example. If the people who are being led think that the leader does not care, then they may not care either; however, if the leader behaves in an upbeat and energetic way, this behaviour may be modelled.

The environment

Think about going to a gym that has grey walls and no decoration; it is cold and there are no staff. Compare this to walking into a gym that is painted brightly and has pictures of athletes achieving great feats, the staff are welcoming and there is upbeat music playing. The second environment is much more appealing to us, and we will be motivated to train there and also to return regularly.

The influence of other people

The motivation of an individual can be affected by social influences, in that other people will offer either approval or disapproval of their behaviour. The support and encouragement an individual receives from their family, friends, teachers and coaches can be vital in maintaining their motivation.

Key learning points 1

- Personality theories focus on whether personality is based in genetics (trait theory) or is learned from our environment (social learning theory).
- Motivation is defined as the direction and intensity of one's effort (Sage, 1974).
- Motivation can be intrinsic (coming from sources within the individual) or extrinsic (coming from sources outside the individual).

Student activity 17.1

1 hour — P1 P2 M1 D1

Choose three performers in three different sports, then fill in the following table to show how their personality affects performance.

Sports performers	Define personality and describe motivation and how they affect sports performance (P1, P2)	Explain the effects of personality and motivation on sports performance (M1)	Evaluate the effects of personality and motivation on sports performance (D1)
1			
2			
3			

Quick quiz 1

Decide whether each of the following statements is an example of intrinsic or extrinsic motivation:

- I want to win medals.
- I want to earn an England cap.
- I want to reach my full potential.
- I want to make money.
- I want to play in a good team.
- I want to play in front of large crowds.
- I want to give the public enjoyment.
- I want to feel good about my performance.
- I want to be recognised by the public for my ability.
- I want to feel mastery in my own ability.
- I want to feel the joy of winning.

17.3 The Relationship Between Anxiety, Arousal, Stress and Sports Performance

P3 P4 M2

Stress

Stress is usually talked about in negative terms. People complain that they have too much stress or are stressed out. Sportspeople claim that the stress of competition is too much for them. However, we should not see stress as an entirely negative thing, because it provides us with the mental and physical energy to motivate us into doing things and doing them well.

Stressors are anything that causes us to have a stress response, and these are invariably different for different people. If we did not have any stress in our lives, we might not bother to do anything all day. We need stressors to give us the energy and direction to get things done. This type of positive stress is called eustress (good stress). If we have too much stress it can become damaging, and we call this distress (bad stress).

- **Eustress** (good stress):
  - gives us energy and direction
  - helps us to be fulfilled and happy.
- **Distress** (bad stress):
  - causes discomfort
  - can lead to illness
  - can cause depression.

Too much stress in our lives over a long period of time can seriously damage our health, causing coronary heart disease, high blood pressure, ulcers, impotence, substance addiction, mental health problems and suicidal tendencies.

Sport is a source of stress for some sportspeople. This is related to the experience of the performer, the importance of the competition, the quality of the opposition, the size of the crowd or previous events. The stress response will be specific to the individual.

The feelings you have are the symptoms of stress, and they can be separated into physical (the effects on your body), mental (the effect on your brain) and behavioural (how your behaviour changed).

Key terms

Stress: any factor that changes the natural state of the body.

The classic definition of stress sees the body as having a natural equilibrium or balance, when the heart rate and breathing rate are at resting levels and blood pressure is at normal level. Anything that changes these natural levels is a stressor. Theoretically, we could say we become stressed as soon as we get out of bed, as our heart rate, breathing rate and blood pressure all rise. Indeed, to some people, the alarm going off is a real source of stress!

The Stress Process

McGrath (1970) sees the stress response as a process and defines stress as 'a substantial imbalance between demand (physical and psychological) and response capability, under conditions where failure to meet the demand has important consequences'.

Stress will occur when the person does not feel they have the resources to deal with the situation and that this will have bad consequences.

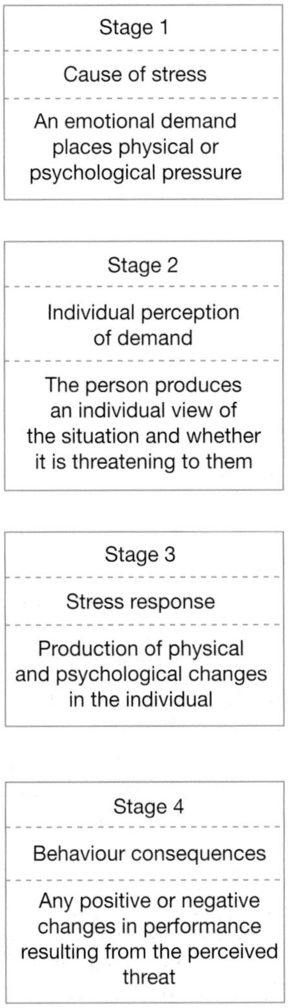
Stage 1
Cause of stress
An emotional demand places physical or psychological pressure
Stage 2
Individual perception of demand
The person produces an individual view of the situation and whether it is threatening to them
Stage 3
Stress response
Production of physical and psychological changes in the individual
Stage 4
Behaviour consequences
Any positive or negative changes in performance resulting from the perceived threat

Fig 17.2 The four stages of the stress process

Causes of Stress

The causes of stress are many and varied, but, crucially, they are specific to an individual. For example, you can have two people in the same event, each with a different stress response.

The sources of stress can generally be divided into four categories:

- internal: things we think about, such as past memories and experiences, current injuries, past injuries, our feelings of self-worth, and so on
- external: things in our surroundings and our environment, such as competition, our opponents, the crowd, the weather, spiders and snakes, transport problems
- personal factors: people we share our lives with, such as friends, family, partners; and life factors such as money and health
- occupational factors: the job we do, the people we work with and our working conditions; in sport, this could include our relationships with teammates and coaches/managers.

Stress levels also depend on personality. Those people who have a predominantly type A personality will find more situations stressful, as will people who have a high N score using Eysenck's personality inventory.

The Physiology of Stress

When we perceive ourselves to be in a situation that is dangerous, our stress response is activated. This has been developed as a means of ensuring our survival, by making us respond to danger. For example, if we are walking home at night through dark woods and we hear noises behind us, the body will instigate physiological changes, called the fight-or-flight response, as the body is preparing to turn and fight the danger or run away as fast as it can.

The response varies depending on how serious we perceive the threat to be. The changes take place in our involuntary nervous system, which consists of two major branches:

- sympathetic nervous system
- parasympathetic nervous system.

The sympathetic nervous system produces the stress response, and its aim is to provide the body with as much energy as it can to confront the threat or run away from it. The sympathetic nervous system works by releasing stress hormones, adrenaline and cortisol, into the bloodstream. The sympathetic nervous system produces the effects listed in Figure 17.3.

The parasympathetic nervous system produces the relaxation response, its aim being to conserve energy. It is activated once the stressor has passed.

It is not healthy for the body to be in a constant state of stress because of the activation of the sympathetic nervous system. The excess production of adrenaline is dangerous because the body requires more cholesterol to synthesise adrenaline. This excess cholesterol production raises blood cholesterol levels and is a risk factor for coronary heart disease.

Sympathetic nervous system	Parasympathetic nervous system
Increased adrenaline production	Decreased adrenaline production
Increase in heart rate	Slowed heart rate
Increase in breathing rate	Slower breathing rate
Increased metabolism	Slower metabolism
Increased heat production	Lower body temperature
Muscle tension	Muscle relaxation
Dry mouth	Dry skin
Dilated pupils	Smaller pupils
Hairs on the skin stand on end (to make us look bigger)	
Digestive system slows down	Digestion speeds up
Diversion of blood away from internal organs to the working muscles	

Table 17.3 Nervous systems

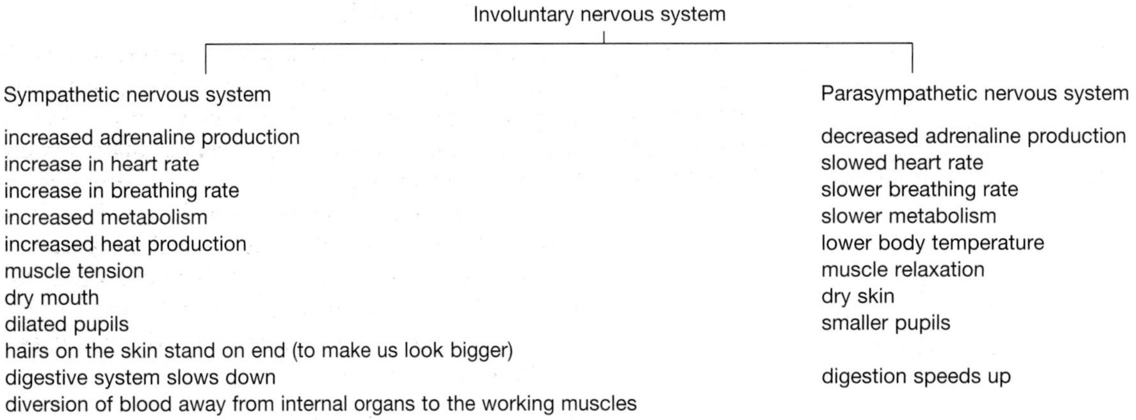

Fig 17.3 The involuntary nervous system

Symptoms of Stress

Stress has a threefold effect on the body, causing cognitive (mental), somatic (physical) and behavioural responses, as outlined in Table 17.4.

Arousal and Anxiety

Arousal and anxiety are terms related to stress. Arousal is a response to stress and shows how motivated we are by a situation. The more aroused we become, the more interested and excited we are by a situation. We can see this when we watch a football match involving a team we support. We are so aroused that we are engrossed in the action to the point that we don't hear noises around us and time seems to go by very quickly. During a match that does not arouse us to the same extent, we find that our attention drifts in and out as we are distracted by things happening around us.

We can look at levels of arousal on a continuum that highlights the varying degrees of arousal:

Deep sleep → Mild interest → Attentive → Absorbed → Engrossed → Frenzied

Cognitive response	Somatic response	Behavioural response
Reduced concentration	Racing heart rates	Talking, eating and walking quickly
Less interested	Faster breathing	Interrupting conversations
Unable to make decisions	Headaches	Increased smoking, drinking and eating
Sleep disturbances	Butterflies in the stomach	Fidgeting
Making mistakes	Chest tightness and pains	Lethargy
Unable to relax	Dry cotton mouth	Moodiness and grudge bearing
Quick losses of temper	Constant colds and illness	Accidents and clumsiness
Loss of sense of humour	Muscular aches and pains	Poor personal presentation
Loss of self-esteem	Increased sweating	Nervous habits
Loss of enthusiasm	Skin irritations	

Table 17.4 Symptoms of stress

Arousal and Attention Span

As arousal levels increase, they can affect a performer's attention span. If a performer has a broad attention span, they are able to pick up information from a wide field of vision. The narrower the attention span becomes, the less information the performer will pick up and the more they will miss. The attention span can be too broad, as the performer may try to pick up too much information.

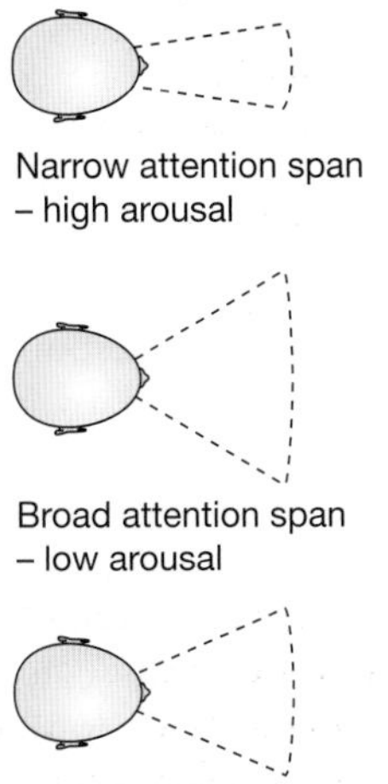

Fig 17.4 Three attention spans

Anxiety

Anxiety can be seen as a negative aspect of stress, and it may accompany high levels of arousal. It is not pleasant to be anxious. It is characterised by feelings of nervousness and worry. Again, the stress and anxiety responses are unique to each individual.

Trait and State Anxiety

Trait anxiety means that a person generally experiences high levels of anxiety as part of their personality. They tend to worry and feel nervous in a range of situations and find them threatening. State anxiety is anxiety felt in response to a specific situation. It is anxiety related to a specific mood state. Usually, a person who has high trait anxiety will also experience higher levels of state anxiety. This is important for athletes because their levels of trait anxiety will determine their state anxiety in competition and, as a result, their performance.

Arousal and Performance

Arousal levels will have an influence on performance, but it is not always clear-cut what this relationship is. The following theories help to explain the relationship.

Drive Theory

Drive theory, initially the work of Hull (1943), states that as arousal levels rise, so do performance levels. This happens in linear fashion and can be described as a straight line.

The actual performance also depends on the arousal level and the skill level of the performer. Arousal will exaggerate the individual's dominant response, meaning that if they have learned the skill well, their dominant response will be exaggerated positively. However, if they are a novice performer, their skill level will drop to produce a worse performance.

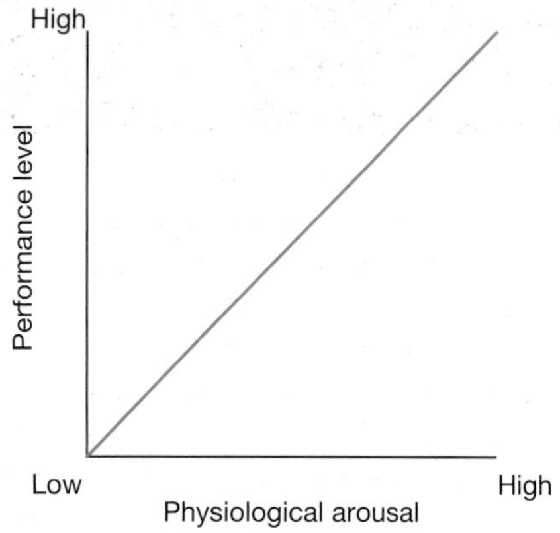

Fig 17.5 Drive theory

The Inverted U Hypothesis

This theory is based on the Yerkes and Dodson law (1908) and seeks to address some of the criticisms of the drive theory. This theory agrees that arousal does improve performance, but only up to a point, and once arousal goes beyond this point, performance starts to decline. Figure 17.6 shows the curve looking like an upside-down U.

This theory's main point is that there is an optimum level of arousal before performance starts to diminish. This is also called the ideal performing state (IPS) and is often referred to as the zone. At this point, the arousal level meets the demands of the task, and everything feels good and is going well.

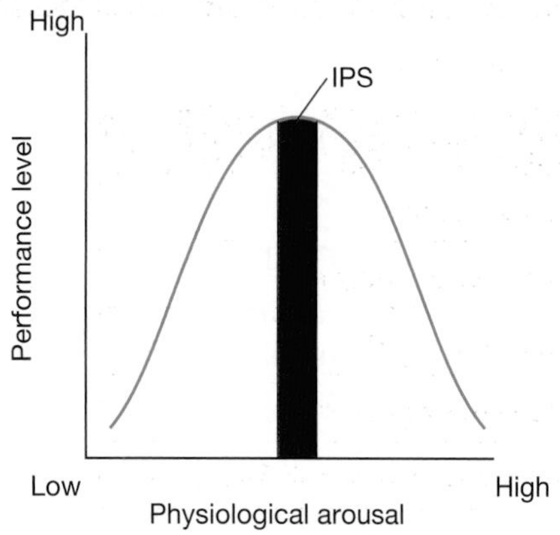

Fig 17.6 The inverted U hypothesis

Catastrophe theory

This theory has been taken a step further by Fazey and Hardy (1988), who agree with the inverted U hypothesis, but say that once arousal level has passed, the IPS will drop off drastically rather than steadily. The point where performance drops is called the point of catastrophe. The Americans refer to this phenomenon, when performance drops, as choking. The history of sport is littered with examples of people or teams throwing away seemingly unassailable positions.

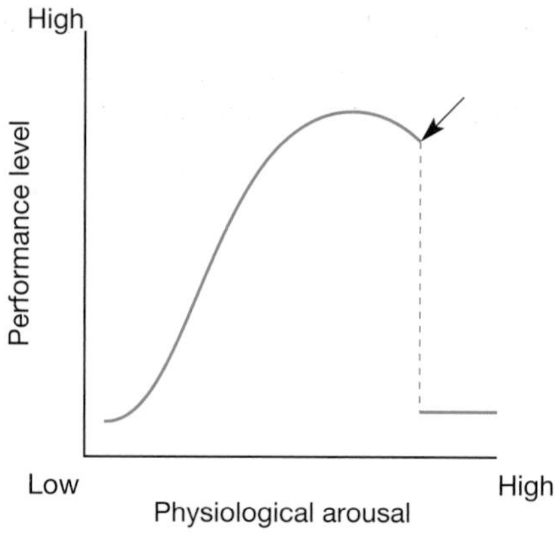

Fig 17.7 Catastrophe theory

Key learning points 2

- Stress is any factor that changes the natural balance of the body.
- Symptoms of stress can be cognitive, somatic or behavioural.
- Arousal is a response to stress that describes how interested and motivated an individual becomes in a situation.
- Anxiety is a negative response to a stressful situation, characterised by nervousness and apprehension.
- The theories of arousal show that changing levels of arousal will influence performance.
- The drive theory of arousal says that increases in arousal level will cause an increase in performance level, while the inverted U hypothesis suggests that increases in arousal level will cause an improvement in performance, but only up to a certain point; after this point, increases in arousal level will cause decrements in performance level.

Student activity 17.2 — 90 minutes — P3 P4 M2

Read the case study and answer the questions below.

1 Using Oliver as an example, describe how stress and anxiety affect him and what their causes are.

2 Describe how Oliver experiences arousal and, using the theories of arousal, what effect changes in arousal have on his performance.

3 Explain how Oliver experiences arousal and, using the theories of arousal, what effect changes in arousal have on his performance.

Oliver is a 16-year-old tennis player whose play is characterised by moments of brilliance mixed with temper tantrums. When Oliver trains in the gym, he loves to lift weights to increase his strength, and he finds that the more up for it he is, the heavier weights he can lift, so he spends time psyching himself up before lifting weights. Oliver loves the excitement of playing a match and feels that it gives him energy and helps to focus his attention. When Oliver plays tennis, he always starts off quite relaxed, but sometimes he is too relaxed to play well and will start to lose points. However, when he is in a losing situation, he starts to become worried and gets butterflies in his stomach, and this spurs him on to play better and get back into the match. Sometimes he wants to win so much that he starts to miss the service box or the base line, often by quite large margins. This can make him really angry, and when he loses his temper he quickly loses the match.

Q Quick quiz 2

1 Match each of the terms in the table below to the appropriate description.

Term	Description
Stress	An individual tends to get worried in most situations
Arousal	Feelings of worry associated with uncomfortable thoughts
Trait anxiety	Any force that changes the natural balance of the body
State anxiety	Racing heart rate and butterflies accompany feelings of worry
Cognitive anxiety	An individual experiences feelings of apprehension in certain situations
Somatic anxiety	Feelings of motivation and excitement produced in a situation

2 Fill in the blanks in the following paragraph.

According to drive theory, increased ________ levels will result in an increase in ________ levels; however, this works best for ________ performers, as arousal will exaggerate the dominant response, while for a novice it can produce a ________ in performance level. The inverted U hypothesis disagrees with drive theory, as it says that increased arousal levels will improve performance, but once arousal gets to a certain point, ________ will start to decline. The point at the top of the curve is called the ________ ________ ________.

17.4 The Role of Group Dynamics in Team Sports

P5 M3 D2

Throughout our sporting and social lives, we are involved in working in groups, such as our families, school groups, friendship groups and the sports teams in which we play. Sports teams have different characteristics – an athletics team will have different teamwork demands to a rugby or cricket team. However, all groups rely on the fundamental characteristic of teamwork.

Defining a group is not easy, but the minimum number of people required is two. A group can be seen as two or more like-minded people interacting to produce an outcome they could not achieve on their own. Groups involve interaction or working with other people in order to influence the behaviour of other people and, in turn, be influenced by them.

Key term

Group: a group should have:

- a collective identity
- a sense of shared purpose or objectives
- structured modes of communication
- personal and/or task interdependence
- interpersonal attraction.

(Weinberg and Gould, 2007)

A Group or a Team?

Generally speaking, an instructor will call people who are involved in an exercise class or dance class a group, and people playing cricket or rugby a team. People involved in the group have a similar sense of purpose and may share common objectives. However, a team's members will actually be dependent on one another to achieve their shared goals and will need to support each other.

So why is the outcome of the group not always equal to the sum of its parts? For example, we can see in football that the teams with the best players do not always get the results they should. In 2006, the very talented Brazil and Argentina teams were knocked out at the quarter-final stage of the World Cup, and in 2004 the European Championships were won by Greece rather than the individually talented Portugal team. In cricket, the England one-day side is continually changing its players, as it seeks to find a team rather than a group of individuals. We can even see the importance of a team when individual players come together in an event such as the Ryder Cup in golf. In 2004 and 2006, the British and European team beat the Americans emphatically, due to the team feeling that had developed.

Stages of Group Development

A group of people coming together does not form a team. Becoming a team demands a process of development. Tuckman and Jensen (1977) proposed a five-stage model of group development:

1. Forming.
2. Storming.
3. Norming.
4. Performing.
5. Adjourning.

Each group will go through the five stages. The length of time they spend in each stage is variable.

Forming

The group comes together, with individuals meeting and familiarising themselves with the other members of the group. The structure and relationships within the group are formed and tested. If it is a team, the coach may develop strategies or games to break the ice between the group members. At this point, the individuals are seeing whether they fit in with this group.

Storming

A period of conflict will follow the forming stage, as individuals seek their roles and status within the group. This may involve conflict between individual members, rebellion against the leader or resistance to the way the team is being developed or managed, or the tactics it is adopting. This is also a period of intense inter-group competition, as group members compete for their positions within the team.

Norming

Once the hostility and fighting have been overcome, by athletes either leaving the group or accepting the common goals and values of the group, a period of norming occurs. Here, the group starts to cooperate and work together to reach common goals. The group pulls together and the roles are established and become stable.

Performing

In the final stage, the group members work together to achieve their mutual goals. The relationships within the group have become well established, as have issues of leadership and strategies for play.

It is unrealistic to see the group as being stable and performing in a steady way. The relationships within the group will change and develop with time, sometimes for the good of the group and sometimes to its detriment. As new members join the group, there will be a new period of storming and norming, as each person is either accepted or rejected. This re-evaluation of the group is often beneficial and stops the group becoming stale. Successful teams seem to be settled and assimilate two or three new players a year to keep them fresh. Bringing in too many new players can disrupt the group and change the nature of the group completely.

Adjourning

Once the group has achieved its goals or come to the end of its useful purpose, the team may break up. This may also be caused by a considerable change in the personnel involved or the management and leadership of the group.

Group Effectiveness

The aim of a group is to be effective by using the strengths of each person to better the effectiveness of the group. However, the outcome is often not equal to the sum of its parts. Steiner (1972) proposed the following model of group effectiveness:

Actual productivity = Potential productivity − Process losses

- Actual productivity = the actual performance achieved.
- Potential productivity = the best possible performance achievable by that group, based on its resources (ability, knowledge, skills).
- Process losses = losses due to working as part of a group (coordination losses, communication problems, losses in motivation).

For example, in a tug-of-war team, each member can pull 100 kg individually, and as a team of four they pull 360 kg in total. Why do you think this would happen?

Social Loafing

One of the problems of working in groups is that it tends to affect motivation. People do not seem to work as hard in groups compared with working on their own. Research shows that rowers in larger teams put in less effort than those in smaller teams:

1 person = 100 per cent effort
2 people = 90 per cent effort
4 people = 80 per cent effort
8 people = 65 per cent effort.

This phenomenon is called the Ringelman effect, or social loafing, and is defined as the tendency of individuals to lessen their effort when part of a group.

Cohesion

Cohesion is concerned with the extent to which a team is willing to stick together and work together. The forces tend to cover two areas:

- the attractiveness of the group to individual members
- the extent to which members are willing to work together to achieve group goals.

To be successful in its goals, a group has to be cohesive. The extent to which cohesion is important depends on the sport and the level of interaction needed.

> **Key term**
>
> **Cohesion:** 'The total field of forces which act on members to remain in the group' (Festinger *et al.*, 1950).

Types of Cohesion

There seem to be two definite types of cohesion within a group:

- task cohesion – the willingness of a team to work together to achieve its goals
- social cohesion – the willingness of the team to socialise together.

It would appear that task cohesion comes first, as this is why the team has formed in the first place. If the group is lucky, they will find that they develop social cohesion as well, and this usually has a beneficial effect on performance. This is because if you feel good about your teammates, you are more likely to want success for each other as well as yourself.

Research says that cohesion is important in successful teams, but that task cohesion is more important than social cohesion. It does depend on the sport being played, as groups that need high levels of interaction need higher levels of cohesion. Research also suggests that success will produce increased cohesion, rather than cohesion coming before performance. Being successful helps to develop feelings of group attraction, and this will help to develop more success, and so on. This can be seen with the cycle of success, in that once a team has been successful it tends to continue being successful – success breeds success.

Leadership in Sport

The choice of a manager, coach or captain is often the most important decision a club's members have to make. They see it as crucial in influencing the club's chances of success. Great leaders in sport are held in the highest regard, irrespective of their talent on the pitch.

Key term

Leadership: 'The behavioural process of influencing individuals and groups towards goals' (Barrow, 1977).

Leadership behaviour covers a variety of activities, which is why it is described as multi-dimensional. It includes:

- decision-making processes
- motivational techniques
- giving feedback
- establishing interpersonal relationships
- confidently directing the group.

Leaders are different from managers. Managers plan, organise, budget, schedule and recruit, while leaders determine how a task is completed.

People become leaders in different ways; not all are appointed. Prescribed leaders are appointed by a person in authority – a chairman appoints a manager, a manager appoints a coach, a principal appoints a teacher. Emergent leaders emerge from a group and take over responsibility. For example, John Terry emerged to become the leader of the England football team, just as Andrew Strauss emerged to become the new England cricket captain. Emergent leaders can be more effective, as they have the respect of their group members.

Theories of Leadership

Sport psychologists have sought to explain leadership effectiveness for many years, and they have used the following theories to help understand effective leadership behaviour.

Trait Approach

In the 1920s, researchers tried to show that characteristics or personality traits were stable and common to all leaders. Thus, to be a good leader, you needed to have intelligence, assertiveness, independence and self-confidence. Therefore, a person who is a good leader in one situation will be a good leader in all situations.

Behavioural Approach

The trait approach says that leaders are 'born', but the behavioural approach says that anyone can become a good leader by learning the behaviour of effective leaders. Thus, the behavioural approach supports the view that leadership skills can be developed through experience and training.

Interactional Approach

Trait and personal approaches look at personality traits. The interactional approach looks at the interaction between the person and the situation. It stresses the following points:

- Effective leaders cannot be predicted solely on personality.
- Effective leadership fits specific situations, as some leaders function better in certain circumstances than others.
- Leadership style needs to change to match the demands of the situation. For example, relationship-orientated leaders develop interpersonal relationships, provide good communication and ensure everyone is feeling good within the group. However, task-orientated leaders are concerned with getting the work done and meeting objectives.

Social Facilitation

Social facilitation is the change in performance that occurs due to the presence of others – whether the presence is an audience or fellow competitors. There is no doubt that our performances change as the result of the presence of other people. Think about how you feel when your parents or friends come to watch you, or when you start to perform in front of an audience.

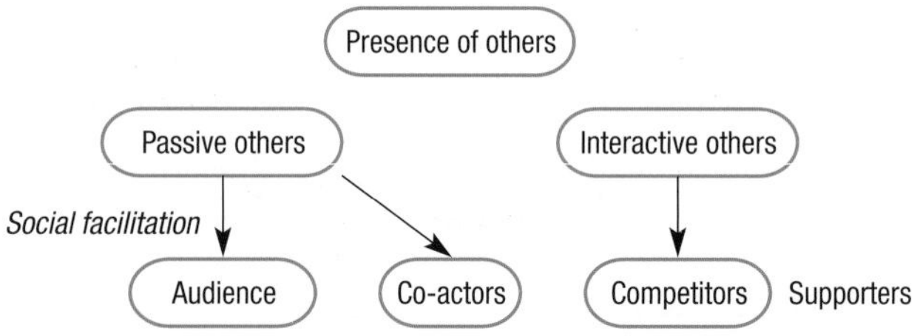

Fig 17.8 Social facilitation model

Zajonc (1965) defined the different types of people present, separating them into those people who are competing against you and those people who are merely present and not competing.

Key term

Social facilitation: 'The consequences upon behaviour which derive from the sheer presence of other individuals' (Zajonc, 1965).

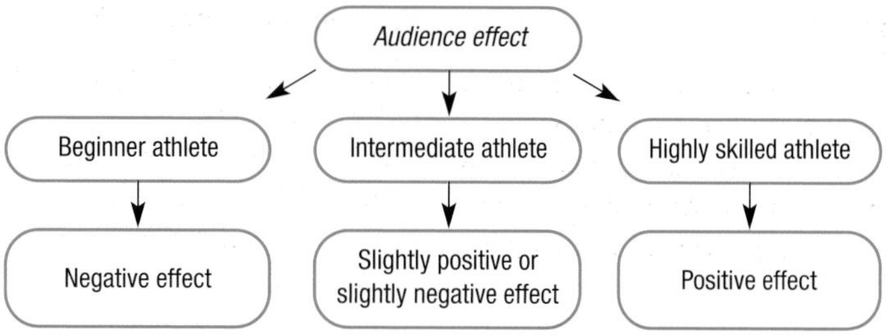

Fig 17.10 Audience effect and the standard of performer

Co-actors are people involved in the same activity, but not competing directly. Triplett (1898) did some of the earliest experiments in sport psychology. He examined co-action in the following three conditions, using cyclists:

1. Unpaced.
2. Paced (co-actor on another bike).
3. Paced competitive (co-actors pacing and competing).

Triplett's findings were that cyclists in condition 2 were 34 seconds per mile faster than cyclists in condition 1, while cyclists in condition 3 were 39 seconds per mile faster than cyclists in condition 1.

The reasons for social facilitation are not always clear. Triplett concluded that in his experiment it was due to the physical effects, such as suctioning and sheltering resulting from travelling behind another rider; and psychological effects, such as encouragement, anxiety, pressure and competitiveness, which are felt as the result of cycling with someone else. Triplett concluded that it did not matter if the cyclists were competing. What was important was that 'the bodily presence of another rider is stimulus to a rider in arousing the competitive instinct'.

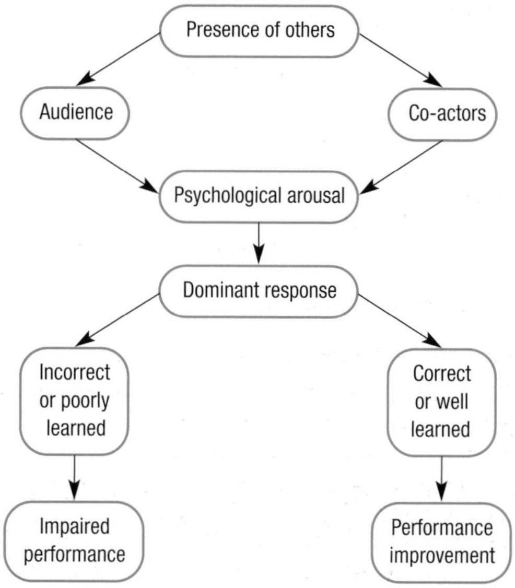

Fig 17.9 Zajonc's expanded model (1965)

Zajonc's expanded model (Figure 17.9) showed that whether the audience or co-actors have a positive or negative effect on performance depends on how well the skill has been learnt. A poorly learnt skill will become worse, while a well-learnt skill will be improved. This links in well with the effect of stress on performance, and it can be seen that the presence of others would cause more stress.

Zajonc also looked at the relationship between the audience effect and the standard of the performer. His results are shown in Figure 17.10.

The effect also depends on the nature of the task – whether it is strength- or skill-related. Strength tasks will usually be enhanced by the presence of others. However, skilled tasks (especially poorly learnt skills) may suffer. Social facilitation effects tend to disappear as the individual gets used to them.

Cottrell (1968) said that it is not the mere presence of an audience that creates arousal, but that the type of audience is also very important. For example, a blindfolded audience had no facilitation effect. The following factors will affect social facilitation:

- audience expertise: an expert audience will increase arousal level
- type of audience: a pro-winning audience will have more of a facilitation effect than a pro-enjoyment audience
- performer's evaluation of the audience: the performer decides what they think the audience wants and is aroused accordingly
- size: a larger audience will have more of a facilitation effect.

Home advantage

Home advantage is the view that the team playing at home has a disproportionately higher chance of winning in relation to the team playing away from home. This phenomenon was apparent in cricket, as home teams are more often successful in test matches. For example, England beat Australia to win the Ashes in 2005 and 2009, yet they were beaten 5–0 in Australia in 2006 when they tried to retain the Ashes. In the football World Cup of 2006, which was held in Germany, all four semi-finalists were European countries.

There are many reasons why home teams are more successful. Some of these are physical and some are psychological:

- familiarity with the surroundings and the surfaces
- a supportive home crowd who give positive approval
- less intimidation from opposing supporters
- the territory is theirs and claimed by display of their playing colours
- there is less travel involved in getting to the match
- travel can cause boredom and staleness
- players do not have to stay in unfamiliar surroundings and eat unfamiliar food
- home teams are more likely to play offensively
- away teams may not be treated well by their opponents
- referees and officials may unconsciously favour the home team to seek the crowd's approval.

Home advantage may be seen as being a disadvantage to the away team rather than an advantage to the home team. It is the job of the coach and psychologist to find ways of minimising this away disadvantage.

Key learning points 3

- A group is defined as two people who have to work together to achieve an outcome they could not achieve individually.
- Members of a team will have greater dependence on each other to achieve their outcome than members of a group.
- The model of group effectiveness states that the actual productivity of a group will equal the potential productivity (best possible outcome of the group) minus process losses (losses due to the problems of working as a group).
- Process losses include problems with coordination, communication and motivation of individuals in the group.
- Social loafing describes the tendency of individuals to exert less effort when working as a part of a group than they would individually.
- Cohesion is described as the total sum of forces that cause individuals to remain in a group.
- The leader in the group can influence its effectiveness, especially if they are able to adapt their personality to the demands of the situation they find themselves in.

Q Quick quiz 3

Match each of the terms in the table below to the appropriate description.

Term	Description
Social loafing	The degree of attraction an individual feels towards a group
Task cohesion	Loss of performance caused by working as part of a group
Leadership	The presence of other people can have a beneficial effect on performance
Social cohesion	The tendency for an individual to give less effort when part of a group
Process losses	The process of influencing individuals or groups towards achieving their goals
Social facilitation	The extent to which team members want to work together

Student activity 17.3 — 1 hour — P5 M3 D2

Read the case study, in which Patrick, a former professional player, talks about two teams he played for in his career, then answer the questions below.

1 From Patrick's explanation, identify four factors that influence group dynamics and performance in team sports.

2 Using Patrick's explanation, explain four factors that influence group dynamics and performance in team sports.

3 Using Patrick's explanation, analyse four factors that influence group dynamics and performance in team sports.

I played for several teams in my career, but when I was a young player I was lucky to have a brilliant manager. At the beginning of the season, he would tell each player what their role was in the team, and then he would bring the team together and tell us how he wanted us to play together. We each knew our individual role, and as long as we performed it we were kept in the team. I remember the manager taking players off early in matches because they were not doing their job. He was a hard manager to please, but his methods worked well and we were very successful. My second team was managed by an ex-player who I knew from the first club, and he put together a team of players that he had played with and trusted. We were never the most talented group of individuals, but once we were on the pitch, we all worked for each other and achieved more than the individual sum of our talents should have achieved. The manager always took us out on Monday nights, when we would go for a meal, go bowling or play darts, which helped to build a solid bond between us, and we cared for each other on and off the pitch. This manager was so successful that he moved to a bigger club; he was replaced by a new manager who was not successful because he didn't understand how the club worked and he could never explain how he wanted us to play.

17.5 Planning a Psychological Skills Training Programme to Enhance Sporting Performance

P7 M4 D3

Assessing Psychological Strengths and Weaknesses

An assessment of an individual's mental strengths and weaknesses can be made in different ways. We will look first at the use of a questionnaire, but it could also be done through performance profiling.

Example Questionnaire

Name:

Sport played:

- Explain any past experience you have of psychological skills training.
- Explain your involvement in sport and any important competitions or events coming up.
- What do you consider to be your psychological strengths and weaknesses?

Below is a list of statements. Circle the answer appropriate to your experience.

1 **I always feel motivated to succeed, whatever activity I am doing.**
Don't know Never Sometimes Usually Always

2 **I always work towards clear goals.**
Don't know Never Sometimes Usually Always

3 **I set myself goals on a weekly basis.**
Don't know Never Sometimes Usually Always

4 **I always make full use of my skills and abilities.**
Don't know Never Sometimes Usually Always

5 **When I am involved in my physical activity, I often find my attention wavering.**
Don't know Never Sometimes Usually Always

6 **I am easily distracted during whatever activity I am involved in.**
Don't know Never Sometimes Usually Always

7 **I perform much better when I am under a lot of pressure.**
Don't know Never Sometimes Usually Always

8 **I become very anxious when I am under pressure.**
Don't know Never Sometimes Usually Always

9 **If I start to become tense, I can quickly relax myself and calm down.**
Don't know Never Sometimes Usually Always

10 **I find it easy to control my emotions, whatever the situation.**
Don't know Never Sometimes Usually Always

11 **I am always able to remain upbeat and positive, whatever the situation.**
Don't know Never Sometimes Usually Always

12 **If I am criticised by a coach or trainer I tend to take it very badly.**
Don't know Never Sometimes Usually Always

13 **I am easily able to deal with unforeseen situations.**
Don't know Never Sometimes Usually Always

14 **I have my own set of strategies for dealing with difficult situations.**
Don't know Never Sometimes Usually Always

Analysing the results:

- Questions 1–4 relate to motivation
- Questions 5–6 relate to concentration
- Questions 7–10 relate to arousal and anxiety
- Questions 11–14 relate to self-confidence.

There is no scoring system as such, but the questions are designed for you to establish areas of strength and areas of weakness.

Identifying the Psychological Demands of a Sport

Each sport will have an individual psychological demand on it which is also constantly open to change. The main categories of psychological demands are listed here:

- Motivation
- Arousal control
- Confidence
- Concentration
- Emotional control

By using techniques such as performance profiling, we can assess why each one of these is important in our sport, how important it is and our current level of competence at the skill. Once our current competence level and the importance of the skill to the sport have been identified, you can lay down the aims of the training programme and begin to identify the content and the techniques needed to address these skills.

Techniques to Influence Motivation: Goal Setting

The main way that sports psychologists develop motivation is through the use of goal setting. In reality, goals are the dreams we have for ourselves, but goal setting gives these dreams legs and starts moving us towards them. A goal usually represents a situation we want to be in, which involves us moving away from the situation we are currently in.

> **Key term**
>
> **Goal:** what an individual is aiming to achieve. It is the outcome they desire from their actions.

Why Does Goal Setting Work?

Goal setting works because it gives our wants and desires a specific outcome and provides us with the steps we need to move towards this outcome. It gives our daily actions a meaning or framework to work within and gives us direction in life. Goals will work to direct our energy and efforts.

What you focus on you will move towards.

Short-term, Medium-term and Long-term Goals

Short-term goals are set over a brief period of time, usually from one day to one month. A short-term goal may relate to what you want to achieve in one training session or where you want to be by the end of the month.

Short-term goals may be:

- one session
- one day
- one week
- one month.

Medium-term goals will bridge the gap between short- and long-term goals and are set from one to three months.

Long-term goals will run from three months to several years. You may even set some lifetime goals, which run until you retire from your sport. In sport, we set long-term goals to cover a season or a sporting year.

Long-term goals may be:

- four months
- six months
- nine months
- one year
- one season
- three years
- lifetime.

Usually, short-term goals are set to help achieve the long-term goals. It is important to set both short-term and long-term goals, particularly short-term goals, because they will give a person more motivation to act now. If you have to give in a piece of coursework tomorrow, it will make you work hard tonight, but if you have to submit it in one month, you are unlikely to stay in tonight and complete the work!

Outcome and process goals

An outcome goal focuses on the outcome of an event or performance, such as winning a race or beating an opponent.

A process goal focuses on the process or actions that an individual must produce to perform well – for example, train three times a week or get eight hours' sleep a night.

Both types of goal are important, and we find that short-term goals are normally process goals, while long-term goals are outcome goals.

The process goals will be the small steps we take towards the big outcome or goal. A marathon race is the result of millions of small steps, and it is each individual step that is most important at that time.

SMART Goals

When goals are set you need to use the SMART principle to make them workable. SMART stands for:

- Specific
- Measurable
- Achievable
- Realistic
- Time-constrained.

Specific

The goal must be specific to what you want to achieve. This may be an aspect of performance or fitness. It is not enough to say, 'I want to get fitter'; you need to say, 'I want to improve strength, speed or stamina, etc.'

Measurable

Goals must be stated in a way that is measurable, so they need to state figures. For example, 'I want to improve my first serve percentage' is not measurable. However, if you say, 'I want to improve my first serve success by 20 per cent', it is measurable.

Achievable

It must be possible to actually achieve the goal.

Realistic

We need to be realistic in our goal setting and look at what factors may stop us achieving our goals.

Time-constrained

There must be a time-scale or deadline on the goal. This means you can review your success. It is best to state a date by which you wish to achieve the goal.

How to set goals

The best way to do this is to answer three questions:

1. What do I want to achieve? (Desired state)
2. Where am I now? (Present state)
3. What do I need to do to move from my present state to my desired state?

Then present this on a scale:

Present state				Desired state
1	2	3	4	5

1. Write in your goal at point 5 and your present position at point 1.
2. Decide what would be halfway between points 1 and 5; this is your goal for point 3.
3. Then decide what would be halfway between your present state and point 3; this is your short-term goal for point 2.
4. Then decide what would be halfway between point 3 and the desired state; this is your goal for point 4.

5 All these goals are outcome goals and must be set using the SMART principle.
6 Work out what needs to be done to move from point 1 to point 2. These are your process goals and, again, must use the SMART principle.

It is best to use a goal-setting diary to keep all goal-setting information in the same place, and to review the goals on a weekly basis.

Techniques to Influence Motivation: Performance Profiling

Performance profiling is a way of getting the athlete to analyse their strengths and weaknesses. It can be a way of monitoring improvements in psychological skills as well as being used to motivate and energise athletes.

The benefits of performance profiling are as follows:

- it considers what the individual feels is important
- the individual is actively involved and will feel some sense of possession of their performances
- it is used to motivate and monitor improvements
- it is specific for each athlete
- the visual display helps to give it more power
- it enables the athlete and coach to identify areas of weakness.

Process of Performance Profiling

Introduce the idea of performance profiling
This may be a new concept for the athlete and a period of explaining the process will be valuable. You will need to cover the following information:

- explain performance profiling
- explain the benefits and how the results can be applied
- emphasise that there are no wrong or right answers and that what is important is the individual's view
- show them examples of completed performance profiles (these should be anonymous).

Elicit the constructs
The sports psychologist will need to ask the athlete to come up with ten psychological factors that are vital to their performance. You may ask a question such as: What psychological factors do you consider to be most important in helping you to achieve your best performance?

The sports psychologist may assist the process by making relevant suggestions if the athlete is struggling to come up with good responses.

The ten factors they come up with are called 'constructs'.

Assess the constructs
The athlete is asked to complete the following tasks:

- Rate themselves on a scale of 1–10 to show their current level of competence at each construct. A rating of 10 would represent their idea of perfection.
- Rate how far they would like to progress towards their idea of perfection; they may feel that a score of 10 is not necessary and they would be happy to get to 7.

Plot the performance profile
Once the above tasks have been completed, you can present the information on a grid, with dark bars showing current levels of competence and lighter bars showing desired levels.

You can then use this information in different ways:

- assess their strengths and weaknesses
- see what they feel is important in their sport
- as their coach, you may have different ideas about what is important and their level of skill. This exercise will highlight any differences in your points of view.

You can identify the following information from the profile:

- areas of perceived strength – where they score 5 or more (e.g. Aggression control)
- areas of perceived weakness – where they score less than 5 (e.g. Arousal control)
- areas resistant to change – where there is little difference between their current rating and the rating they would like to achieve (e.g. Attitude).

Imagery

Imagery is one of the most important techniques in sports psychology because the pictures and thoughts that we have in our head will influence how we feel and how we behave. If we can have positive thoughts and images, they are going to be beneficial to our performance.

What Is Imagery?

Imagery is the creation or re-creation of an image or experience in your mind rather than physically practising the skill. It will involve the employment of all the senses in actually re-creating the experience. Imagery is used extensively by many athletes, particularly golfers and track and field athletes. Jack Nicklaus, one of the most successful golfers of all time, explains how he uses visualisation:

> Before every shot I go to the movies in my head. Here is what I see. First I see the ball where I want

it to finish, nice and white, sitting up high on the bright green grass. Then I see the ball going there – its path and trajectory and even its behaviour on landing. The next scene shows me making the kind of swing that will turn the previous image into reality. These home images are the key to my concentration and to my positive approach to every shot. (Nicklaus, 1976)

Imagery is a skill and some people will be better at it than others. If you find developing images difficult, you will need to use the practices later to help you with this skill.

Why does imagery work?

Imagery works because when you imagine yourself performing a skill, the brain is unable to differentiate between a real experience and an imagined experience. As a result, the brain sends impulses to the muscles via the nervous system; these impulses are not strong enough to produce a muscular contraction, although you may see twitches. As the impulses are passed down the nervous system, so the pattern becomes imprinted on the nervous system and is there for whenever you physically perform the skill. It is as if you have been there without actually going there.

Imagery can be used for the following skills:

- management of mental state
- mental rehearsal
- relaxation techniques
- developing confidence
- concentration skills.

Mental Rehearsal

Mental rehearsal is taking time to sit down and think about your sport. It is seeing, feeling and hearing yourself playing your sport. It can be utilised in different ways:

- developing and practising skills
- reducing anxiety about an event.
- practising 'what if…' scenarios
- developing confidence before an event
- replaying and reviewing performance.

Rather than just physical practice, mental rehearsal can complement your skill development. However, you need to have well-developed imagery skills to be able to perform mental rehearsal effectively.

Developing and Practising Skills

Mental rehearsal can be used before, during and after competitions to ensure the best performance. Roger Black, who won the 400 m silver medal in the 1996 Olympics, talks about the power of mental rehearsal:

For the Olympic Games I walked around the stadium four months prior and I kept that picture in my mind every day. I ran it from every lane. I could close my eyes now and run the 400 m race and I would feel how I would feel. (Black, in Grout and Perrin, 2004)

Here are some guidelines for mental rehearsal:

- Precede the session with a short relaxation session.
- Bring up the picture and make sure it is big, colourful, sharply focused and as bright as a film.
- Employ all your senses, by hearing the sounds and experiencing the feelings associated with performing.
- Visualise at the correct speed (same speed as the action).
- Always visualise yourself successfully executing the skills.
- Visualise from inside your head looking out.
- Practise in intervals of five to ten minutes a day.

Developing Confidence Before an Event

Self-confidence is the extent to which you expect to be successful. If you can, use imagery to recall times when you were sure about being successful, or you can use the following techniques to help you experience what it would be like to be completely self-confident.

Techniques to Control Arousal Levels

According to the inverted U hypothesis, our performance is related to our arousal level. If we are over-aroused, we need to reduce arousal by using relaxation techniques; conversely, if we find ourselves under-aroused, we need to use energising techniques to raise our arousal level.

Relaxation Techniques

There is a range of relaxation techniques which addresses different aspects of the effects of stress and anxiety. These techniques are:

- progressive muscular relaxation (PMR)
- mind-to-muscle techniques (imagery)
- breathing control.

Certainly, relaxation techniques will control arousal before and during performance, and they can also be used for other purposes:

- to lower levels of trait and state anxiety
- to help the athlete fall into a deep sleep before or after a competition
- to keep the athlete calm and reduce energy lost through nervous worry before a competition

- to relax and recover during breaks in play or between races or matches
- to help recovery from illness and injury
- to help them enjoy their life in general.

When performing relaxation techniques, it is important to follow these instructions:

1 Find a place where you will not be disturbed.
2 Sit or lie down in a comfortable place.
3 Close your eyes and turn down the lighting.
4 Put on some relaxing music.
5 Enjoy the experience.

Progressive muscular relaxation (PMR)
This technique is excellent for people who are experiencing the symptoms of somatic anxiety, such as tension in the muscles and butterflies in the stomach. PMR involves listening to a recording of a script, or a psychologist reading out a script where muscle groups are sequentially contracted and then relaxed. This starts from the hands and arms, up to the face, upper body and then the lower body.

Mind-to-muscle techniques (imagery)
These techniques will work with a person who is experiencing cognitive anxiety. It works best with people who have well-developed imagery skills. This technique involves listening to a recording of a script or a psychologist reading out a script where you develop pictures in your head. These pictures will be of a relaxing place or room where you can go to rest and relax when you need to.

Breathing control
Breathing control is a method often used by athletes to reduce muscle tension and lower anxiety levels. When we become stressed and anxious, we experience short and shallow breathing; when we are relaxed, our breathing deepens.

To aid relaxation, we can teach the athlete to breathe deeply and slowly from the diaphragm to produce mental and physical relaxation. If they are focusing on their breathing, it will shift their attention from whatever is causing them stress. It can be done in a standing or sitting position. Get the individual to place their hands on their stomach and see how the hands move out and fall back as they breathe in and out.

Once they have learnt how to breathe properly, they can use it at the appropriate time during a competition.

Energising techniques

If the athlete is feeling under-aroused, there are ways of raising the arousal level. For example, many coaches will use music to psych up their athletes and raise their energy levels. This can be a personal choice or a team may develop a theme tune that they play before performing in order to lift them. Also, scripts, similar in style to relaxation scripts, can be employed to raise arousal and energy levels.

Self-talk to develop confidence

Self-talk is what we say to ourselves when we have internal conversations, and this affects our mental state at any time. If we have positive thoughts and say positive things to ourselves, we will maintain high levels of confidence. However, if we say to ourselves that we are useless and no good, that is how we will act and we will get poor outcomes as a result. We need to keep building our confidence by reframing any negative thoughts we have in a positive way. For example, rather than saying, 'I always perform poorly against Sheena', you might say, 'Playing Sheena is a good challenge for me'.

Key learning points 4

- Before looking at techniques to improve performance in sport, you need to identify the psychological demands of the sport.
- Goal setting and performance profiling can be used to influence motivation.
- Imagery can be used for mental rehearsal, developing confidence and to promote relaxation.
- Relaxation techniques can be used to lower arousal levels, while energising techniques can increase them.

Student activity 17.4 — 2 hours — P6 P7 M4 D3

Choose a sports performer from your fellow students and then plan and carry out a consultation with this performer. You could use the sample questionnaire provided and any other methods you feel are important. You might watch them perform to see how they behave during competition or plan an interview with them.

Once you have found out as much information as you can, use the following template to plan a six-week psychological skills training programme.

Current situation: [Write a description of the athlete and what sport they play, and summarise their main issues/problems, as in the case study of Sarah] Aims of the psychological skills training: [What areas are you going to address/improve?] 1 2 3
Action plan: [The steps you will take to achieve the aims (e.g. set goals or teach relaxation skills)] 1 2 3 4
Training plan: [What you will do week by week] Week 1: Week 2: Week 3: Week 4: Week 5: Week 6:
Comments on progress:

(To achieve M4, explain why you have planned the training programme for your selected performer. To achieve the first part of D3, you need to justify your training programme. You can do this by showing why you have chosen each technique you recommended. To achieve the second part of D3, you need to review your training programme and make suggestions for its improvement.)

References

Barrow, J. (1977) The variables of leadership: a review and conceptual framework. *Academy of Management Review*, 2, 231–51.

Bowers, K.S. (1973) Situationism in psychology: an analysis and a critique. *Psychological Review*, 80, 307–36.

Cattell, R.B. (1965) *The Scientific Analysis of Personality*, Penguin.

Cottrell, N.B. (1968) Performance in the presence of other human beings: mere presence, audience and affiliation effects, in E. Simmell, R. Hoppe and G. Milton (eds), *Social Facilitation and Imitative Behaviour*, Allyn & Bacon.

Cox, R. (2007) *Sports Psychology: Concepts and Applications*, Wm C. Brown Communications.

Eysenck, H. (1964) *Manual of Eysenck Personality Inventory*, University of London Press.

Fazey, J. and Hardy, L. (1988) *The Inverted U Hypothesis: A Catastrophe for Sport Psychology?* British Association of Sports Sciences Monograph, no. 1, NCF.

Festinger, L.A., Schachter, S. and Back, K. (1950) *Social Pressures in Informal Groups: A Study of Human Factors in Housing*, Harper.

Friedman, M. (1996) *Type A Behaviour: Its Diagnosis and Treatment*, Plenum Press.

Gill, D. (2000) *Psychological Dynamics of Sport and Exercise*, Human Kinetics.

Grout, J. and Perrin, S. (2004) *Mind Games*, Capstone.

Hull, C.L. (1943) *Principles of Behaviour*, Appleton-Century-Crofts.

Jarvis, M. (2006) *A Student's Handbook*, Routledge.

McClelland, D.C., Atkinson, J.W., Clark, R.W. and Lowell, E.J. (1953) *The Achievement Motive*, Appleton-Century-Crofts.

McGrath, J.E. (1970) Major methodological issues, in J.E. McGrath (ed.), *Social and Psychological Factors in Stress*, Holt, Rinehart & Winston.

Nicklaus, J. (1976) *Play Better Golf*, King Features.

Sage, G. (1974) *Sport and American Society*, Addison-Wesley.

Sage, G. (1977) *Introduction to Motor Behaviour: A Neuropsychological Approach*, Addison-Wesley.

Schurr, K., Ashley, M. and Joy, K. (1977) A multivariate analysis of male athlete characteristics: sport type and success. *Multivariate Experimental Clinical Research*, 3, 53–68.

Steiner, I.D. (1972) *Group Processes and Productivity*, Academic Press.

Triplett, N. (1898) The dynamogenic factors in pacemaking and competition. *American Journal of Psychology*, 9, 507–33.

Tuckman, L. and Jensen, M. (1977) *Stages of Small Group Development Revisited*, Group and Organisational Studies.

Weinberg, R.S. and Gould, D. (2007) *Foundations of Sport and Exercise Psychology*, Human Kinetics.

Williams, J.M. (1980) Personality characteristics of the successful female athlete, in W.M. Straub, *Sport Psychology: An Analysis of Athlete Behavior*, Movement.

Yerkes, R.M. and Dodson, J.D. (1908) The relationship of strength and stimulus to rapid habit formation. *Journal of Comparative Neurology and Psychology*, 18, 459–82.

Further reading

Cox, R. (2007) *Sports Psychology: Concepts and Applications*, Wm C. Brown Communications.

Thatcher, J., Thatcher, R., Day, M., Portas, M. and Hood, S. (2009) *Sport and Exercise Science*, Learning Matters.

Weinberg, R.S. and Gould, D. (2007) *Foundations of Sport and Exercise Psychology*, Human Kinetics.

Useful websites

www.bbc.co.uk/wales/raiseyourgame

Online articles and short videos featuring famous sports people to help you improve on specific aspects of your sports psychology

www.5min.com/Video/How-to-Develop-Motivation-for-Sport-34094922

Short video to help you develop your personal motivation for sport

19: Analysis of Sports Performance

19.1 Introduction

Every sportsperson is aiming to improve their performance in terms of their technical ability, physiological fitness, psychological strength and biomechanical efficiency. We tend to become even more reflective and ask more questions when things are not going well and we are losing competitions. In order to analyse our performances we need a structure or framework in which to work. This unit provides a structure for athletes to interpret their performances and their successes and failures.

By the end of this unit you should:

- know the performance profile of a sporting activity
- be able to analyse sporting performance
- be able to provide feedback to athletes regarding performance
- understand the purpose and resources required for analysing different levels of sporting performance.

Assessment and grading criteria		
To achieve a PASS grade the evidence must show that the learner is able to:	**To achieve a MERIT grade the evidence must show that, in addition to the pass criteria, the learner is able to:**	**To achieve a DISTINCTION grade the evidence must show that, in addition to the pass and merit criteria, the learner is able to:**
P1 describe the performance profile of a selected sporting activity	**M1** explain the performance profile of a selected sporting activity	**D1** analyse the performance profile of a selected sporting activity
P2 describe five factors that may influence the performance of an athlete		
P3 perform an assessment of a selected athlete undertaking sporting activity using three components of their performance profile, with tutor support	**M2** explain the function of the cardiovascular system	**D2** analyse the performance of a selected athlete using three components of their performance profile.
P4 provide feedback to the athlete based on the assessment of their performance, with tutor support	**M3** independently perform an assessment of a selected athlete undertaking sporting activity using three components of their performance profile.	
P5 explain the purpose of, and the resources required for, analysis at two different levels of sports performance.		

19.2 The Performance Profile of a Sporting Activity

P1 P2 P3 M1 M2

The performance profile is a visual method of looking at performance in a broad manner. It is used by the athlete and coach to pinpoint strengths and weaknesses and this information is then used to design future actions. When a coach works with an athlete the coach can make decisions on techniques and changes, with the methods being imposed on the athlete by the coach. In this method the success or failure of the training programme is viewed by the athlete as being dependent upon the effectiveness of the coach in meeting their needs.

However, the coach only has the 'outsider' view. Butler and Hardy (1992) identified that this was a major weakness as it affected an individual's intrinsic motivation. Bull (1991) agreed that an athlete's commitment to their training schedule and the accompanying educational work would be affected if the coach who had imposed the schedules was not always present. It would seem to be a more productive relationship if the expertise of two people was utilised. The coach is the expert in terms of 'the outsider' view of the athlete's performance, while the athlete is the expert in terms of 'the insider' view of their experiences and how they are feeling.

Butler (2000) described the athlete's role as follows:

> 'The athlete's assertions, discriminations and insights are not only valid but valuable. They make a significant contribution to the development of an effective training programme.'

The performance profile gives the coach and athlete a tool to provide a visual display of the areas of performance that are perceived to be important in working towards a top performance, and their assessment of the current position in relation to this.

Using a Performance Profile

First, you need to choose the sporting activity you want to examine and then you can look at any of the following:

- technical and tactical (shooting, passing, tackling)
- physiological fitness (strength, power, flexibility)
- psychological (motivation, arousal, confidence)
- biomechanical (speed, motion, momentum).

To construct a performance profile you would do the following:

- The athlete is asked to think about the qualities or skills that are shown by those athletes who perform at the top level of their sport in the same position, role or event as themselves.
- These qualities or skills are called the 'constructs', and they are placed on the performance profile.
- The athlete then describes their current position in terms of their competency by giving themselves a mark out of 10. This score of 10 is in comparison to an athlete they consider to be excellent in their chosen sport.
- The coach may do the same exercise to provide the 'outsider viewpoint'.

These scores can be filled in on the performance profile and used to:

- identify their current level of competence
- identify areas of strength and weakness
- monitor progress and any changes occurring
- monitor effectiveness of training programmes
- identify any differences in the viewpoints of athlete and coach
- provide a basis for designing a training programme.

Technical Analysis of a Sporting Activity

You can analyse a sporting activity in terms of the whole activity, an individual position or an individual aspect of the game.

Whole Activity

Snooker, for example, can be broken down into the following constructs:

- stance
- snookering
- cueing action
- back spin
- bridging
- top spin
- striking
- side spin
- long potting
- deep screw
- short potting
- follow through
- cushion shots.

Positional Activity

A midfielder in football would perform the following techniques:

- short passing
- blocking
- long passing
- long-range shooting
- crossing
- close-range shooting
- dead ball work
- defensive heading
- throwing in
- attacking heading
- tackling.

Individual Aspect of an Activity

A tennis player would perform the following backhand shots:

- smash
- lob
- volley
- flat drive
- half volley
- topspin drive
- drop volley
- slice.

	1	2	3	4	5	6	7	8	9	10
Short passing										
Long passing										
Crossing										
Dead ball work										
Throwing in										
Tackling										
Blocking										
Long-range shooting										
Close-range shooting										
Defensive heading										
Attacking heading										

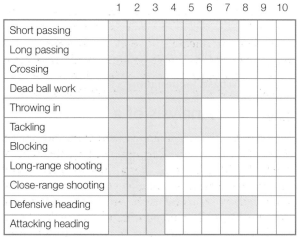

Fig 19.1 Performance profile for a midfielder

Physiological Analysis of a Sporting Activity

This is completed in the same manner as the technical analysis except the constructs will be different (see Figure 19.2).

Psychological Constructs

This is also completed in the same manner as the technical analysis, except the constructs will be different (see Figure 19.3).

	1	2	3	4	5	6	7	8	9	10
CV fitness										
Anaerobic fitness										
Speed										
Strength										
Power										
Muscular endurance										
Flexibility										
Lung function										
Body composition										
Agility										
Reaction times										
Core stability										

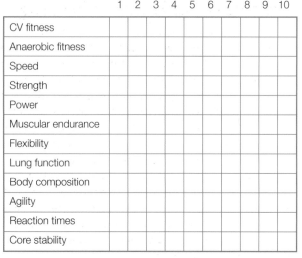

Fig 19.2 Physiological constructs for a tennis player

	1	2	3	4	5	6	7	8	9	10
Intrinsic motivation										
Extrinsic motivation										
Arousal control										
Anxiety levels										
Attentional focus										
Confidence										
Controlling agression										
State management										
Concentration skills										
Relaxation skills										
Emotional well-being										
Mental rehearsal										
Imagery skills										

Fig 19.3 Psychological constructs for a boxer

Biomechanical Constructs

A fourth analysis can be completed of the biomechanical demands of a sporting activity (see Figure 19.4).

	1	2	3	4	5	6	7	8	9	10
Development of velocity										
Velocity at release										
Acceleration										
Application of force										
Use of levers										

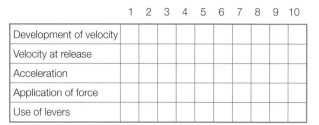

Fig 19.4 Biomechanical constructs for a javelin thrower

Benefits of Performance Profiling

As a technique for analysing performance, profiling works very well because it can take into account a vast amount of information for analysis by coach and athlete. It also considers the roles of coach and athlete as equally important with their different viewpoints on performance. Crucially, it takes into account the opinion of the athlete and gives them an active role in the analysis process, allowing them to take ownership of their performance and outcomes. It also allows the coach and athlete to identify any areas of mismatch where there is a differing opinion, and provides a basis for discussion. It can act as a process of education for the athlete as they become self-aware of the varying demands on them as well as their relative importance.

Performance profiles can form the basis of a review of progress on a monthly basis as the athlete and coach track their progress. They can also inform the process of goal setting to set the way forward.

Key learning points 1

- Performance profiling is a way of looking at performance in a broad sense.
  - It involves the opinion of the athlete as well as that of the coach.
  - It can be used to identify strengths and weaknesses.
- Performance profiling can be applied to technical, physiological, psychological and biomechanical components of performance.

The effectiveness of an individual's sporting performance comes down to a range of factors, which can be split into two categories:

- intrinsic – factors within the body
- extrinsic – factors outside the body.

Intrinsic factors would include:

- age
- health
- diet
- previous training
- motivation
- confidence
- ability level.

Extrinsic factors would include:

- group dynamics
- group cohesion
- temperature
- time of the day.

Intrinsic Factors

Age

It is generally accepted that performance declines after the age of 35. Up to the age of 35 the body is building up in terms of bone and muscle strength and cardiovascular fitness. After the age of 35 these structures of the body slowly start to lose their efficiency with a resulting performance decrement, although, having said that, training will slow down this decline and maintain strength, flexibility and cardiovascular fitness. We have seen many sportspeople remain at the top level despite being over the age of 35. Martina Navratilova was winning tennis titles into her fifties. Ryan Giggs, Simon Shaw (Rugby Union), Ricky Ponting (cricket), Lee Westwood (golf) are all still able to perform at the top level in their sports despite their age.

Health

The health of an individual's organs and systems are all vital in gaining their adaptations from training and then producing top-level performances. The body functions as a whole organism made up of many systems and organs, and poor function in one area will affect the functioning of the whole organism.

Diet

There is a clear link between nutrition and health. When we eat we are ultimately feeding the cells of the body with nutrients to allow them to function and give them the basic building blocks to remain healthy. If we feed our cells with fresh, nutritious foods we will have healthy cells, contributing to our health. But if we feed our cells with poor-quality nutrients from processed or fast foods we will end up with unhealthy and ultimately diseased cells, contributing to illness.

Previous Training

Our current position is the result of all the activity we have or have not done in our lives. The performance the athlete is able to produce depends upon the quality of their training programme and the fine balance between training and rest periods.

Motivation

Motivation is the amount of drive and energy that we possess at any point in time. It influences our desire to win. If we have trained hard and looked after our nutrition and rest patterns, we will feel better and subsequently more motivated.

Confidence

Our confidence is the extent to which we feel we will be successful; it is affected by a range of factors.

These will include our previous experiences and our perception of these experiences as either successful or otherwise. In addition, there is our perception of our opponents and our ability to deal with the environment in which we are placed. For example, we may feel more confident when we compete on our home territory and slightly intimidated when we go away. Our confidence level is closely related to our anxiety levels and if we are anxious about our performance this will start to erode our confidence levels.

Ability Level

Our ability is the natural level of skills we possess and is the basis for developing further skills. Our performance is clearly the result of the ability and skills we possess.

Extrinsic Factors

Group Dynamics

Group dynamics refers to the sum of the processes occurring within the group that will influence its effectiveness. The most successful groups have a high level of attractiveness for the individual members, and the members will also share the same goals and work towards achieving these objectives.

Group Cohesion

Group cohesion is the extent to which the individual members of the group have an attraction to the group and keep the group together. Cohesion can be task-related or socially related. Task cohesion is the extent to which you are willing to work together in the sporting environment, and social cohesion is how well you get on away from the sporting field. Task cohesion is the most important factor but it can be boosted by social cohesion.

Temperature

Extremes of temperature can have a negative effect on performance due to the effect on the physiological systems of the body. Heat can cause excess sweating, dehydration and heat exhaustion, while cold can make it difficult for the cardiovascular and muscular systems to achieve the correct temperature for optimal functioning.

Time of Day

The time of day can influence performance in terms of nutritional and fatigue status. In the morning before a person has eaten they will be in a dehydrated state with low blood sugar and in a far from optimal state to perform effectively. Depending upon when they eat and drink they will fluctuate in terms of their nutritional status through the day. Other physical factors can change through the day. Mobility and flexibility will be lowest in the morning due to the inactivity of the joints and the lack of synovial fluid that has been excreted into the joint.

Q Quick quiz 1

Decide whether each of the following constructs for a netball player should be categorised as technical (T), physiological (Ph) or psychological (Ps)

- confidence
- passing
- speed
- aerobic fitness
- blocking
- arousal control
- aggression control
- movement
- power
- shooting.

Student activity 19.1 — 45 minutes — P1 P2 M1 D1

Example of a performance profile

CASE STUDY: WILLIAM

William is a 16-year-old rugby player who plays number 8 for his college U17 team. He is a very promising player, but has only been playing for about 18 months and is still learning about the game. To help him to improve his performances he has agreed to have a performance profile constructed. The results of the performance profile are shown below:

	1	2	3	4	5	6	7	8	9	10
Tackling							7			
Strength				4						
Power			3							
Rucking			3							
Aggression control		2								
Concentration			3							
Passing								8		
Aerobic endurance							7			
Arousal control		2								
Scrummaging					5					

Part 1

1 Describe the performance profile for William.

P1

2 Explain the performance profile for William.

M1

3 Analyse the performance profile for William.

D1

Part 2

Describe how the following factors may influence performance:

P2

Factor	How it may affect performance
Diet	
Motivation	
Confidence	
Group dynamics	
Temperature	

19.3 Analysing Sporting Performance

D1 D2

Performance Profile Assessment

The performance profile relies on the respective viewpoints of the athlete and coach. It is also useful to gather information to be used in rating the score for each construct. The opinions of the athlete and coach would be qualitative data, while the information gathered from testing would be quantitative data.

The four aspects of the performance profile could be analysed using the following quantitative data

Technical constructs:

- notational analysis
- tally charts.

Physical constructs:

- multi-stage fitness test
- 40-m sprint
- 1 rep max
- 15 rep max
- sit and reach test
- peak flow test
- skinfold calipers
- T-test.

Psychological constructs:

- questionnaires
- interviews
- observation of behaviour.

Biomechanical analysis:

- video recording
- computer packages.

Notational analysis

Notational analysis is the tracking of the actions of an individual performer through the course of a game or match to see the frequency with which they perform a particular technique. It can be done through a computer package or by hand using tally charts.

A tally chart for football is reproduced in Figure 19.5:

Tally chart: football		
Skill	**Successful completion**	**Unsuccessful completion**
Short-range pass (< 5m)		
Medium-range pass (5–15m)		
Long-range pass (> 15m)		
Dribble		
Short-range shot (< 6m)		
Medium-range shot (7–18m)		
Long-range shot (> 18m)		
Tackle		
Block		
Defensive header		
Attacking header		
Throw-in		
Free kick		
Corner		
Penalty kick		

Fig 19.5 A tally chart for football

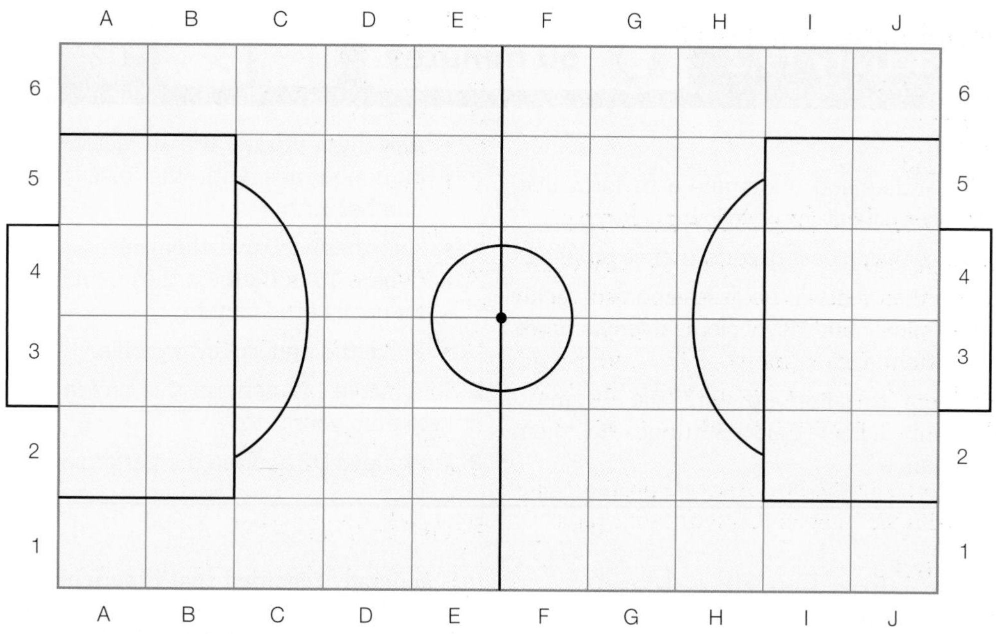

Fig 19.6 Football pitch sectionalised into areas

Passing record		
Skill	**Successful completion**	**Unsuccessful completion**
Short-range pass (< 5m)	G5–F5 D3–D2 I6–J5	F4–F3 C3–C4
Medium-range pass (5–15m)	G2–E4 C6–A6 H1–F3	D5–B4
Long-range pass (> 15m)	I4–E3 C1–B5	F6–D1 I5–D3 F1–C4

Fig 19.7 A passing record for football

This information is of limited value as you also need to look at where this action occurs. This can be done by sectionalising the area of play (see Figure 19.6) and giving each area a label. This will elicit more valuable information.

This can be done with a cricket pitch, tennis or netball court. You can then track where each type of skill occurs and its outcome.

An example of tracking the passing of a footballer is also reproduced in Figure 19.7.

The uses of notational analysis are to:

- identify individual strengths and weaknesses
- analyse all the actions of a player
- build up information to rate score on performance profile
- develop an action plan to improve performance.

Student activity 19.2 — 60 minutes — P3 M2 D2

Task

1 Select an athlete and undertake a performance profiling assessment in the following way:
- Introduce the process of performance profiling.
- Explain that you will be assessing technical, physiological and psychological aspects of their performance.
- Ask them to come up with the 10 most important factors that contribute to their performance.
- Ask them to rank the 10 factors in the order of importance with the most important at number 1.
- Ask them to give themselves a score of 10 (where 10 is the best they could possibly be) for each of the factors.
- Fill in the performance profile.

2 To achieve M2 perform this profile without any help from your tutor.

3 To achieve D2 analyse the performance profile.

19.4 Providing Feedback on Performance

P4 M3

It is impossible for anyone to improve or change unless they receive feedback.

Key term

Feedback: information about performance.

It has no value judgement attached to it as it is not positive or negative. It is simply information. The information is provided and the athlete has the choice of doing something about it or not.

Types of Feedback

There are different categories of feedback regarding its timing and the type of feedback given. They are:

- knowledge of performance and results
- immediate and delayed
- internal and external
- concurrent and terminal.

Knowledge of Performance and Results

Knowledge of performance (KP) is information regarding how well skills were performed in a technical sense and will involve qualitative judgements. Knowledge of results (KR) is information regarding the outcome of the skill – whether the action produced success or failure – this is a quantitative judgement. It is possible to perform a skill well (KP) and have a negative outcome (KR) or have a poor performance (KP) and a positive outcome (KR).

It is generally regarded that experienced performers are more interested in knowledge of performance, while novices are more interested in knowledge of results.

Immediate and Delayed

Immediate means that the feedback is given immediately after the skill has been performed, while delayed means feedback is provided at a time after the event – this could be a day or an hour later. The coach needs to consider the impact that the feedback will have on the athlete's motivation and how important it is for the athlete to receive it. Once they have considered those two questions they can decide when to give the feedback.

Internal and External

Internal feedback is generated within the body of the athlete. As you perform a skill you will feel whether you have performed it correctly or not due to the nervous pathways you have set down to produce the movement and judge its correctness. As we hit a tennis ball we feel whether we have struck it sweetly or not. External feedback is provided by an external party, who observes the performance. For example, the coach will observe the performance of the skill and offer feedback as to how it looked and how effective it was. External feedback may also be provided by using camcorders or other recording devices.

Concurrent and Terminal

Concurrent means literally 'running together'. This type of feedback is provided during the performance of the skill in terms of how it feels and often the outcome as well. Concurrent feedback is usually internal in nature and clearly immediate in when it is provided. Terminal means 'at the end'. This type of feedback is provided at the end of the performance. It is usually external and is always delayed.

Delivering the Feedback

Once the coach has decided on what feedback is necessary to address the individual's strengths and areas for improvement, they will need to decide when, where and how to deliver it. How the feedback is received depends upon how it is delivered.

Structure

When giving feedback you should use the sandwich technique. Feedback should have this structure:

- tell them what they are doing right
- tell them what they need to improve on
- tell them something else they did right.

This means that the feedback ends on a high note and the athlete understands what needs to be improved.

Non-verbal Communication

Feedback can be given visually and through gestures as well as verbally. The use of facial expressions, posture and hand gestures will convey more than the actual words used. The delivery of the message should match the message being given. This is called being 'congruent'. Also, gestures such as a pat on the back or a hand on the arm will convey information that cannot be imparted in words.

Avoiding Negative Approaches

Avoid any negative approaches or comments.

- Intimidation: 'If you don't improve you can find a new coach.'
- Sarcasm: 'My granny could have caught that!'
- Physical abuse: 'Unless you listen to what I say, you will be doing press-ups.'
- Guilt: 'You should be ashamed of yourselves the way you played out there. It was gutless and you let your supporters down.'

Private and Confidential

Ensure feedback is given in a private area as it may be sensitive and is not relevant for anyone else.

Focus on Behaviour

Focus on the behaviour rather than identity. This is the difference between a coach saying 'You are an aggressive person and this is not acceptable' and 'Your aggressive actions are not acceptable.' One addresses the behaviour, which can be changed, and the other addresses the identity of the person, which is long term and relatively stable.

Using the Feedback Provided

Once the feedback has been received and processed by the athlete, they have to decide how to use the information. It may be used in the following ways:

- to set SMART targets combining short-, medium- and long-term goals
- to develop or change a training programme to include technical, physiological and psychological components of performance
- to inform the process of performance profiling and assessment of scoring the individual constructs.

Key learning points 2

- Feedback is information about an individual's performance.
- Feedback can be categorised in two ways: knowledge of performance (KP) and knowledge of results (KR). KP is information about how well the skill was performed and KR is information about the outcome of the skill.
- Immediate feedback is given as soon as the skill has been performed, while delayed feedback is given at a period after the performance.
- Internal feedback is derived from sources inside the body and external feedback comes from sources inside the body.
- Concurrent feedback occurs as the skill is being performed and terminal feedback occurs after the completion of the skill.
- When providing feedback keep in mind the following:
  - using the sandwich approach of positive/negative/positive
  - providing it visually as well as verbally through body language
  - avoiding sarcasm, intimidation, abuse and guilt
  - ensuring it is delivered in a private area
  - focus on behaviour rather than identity.

Quick quiz 2

Match the type of feedback to its correct definition.

Type of feedback	Choice of definitions
Knowledge of results	Information given immediately after a skill has been performed
Knowledge of performance	Information generated from sources within the body
Immediate	Information about the outcome of the skill
Delayed	Information generated from sources outside the body
Internal	Information about how well skills are performed
External	Information provided at a period after the skill has been performed

Student activity 19.3

30 minutes P4 M3

Task

Based on the performance profiling exercise that you conducted in Activity 19.2 provide feedback to your selected athlete in the following way:

- Make written notes about the strengths and areas for improvement for your selected athlete
- Conduct a feedback session with your selected athlete.

To achieve M3 this feedback should be provided independent of tutor support.

19.5 The Purpose and Resources Required for Analysing Different Levels of Sporting Performance

P5

Sport England has identified four different levels of sporting performance, as follows.

Foundation Level

At foundation level focus is on the participants learning and understanding basic movement skills and developing a positive attitude to physical activity. This level is concerned with giving school children positive and meaningful experiences of sport.

Beginner or Participation Level

At participation or beginner levels the participants will be taking part in sport for a range of reasons, such as health, fitness and social. They may also be attracted by the competitive aspects of sport. This level of participation would involve out-of-school sports teams and Saturday league players.

Performance Level

At performance level the participants will be active in improving standards of performance through coaching, competition and training. This would involve the participants playing at county or national standard.

Elite or Excellence Level

Elite and excellence levels involve the participants reaching national standards of performance up to Olympic or world-class performances.

Purpose of Analysis and Resources Required

Foundation Level

At this level the emphasis is on fun and enjoyment, and learning the basic skills and techniques. Analysis will be limited to identifying the strengths and weaknesses of the children and giving them feedback to improve their enjoyment of the sports. The resources required are limited to support from teachers and parents.

Beginner Level

At beginner level there is an emphasis on developing techniques and improving weaknesses along with developing strengths. This is a point where talent may be assessed for further development through coaching and physical training. Analysis is again done in a fairly informal manner through recommendations or even talent scouting.

Performance Level

Analysis starts to become very important at this level as it is about achieving standards of performance to reach county or national level. Analysis will be conducted to:

- identify talent
- form the basis for squad selection at county and national level
- assess current level of performance
- identify strengths and weaknesses
- assess fitness level and health status
- inform the process of goal setting.

In terms of resources required there is a need to put in time and effort on behalf of personnel. This is a key stage in moving people towards becoming athletes and to ultimately developing elite potential. Equipment required will include fitness testing equipment, sport science facilities, expertise from sport scientists and time devoted to each individual.

Elite Level

At elite level every aspect of an athlete's performance is analysed to the smallest degree as they seek to gain all the advantages they possibly can to improve their chances of success. At this level, aspects of health, fitness and performance are analysed on a daily basis. Indeed, the athlete may be professional or training on a full-time basis. The purpose of analysis at this level is to:

- assess current health and fitness status
- identify strengths and weaknesses
- assess current level of performance
- inform the process of goal setting
- identify any future issues or problems.

As athletes at this level may have contact with their support team at facilities such as a national sports centre, they are heavily dependent on resources. These resources are human in terms of sport scientists with various expertise, and physical resources for assessing fitness levels and analysing skills and techniques.

Key learning points 3

- At foundation level focus is on the participant's learning and understanding basic movement skills and developing a positive attitude to physical activity. Analysis is provided at this level to help participants improve their skills.
- At participation or beginner levels the participants will be taking part in sport for a range of reasons, such as health, fitness and social and competitive reasons. Analysis is used at beginner level to improve performance and identify talent.
- At performance level the participants will be active in improving standards of performance through coaching, competition and training. Analysis is provided to assess current level of performance and how to improve it, as well as identify talent to move to a higher level.
- Elite and excellence levels involve the participants reaching national standards of performance up to Olympic or world-class performances. Analysis is done at elite level to identify any area where the athlete could improve so they can compete at the very highest level.

Student activity 19.4 — 30 minutes — P5

Task

Fill out the following table to explain the purpose and resources required for analysis at two different levels of sport.

	Participation level	Elite level
Purpose of analysis		
Resources needed		

References

Bull, S. J. (1991) *Sport Psychology: A Self-help Guide*, Crowood.

Butler, R. J. (2000) *Sport Psychology in Performance*, Arnold.

Butler, R. J. and Hardy, L. (1992) 'The performance profile: theory and application', *The Sport Psychologist*, 6, 253–264.

Further reading

Hughes, M. and Franks, I. (2004) *Notational Analysis of Sport*, Abingdon: Routledge.

Martens, R. (2004) *Successful Coaching*, Champaign, IL: Human Kinetics.

Weinberg, R.S. and Gould, D. (2007) *Foundations of Sport and Exercise Psychology*, Champaign, IL: Human Kinetics.

Useful websites

www.brianmac.co.uk/eval.htm

Provides details of how to evaluate and test sports performance

www.pponline.co.uk/encyc/sports-performance-analysis-coaching-and-training-39

Article detailing how sports analysis can help coaching and training

24: Physical Education & the Care of Children & Young People

24.1 Introduction

Physical education is a compulsory activity in the national curriculum. Children from the age of 5 to 16 will have PE lessons scheduled into their timetable. PE lessons include a variety of activities, such as games, gymnastics, athletics, swimming and racket sports. In these lessons, children work as both individuals and members of a team, and as such learn a variety of different skills as well as the importance of healthy, active lifestyles.

If you are thinking of working as a PE teacher, this unit will provide you with the basic theoretical knowledge and practical activities that are required for effective sports teaching as well as classroom management strategies.

The unit explores PE across the different Key Stages as well as the role and values of PE in a wider social context.

The importance of safeguarding the needs of children and young people in education is also examined, including the 'Every Child Matters: Change for Children' agenda, which will enable you to identify ways of safeguarding children and young people in the learning context.

By the end of this unit you should:

- know the structure of physical education within the curriculum
- understand the importance of physical education in society
- be able to structure a lesson of physical education
- know the responsibilities of those who work with children to safeguard and promote their welfare, and strategies for safeguarding children, young people and self.

Assessment and grading criteria

To achieve a PASS grade the evidence must show that the learner is able to:	To achieve a MERIT grade the evidence must show that, in addition to the pass criteria, the learner is able to:	To achieve a DISTINCTION grade the evidence must show that, in addition to the pass and merit criteria, the learner is able to:
P1 describe the structure of the physical education curriculum		
P2 describe the impact of stakeholder views on the development of the physical education curriculum		
P3 describe the ways in which the curriculum is implemented	**M1** explain the different ways that learning providers meet national curriculum requirements	
P4 explain the importance of physical education to children and young people's educational attainment		
P5 outline the importance of physical education to society in general		
P6 plan a lesson of physical education describing how learning is supported	**M2** plan a lesson of physical education explaining how learning is supported	**D1** plan a lesson of physical education analysing support for learning
P7 describe strategies for supporting the safety of children and young people		
P8 describe the legislation, policies and procedures that safeguard children and young people in a learning context	**M3** explain how procedures keep children, young people and those working with them safe.	**D2** evaluate procedures in terms of how they keep children, young people and those working with them safe.
P9 describe strategies to ensure own protection when working with children and young people.		

24.2 Physical Education and the National Curriculum

P1 P2 P3 M1

The national curriculum (NC) attempts to raise standards in education and sets out a range of learning experiences that the government has decided is essential for all young people in education.

The national curriculum is administered by the Qualifications and Curriculum Development Agency (QCDA), which is part of the Department for Children, Schools and Families (DCSF). The QCDA's main role and responsibility is to advise and support schools and colleges to deliver and develop the national curriculum, a variety of tests and a range of examinations.

Structure of the National Curriculum

Education in England, Wales and Northern Ireland is structured into Key Stages (see Table 24.1).

Physical education is a core subject at all Key Stages, which means it continues to be one of only five subjects that pupils of all abilities must pursue, from their entry into school at the age of five until the end of compulsory schooling at age 16.

Physical education: KS 1 ✓ KS 2 ✓ KS3 ✓ KS4 ✓

The education system in Scotland also makes physical education a compulsory subject at all stages. The structure of the Scottish curriculum runs from ages 3–18, and is organised into Early, First, Second, Third and Fourth stages.

Stakeholders in Education

The government and the QCDA make use of a large network of experts to advise them in educational matters and in the design of the national curriculum. These include people, groups and organisations with an interest in education, who are called 'stakeholders'.

Stakeholders might represent business, industry, commerce and universities, all areas into which young people may wish to progress when they leave compulsory education. These stakeholders are naturally keen to ensure that state education and the national curriculum provide all young people with the opportunities to develop the abilities and skills needed in modern life.

Sector Skills Councils (SSCs) are state-sponsored, employer-led organisations that cover specific economic sectors in the United Kingdom. They have four key goals:

- To reduce skills gaps and shortages
- To improve productivity
- To boost the skills of their sector workforces
- To improve learning supply.

Examples of stakeholders in physical education, sport and recreation include the following:

1 **SkillsActive**
This is an organisation that works across the UK to help the government achieve its key objective of developing a healthier, fitter nation.

'SkillsActive is committed to increasing the number of industry-recognised qualifications for the active leisure and learning sector. It aims to work with industry and higher education experts, partners and employers to develop tailor-made qualifications that will assist the growth of a highly committed and competent workforce. In doing so, SkillsActive aims to professionalise and upskill the sector in the run up to, and beyond, the London 2012 Olympic Games and Paralympic Games.'
Source: www.skillsactive.com

2 **National occupational standards**
Again led by employers, this is an example of an independent body that acts as a stakeholder in education. It states its main objectives as follows:

Key Stage	Year groups	Ages
Foundation Stage	Preschool – end of Reception Year	3–5
Key Stage 1	Years 1–2	5–7
Key Stage 2	Years 3–6	7–11
Key Stage 3	Years 7–9	11–14
Key Stage 4	Years 10–11	14–16

Table 24.1 Key Stages in education (England & Wales)

- Identify skills and knowledge needed for occupations
- Provide a reference to assess ability and training needs
- Identify and support career paths.

3 **National governing bodies**

National governing bodies (NGBs) are the organising bodies for individual sports. There are 130 national governing bodies of sport that are recognised by UK Sports Councils.

As sporting stakeholders, NGBs play a central part in the national drive to increase participation in sport. The opportunities and challenges of major forthcoming sporting events such as London 2012 and Glasgow 2014 are also a key focus for all sports.

Funded by Sport England, NGBs set the strategic direction for the development of their sport. These plans include Children and Young People plans (CYP) through which NGBs will deliver coaching courses for teachers and students.

NGBs also play an important role in supporting recent government initiatives, which influence curriculum design for PE.

4 **Youth Sport Trust**

The Youth Sport Trust is a charity that strives to improve the quality and quantity of PE and sport for young people. It operates throughout the UK and works closely with the UK Sports Councils.

Its core work can be divided into a number of key areas:

- Raising the standards of PE and school sport
- Improving educational standards through sport
- Getting more young people involved in sport
- Creating opportunities for young leaders and volunteers
- Supporting sporting talent in young people.

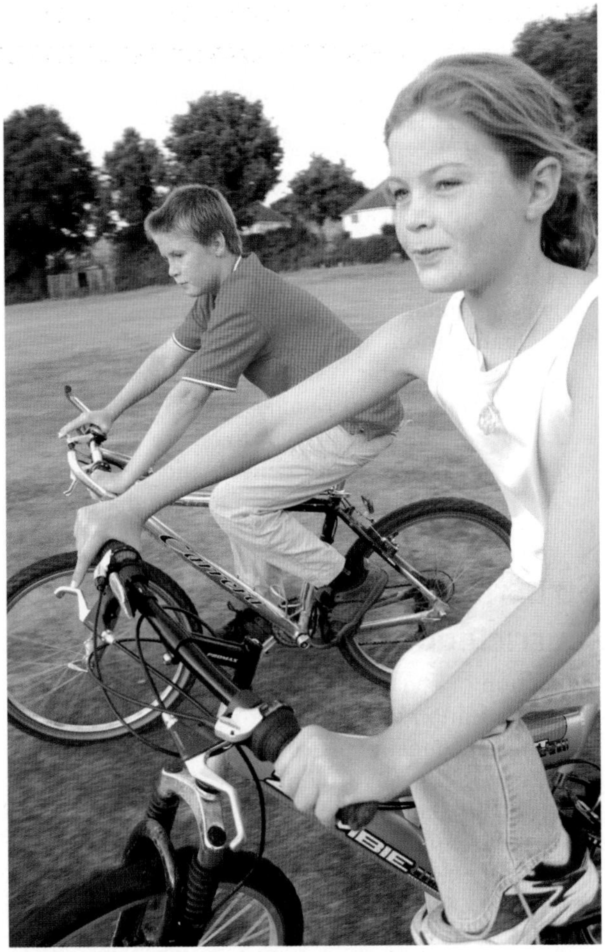

Fig 24.1 Children enjoying exercise

Physical Education in the National Curriculum

Children are required to demonstrate skills, knowledge and understanding in a variety of physical activity areas, which include games, dance, gymnastics, athletics, swimming and outdoor and adventurous activities.

The national curriculum sets out attainment targets, which describe expected levels of performance at the end of each Key Stage.

Pupil progress is measured by teachers, based on four strands of assessment:

- Acquiring and developing skills
- Selecting and applying skills, tactics and compositional ideas
- Evaluating and improving performance
- Knowledge and understanding of fitness and health.

CASE STUDY OF A GOVERNMENT INITIATIVE
PHYSICAL EDUCATION AND SPORT STRATEGY FOR YOUNG PEOPLE (PESSYP)

The Youth Sport Trust plays a central role in supporting the Department for Children, Schools and Families (DCSF) and the Department for Culture, Media and Sport (DCMS) in the delivery of the PE and Sport Strategy for Young People. The strategy sets out how the Olympic legacy aim to get more children and young people taking part in high-quality PE and sport will be reached, through the delivery of the 'five-hour offer'.

The Youth Sport Trust and Sport England are working with the DCSF and the DCMS on ways to help local delivery partners offer all young people aged 5 to 16 the opportunity to participate in five hours a week of PE and sport (three hours for 16 to 19-year-olds). The first outcome of this work is the new 'Guide to Delivering the Five-Hour Offer', a document which outlines the vision for the strategy and the five-hour offer in particular.

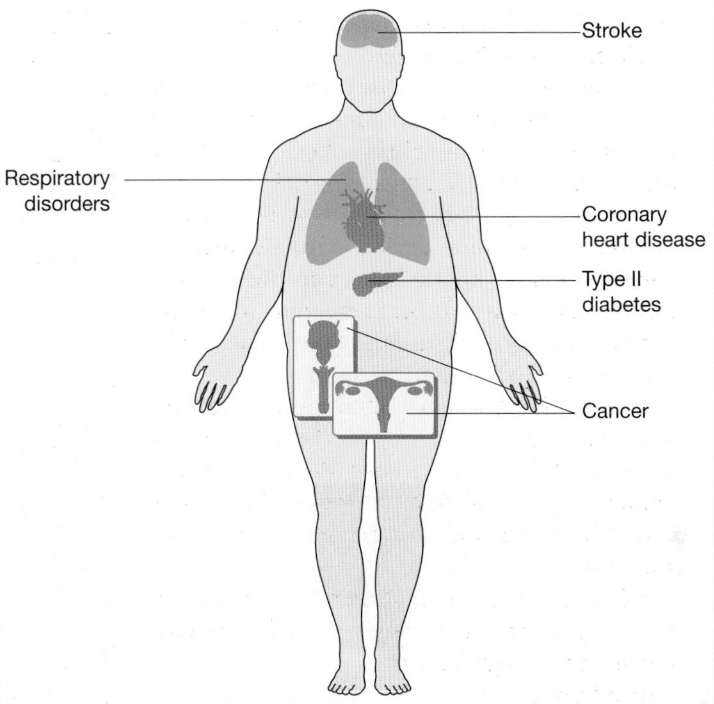

Fig 24.2 Medical conditions brought on by obesity

PESSYP has two main aims:

1 To improve the quality and quantity of curriculum PE in schools.
2 To improve the quality and quality of sport accessible and available to young people in schools, colleges and the wider community.

'All children and young people aged between 5–16 years should have the opportunity to participate in five hours of sport per week by 2011 (including two hours of high quality PE and sport at school).'
Source: www.youthsporttrust.org

The 'five-hour offer' is to be developed by School Sports Partnerships and local club links in the following way:

Two hours of curriculum PE + one hour of school sport + two hours of community sport = five hours

PE must provide support for whole school delivery of two key initiatives:

- Every Child Matters (ECM)
- Personal, Learning and Thinking Skills (PLTS).

Key Stage Implementation

Early Years Foundation Stage (ages 3–5)

Physical development is the main objective at this stage.

Very young children use play to develop physical skills and coordination, and to learn how to be creative and how to share and cooperate in social groupings.

Key Stages 1 and 2 (ages 5–11)

PE in primary schools aims for pupils to enjoy being active and to learn new skills as a foundation for 'physical literacy'.

At this stage, children will:

- Enjoy being active, showing what they can do
- Practise new skills across a range of activities that should include dance, gymnastics, games,

swimming, athletics and outdoor and adventurous activities
- Learn consistency by repeating their movements and linking their skills until their performance is clearer, more accurate and controlled over time
- Pace themselves in challenges in activities such as swimming and athletic activities
- Use their creativity in performing dances, making up their own games, planning gymnastic sequences, and responding to problem-solving and challenge activities
- Know how to improve aspects of the quality of their work, using information provided by the teacher and information and communication technology (ICT) opportunities, and increasingly help themselves and others perform effectively
- Know why activity is important to their health and well-being.

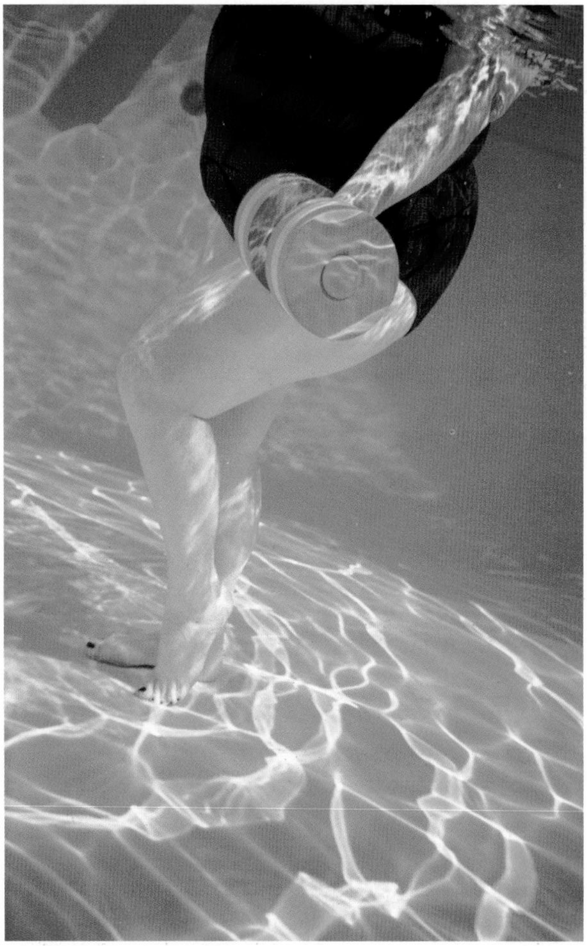

Fig 24.3 Exercising in water

Key Stages 3 and 4

At Key Stages 3 and 4, PE is currently undergoing changes brought about by the introduction of the revised national curriculum (2008–2011).

Greater Flexibility and Coherence

To give schools greater flexibility to tailor learning to their learners' needs, there is less prescribed subject content in the new programmes of study. Pupils will still be taught essential subject knowledge. However, the new curriculum balances subject knowledge with the key concepts and processes that underlie the discipline of each subject.

Key Concepts

There are a number of key concepts that now underpin the study of PE:

- Competence
- Performance
- Creativity
- Healthy and active lifestyles.

Key processes: these are the essential skills and processes in PE that pupils need to learn to make progress:

- Developing skills in physical activity
- Making and applying decisions
- Developing physical and mental capacity
- Evaluating and improving
- Making informed choices about healthy, active lifestyles.

Range and Content

The study of PE should include activities that cover at least four of the following:

1. Outwitting opponents, as in games activities.
2. Accurate replication of actions, phrases and sequences, as in gymnastic activities.
3. Exploring and communicating ideas, concepts and emotions, as in dance activities.
4. Performing at maximum levels in relation to speed, height, distance, strength or accuracy, as in athletic activities.
5. Identifying and solving problems to overcome challenges of an adventurous nature, as in life saving and personal survival in swimming and outdoor activities.
6. Exercising safely and effectively to improve health and well-being, as in fitness and health activities.

Curriculum Opportunities

The curriculum should provide opportunities for pupils to:

- Get involved in a broad range of different activities that, in combination, develop the whole body
- Experience a range of roles within a physical activity

- Specialise in specific activities and roles
- Follow pathways to other activities in and beyond school
- Perform as an individual, in a group or as part of a team in formal competitions or performances to audiences beyond the class
- Use ICT as an aid to improving performance and tracking progress
- Make links between PE and other subjects and areas of the curriculum.

Qualifications in PE at Key Stage 4

Most pupils now are able to gain some form of qualification or accreditation in Years 10 and 11. Some qualifications have an academic focus, while others take a more vocational approach. All provide the basis for future study and progression. The most popular routes to PE and sport qualifications at Key Stage 4 are:

- GCSE PE and Dance
- Short Course PE
- BTEC First Certificate in Sports Leadership
- BTEC First Diploma in Sports Science
- 14–19 Diploma in Sport and Active Leisure
- Level 1 Sports Leadership award
- OCR Nationals in Sport.

Criteria and Specifications

Examination specifications describe the syllabus content, aims, assessment methods and objectives and how the qualification is graded. Specifications are designed by examination boards rather than the QCA. Each examination board offers a slightly different specification, which gives schools and colleges a choice of qualification to best suit their learners.

Key learning points 1

- Purpose and structure of the national curriculum.
- Stakeholders have a significant influence on curriculum design and content.
- Programme of study for PE at each Key Stage.
- PESSYP as a government initiative.
- There have been recent changes to PE at Key Stages 3 and 4.
- There is now a choice of qualification routes available at Key Stage 4.

Q Quick quiz 1

1 What do the initials 'DCFS' and 'QCA' stand for?
2 Steve is 8 and Lucy is 15. Which Key Stages are they in?
3 Summarise the main objectives of 'SkillsActive'.
4 Describe the twin aims of the PESSYP strategy.
5 At Key Stages 3 and 4, 'games' has changed to 'outwitting opponents, as in games activities'. Explain possible reasons for this change.

Student activity 24.1 — 90–120 mins — P1 P2 P3 M1

Physical education plays an important part in every child's development and is a compulsory subject in the national curriculum.

Task 1

Prepare a leaflet that describes the structure of the physical education curriculum. You should include details of the Early Years Foundation Stage and Key Stages 1–4.

Task 2

- Draw a spider diagram to show the different stakeholders involved in the development of the physical education curriculum.
- Prepare a written report that describes the impact of these stakeholders on the development of physical education in the national curriculum.

Task 3

Prepare and deliver a PowerPoint presentation that describes and explains the different ways that the curriculum is implemented by different learning providers.

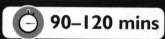

24.3 The Importance of Physical Education in Society

P4 P5

Importance of Curriculum PE

Physical education is a vital element in a comprehensive, well-balanced curriculum and can be a major contributing factor in the development of an individual in all aspects of life: physical, emotional, mental and social.

Through a high-quality physical education experience, an individual has the opportunity to:

- Understand the importance of obtaining and maintaining a high level of physical fitness
- Participate in a wide variety of physical activities, which helps to maintain an active and healthy lifestyle
- Become a skilful, intelligent and independent performer and leader
- Develop fair play, teamwork and socially desirable behaviour
- Gain in self-confidence and self-esteem.

Key term

Physical literacy: having the motivation, confidence, physical competence, knowledge and understanding to maintain physical activity throughout life. This definition reflects the learning outcomes of high-quality teaching and learning in PE.

Physical literacy and an active lifestyle remain the cornerstone of the PE objectives for all pupils, but so much more can be achieved with a broad and balanced curriculum.

Research findings show that pupils striving for academic success at school are far more likely to succeed if they take a full and active part in PE lessons.

- Regular participation in physical education, even if you are not naturally good at games, can make a big difference to academic results at all Key Stages.
- Research shows PE can improve literacy, numeracy and technology skills.
- PE sessions help youngsters improve their communication skills, which in turn helps in the classroom. Pupils are also using technology and IT to support and enhance their work in PE lessons.

Head teachers also report that there has been a noticeable improvement in pupils' key personal, social and learning skills.

Primary school head teachers speak enthusiastically about the positive impact PE can have on pupils' behaviour and their attitudes to work.

High-quality PE will support pupils' cognitive development so that they improve at:

- Creating conditions for personal success
- Taking more responsibility for own learning
- Thinking for themselves
- Solving problems.

Summary

High-quality and enjoyable physical education will enable children to develop a range of abilities:

- **Technical** ability, in a range of skills
- **Physiological** ability, in terms of fitness
- **Social skills,** in group and team settings
- **Cognitive** ability, in terms of thinking skills and problem solving.

Importance of Extracurricular PE and Sport

The PE and Sport Strategy for Young People (PESSYP) aims to offer children and young people in England at least five hours of high-quality PE and sport every week (for those aged 5–16 years). This begins in school with curriculum PE and by participating in after-school clubs.

By building on and improving the quality of existing PE and school sport opportunities available to young people, it is hoped that an increasing proportion of children will be guided into local sports, physical recreation and physical activity, both in school and in the local community. The strategy aims to promote a culture that enables and values the full involvement of every child and young person, whether as a competitor, volunteer, official or organiser. It is hoped that this will lead to a significant increase in the number of young people taking part in high-quality club sport on a regular basis.

The strategy is delivered on a local level through collaboration between schools, school sport partnerships, county sports partnerships (CSPs) and NGB-accredited sports clubs.

Extracurricular activities have been identified as a rich source of personal development for children and young people.

Benefits of regular involvement in physical activity and sport outside the curriculum can help young people to:

- Develop various sports skills

- Develop skills needed to socialise with their peers as well as adults
- Develop independence and confidence
- Develop a sense of achievement, which helps develop a positive self-image
- Develop leadership skills and qualities
- Learn how to cooperate and compete
- Develop agility, coordination, endurance, flexibility, speed and strength
- Develop the ability to make decisions and accept responsibilities
- Develop an interest in continuing sports participation as an adult.

However, the progression from school to club and community sport can be a daunting step for many young people. Traditionally, there has been a sharp decline in participation in sport and physical recreation in the 16–19 age group.

Crucial support is needed from schools, community sport and parents if this decline is to be arrested. Equally, this is an issue that both central and local government take very seriously and spend considerable time and money on.

Importance of PE and Sport in Society

The government believes that high-quality PE and sport:

- Raises standards
- Improves the health of the nation
- Helps ensure that the UK competes successfully on the world stage.

Sporting Benefits

Success in sport has a positive effect on the nation.

- We feel good when we win trophies and competitions. This 'feel good' factor is reputed to help us forget other problems, and can bring together different groups in society. This is known as 'social cohesion'.
- More people playing sport at foundation or 'grass roots' level means there is a larger pool of talent available for talent identification and future development.

Social Benefits

The social benefits of participation in sport are as follows:

- Safer communities with reduced crime rates
- Stronger social networks (social cohesion)
- Purposeful activity improves quality of life.

Economic Benefits

- Healthy and active population.
- Reduction in healthcare costs.
- Increased productivity at work.
- Productive use of leisure time stimulates economic demand.

Mass participation in sport and active leisure is an important aspect of government policy for the sporting, social and economic benefits shown above.

A healthy, active population will cost less, spend more on leisure, develop sporting and artistic interests, and generally cause far fewer problems.

Just what every government wants!

Key learning points 2

- PE promotes physical literacy.
- PE can promote higher attainment in a variety of abilities.
- PE and an active and healthy lifestyle provide a number of health benefits.
- The government values PE and sport for a variety of reasons.

Q Quick quiz 2

1 Explain the term 'physical literacy' in your own words.

2 Give examples of how PE and sport has helped you develop.

3 Describe how PE and sport can promote leadership.

4 Outline two reasons why the government believes in PE and sport.

5 Explain possible reasons for lower participation in the 16–19 age group.

Student activity 24.2 — 60–90 mins — P4 P5

Physical education provides many health, education and social benefits and is encouraged by many different organisations.

Task 1

In pairs, discuss how physical education has benefited you in your:

- Educational attainment
- Role in society.

Task 2

Design a poster with illustrations and text that:

- Explains the importance of physical education to children and young people's educational attainment
- Outlines the importance of physical education to society in general.

24.4 Structure of a Physical Education Lesson

P6 M2 D1

There is a saying: 'Fail to plan, plan to fail'. This is very true in teaching and very true in teaching physical education!

This section will take you through the process involved in planning a physical education lesson.

Key Terms in Lesson Planning

Teaching is the formal process and describes what the teacher says or does.

Learning takes place when the pupils can do, know or understand something that previously they could not achieve or did not know.

Learning outcomes are what it is intended that pupils will achieve, know and understand at the end of each lesson.

Assessment is the gathering of evidence to show pupil progress.

Normal Structure of Lessons

- A **lesson plan** sets out the objectives and content of one lesson.
- A **lesson** is a single part of a unit of work.
- A **unit of work** is part of a programme of study.
- **Programmes of study** make up each Key Stage of the national curriculum.

Each individual lesson contains key elements:

- **Purpose** – what are your intentions for this lesson?
- **Prior learning** – how can you build on learning in previous lessons?
- **Learning outcomes** – what do you want pupils to achieve, learn, and understand?
- **Pupil activities** – how pupils will achieve the learning outcomes.
- **Teaching points** – guidance, feedback and advice for pupils.
- **Assessment** – did most pupils achieve the learning outcomes?
- **Evaluation** – was the lesson successful? Why? Why not?

Every class is a group of individual children. Each pupil is an individual with different needs and learning preferences and each pupil will respond differently to learning situations. Successful teachers can vary their teaching styles and are able to adapt the activities and resources used in lessons to meet the needs of individual pupils or groups of pupils.

Successful lessons are normally introduced by teachers or adults, who guide the direction and pace of the lesson, while the activities and lesson content are based on child-centred principles and appropriate learning outcomes.

Successful lessons are characterised more by learning than by teaching. Skilled teachers will maximise pupils' learning potential by making use of a range of strategies such as:

- Inclusion
- Differentiation
- Questioning rather than telling
- Progression through structured learning situations
- Observation
- Individual feedback
- Praise and encouragement.

Key terms

Inclusion: this ensures equal opportunity for all pupils, irrespective of ability.

Differentiation: making use of a variety of teaching and learning styles and tasks to meet the needs of all pupils.

Lesson Planning in PE

Lesson planning in PE shares the same basic structure and characteristics as all other subjects in the school curriculum. However, on account of its practical nature, there are other considerations and safeguards that teachers of PE must include in all lesson plans.

- **Health & safety.** All schools are required to have 'risk assessment' policies in place – especially important in practical subjects like PE.
- **Special needs and medical conditions.**
- **Parental consent** is often required for lessons such as swimming, as well as after-school clubs and off-site activities.
- **First-aid resources.**
- **Appropriate kit and equipment.**

The structure of a PE lesson often follows a traditional pattern:

- **Warm-up** – teacher-directed or pupil-led
- **Specific focus** – skill-based or situation-based
- **Main activity** – appropriate event, game, etc
- **Cool-down and conclusion.**

This structure concentrates on pupil activities, but there is far more to lesson planning than just the activities. Lesson planning takes time, especially for people new to teaching. You will find detailed examples of lesson planning templates with accompanying notes below and on pages 300–301.

When you have the opportunity to teach a lesson or coach a session, try to make use of the **STEP** formula, which aims to manipulate four key factors to provide the best possible conditions for learners.

The STEP Formula

- **S** stands for **SPACE** – how can you make best use of space?
- **T** stands for **TASK** – are the tasks appropriate for pupils?
- **E** stands for **EQUIPMENT** – is the equipment suitable for pupils?
- **P** stands for **PUPILS** – how can pupils be best grouped?

Lesson Plan – Part One

SUBJECT: CLASS: DATE:
PURPOSE OF LESSON These are your **teaching intentions** for this lesson, e.g. to introduce a new topic or skills to consolidate previous learning.
PRIOR LEARNING (from previous lesson evaluations and pupil assessments) How does information you have obtained about **pupils' learning** in previous lessons inform the planning of this lesson? **Teacher action** (e.g. strategies for pupil and class management, choice of teaching and learning strategies) How will this inform the planning of this lesson?
LEARNING OUTCOMES FOR THIS LESSON **State what you intend pupils to learn.** There might be one key learning objective or there might be a number of them. You may need to identify different learning objectives for different pupils. In addition to the main PE subject focus, there may be cross-curricular learning objectives, e.g. a maths learning objective or a social objective, such as teamwork and cooperation.
CLASSROOM OBJECTIVES Learning objectives expressed in a form that **could be shared with pupils.**
SUCCESS CRITERIA These relate to the learning objectives. They should provide evidence of learning. Express them in a form that could be shared with children.
MONITORING AND ASSESSMENT Tell pupils who, what, how and when you will be monitoring pupils' progress and assessing their learning during this lesson, e.g. 'I will assess your performance as a defender; I will question the whole class during the plenary'.
KEY VOCABULARY Explain the **key subject-specific vocabulary** that the children will need or you intend to introduce/consolidate.
RESOURCES AND PREPARATION (including health and safety considerations) List resources, including ICT, needed by (a) you, (b) the pupils, and (c) any other adults. State how these will be organised. State any safety precautions that are necessary.

Lesson Plan – Part Two

LESSON STRUCTURE			
PHASE TIMING	**TEACHER'S ACTIONS**	**PUPIL ACTIVITIES**	**RESOURCES**
Introduction Estimated time:	State how you will introduce the lesson, e.g. by referring to the lesson objectives. State how you will introduce activities that the pupils are going to carry out. Main teaching points/any questions you might ask. Giving instructions (state key ideas). Explain what comes next.	Explain how pupils (individuals, groups and/or whole class) will be involved. Identify opportunities for pupil contributions, discussion, questions and assessment. Indicate how teaching and learning will be assessed.	Identify resource needs.
Main Activities Estimated time:	This part of the lesson should normally take the greatest proportion of time. You may decide to work with small groups or the whole class. Show how you will: • Monitor their progress to ensure that all are learning • Ensure that all pupils are being challenged and that interest/pace is maintained • Ensure that all pupils understand what they are doing • Decide when to make whole-class interventions • Provide formative feedback • Set targets for individuals and groups for the remainder of this part of the lesson • Assess pupils' learning.	Show how pupils will be organised – individually, in pairs or in groups? Plan activities for pupils to facilitate the learning objectives. Show how these activities will permit inclusion and differentiation.	Identify resources needed for different activities.
Plenary or Conclusion Estimated time:	Time must be planned to allow every lesson to be brought to an appropriate conclusion: • To check and reinforce what has been learned (with reference to the learning objectives) • To question/assess the pupils about what they have learnt • To praise and give feedback • To preview next lesson • To allow time for tidying up and changing.	Indicate how pupils (individuals, groups and/or whole class) will be involved – targeting specific individuals where necessary. Give opportunities for pupil discussion, questions, and self-assessment.	

Lesson Plan – Part Three

LESSON OUTCOMES AND EVALUATION
PUPIL ASSESSMENT NOTES Make brief notes about any significant pupil achievements or difficulties. You may refer to the class as a whole or to individuals.
NEXT STEPS for support of pupils' learning (based on pupil assessment notes) How might you need to change your planning for the whole class or for individuals? (Show this in later lesson plans)
LESSON EVALUATION This involves you analysing your performance as a teacher to identify how you can improve. Evaluation should focus on the reasons for both successes and problems encountered in the lesson. How well did children learn, and how effective were you as a teacher? In order to improve, it is important that you analyse why some aspects were or were not successful, rather than simply describing what happened. The key question is**: 'How can I help children to learn more effectively?'** Evaluate specific aspects of your teaching. For example: • Introductions, use of resources • Questioning skills, feedback to children • Monitoring individuals' work • Behaviour management, pupil attainment, etc.
NEXT STEPS for you as teacher (based on your lesson evaluation) Evaluation is more than a purely descriptive process; it should include proposals for action in the immediate future. What are you going to improve or adapt? Changes should be evident in later lesson plans.

Key learning points 3

- Know the main terms used in lesson planning: purpose, prior learning, learning outcomes, pupil activities, teaching points, assessment and evaluation.
- Know the importance of inclusion and individual needs.
- Specific considerations in planning PE lessons include: health and safety, special needs and medical conditions, parental consent, first-aid resources, and appropriate kit and equipment.
- The structure of a PE lesson follows a traditional pattern: warm-up, specific focus, main activity and cool-down.

Q Quick quiz 3

1 Explain the difference between 'learning outcomes' and 'pupil activities'.
2 What does STEP stand for?
3 Outline three planning considerations specific to PE.
4 Explain the following forms of assessment: teacher assessment, peer assessment and self-assessment.

Student activity 24.3 — 60–90 mins — P6 M2 D1

You have seen the outline plans for a physical education lesson and may one day be expected to plan your own lesson, either as a teacher or on work placement.

Task 1

Design and prepare a physical education lesson for a sport and Key Stage of your choice.

Task 2

Once your lesson plan is complete, write a report that describes, explains and analyses how learning is supported.

24.5 The Responsibilities of Those who Work with Children to Safeguard and Promote their Welfare

P7 P8 P9 M3 D2

Safeguarding Children and Young People

Children have many needs to help ensure they grow up to be happy and well-balanced adults. School, family, and the community in which they grow up are the three major contexts in which children grow and develop. Children learn from all of these environments.

Children need to have some form of education throughout their childhood. This will usually start at home and then progress into pre-school playgroups and then into school. Both physical and social skills are learnt through teaching and through play. The ability to catch and throw a ball is a physical skill that takes time to learn. This is because children need to build 'motor programmes' of performing that activity. This means that a child's brain needs to be able to send the right signals to move the appropriate body parts in the right way in order to perform an action. The more a child practises the activity, the stronger the motor programme becomes and the more likely the child is to catch or throw the ball effectively.

Research has also shown that regular sports participation is strongly linked to improvements in pupil behaviour, school attendance and attainment. Sports participation has also been shown to help children to develop social skills, including teamwork and leadership skills.

Sporting activities allow children to mix with different children. Rather than always spending their time with their 'best friend', children will be placed into different sports teams and will 'mark' different players, which will help them to mix with and to meet new friends. This can help to break down barriers between individuals and groups of young people.

Sports participation can also help children to develop self-esteem and increase their self-confidence. This will help them to stand up for themselves and will therefore make them less likely to be bullied or feel pressured to take part in things they do not want to do – for example, some children may feel pressured to smoke because their friends smoke. Sports participation will also give children a place to go in their free time, which helps to combat anti-social behaviour. Taking part in sports can also help to increase the safety of children – for example, children who are taught how to swim will be less likely to drown.

Sports participation will also help children to remain healthy: it will help to strengthen the immune system, reduce the risk of the child becoming obese, and reduce the risk of coronary heart disease and cancers in later life. Taking part in high-quality and fun sports from an early age will motivate the child to develop good habits, which they will hopefully continue with into their adult life.

Social and Psychological Effects

Children's participation in sport is strongly believed to help them learn how to socialise with other people and it also introduces them to the values and beliefs of society. The basis for this belief is the fact that sport introduces children to other children, rules, social values and the desire to improve their own skills in order to stay in the game and enjoy it. Children will learn to respect other children through sports participation. Research has shown that children automatically admire others who have a greater sporting ability than themselves; however, a good teacher or coach will ensure that all participating children with differing abilities are accepted and respected.

Other valuable social skills can be learnt through sport – these include leadership, communication, cooperation, independence and confidence. There has also been a significant amount of research that implies sports participation can help children to perform better academically.

Sports participation will help children to deal with failure. In most sports, there are winners and losers, and a good coach or teacher will help to ensure children are placed on teams that will have their fair share of wins and losses. This will allow children to increase their confidence and self-esteem when on the wining team and then to accept failure and develop good sportsmanship skills when they are on the losing team.

Legislation, Policies and Procedures

All children, whatever their circumstances or abilities, should be able to participate in and enjoy physical education and sport. A number of laws and regulations are in place to help ensure all children have access to appropriately run sporting activities.

Every Child Matters

This is a government scheme devised to support children. Its main aims are to ensure that all children should have the support they need to:

- **Be healthy** – this includes physical health, sexual health, mental health, emotional health
- **Stay safe** – safe from abuse or neglect, accidental death, bullying, discrimination, anti-social behaviour
- **Enjoy and achieve** – attend and enjoy school, personal and social development, meet national standards or higher
- **Make a positive contribution** – support their community and environment, adopt positive behaviour in and out of school and develop self-confidence
- **Achieve economic well-being** – progress into further education, employment or training, and live in decent homes with access to transport and material goods.

(Adapted from www.everychildmatters.gov.uk, 30.11.06)

The UN Convention on the Rights of the Child

This is a set of legal instructions that promotes the rights of children. Although all humans have rights, children are more vulnerable than adults so they have this set of rights that takes into account their particular right for protection. It recognises the fact that children are human beings with their own rights and responsibilities that will develop as the child gets older. The convention promotes the fact that all children, regardless of race, gender, religion, ability or wealth, should be entitled to a basic quality of life, including shelter and food, and that children should all be encouraged to reach their full potential.

This convention means that any organisation working with children or providing services for children will be able to share information and work together to protect children. In 2005, a children's Commissioner for England was appointed, which means that children's views will be sought and considered in relation to the organisations that work with them.

United Nations Children's Fund (UNICEF)

This is an international charity that promotes the protection of children's rights, and campaigns to help all children receive their basic needs and reach their full potential.

Playing for Success

Another government initiative, from the Department for Children, Schools and Families, is called Playing for Success. This has helped to set up after-school clubs and weekend clubs held within top sports clubs. Through a sports medium, these clubs help to teach numeracy, literacy and ICT.

The Children Act 1989

This act puts the child first by promoting and safeguarding their welfare. It sets out rules and regulations for how a child should be treated, which any person working with children should adhere to.

The Child Protection in Sport Unit (CPSU)

This unit was founded in 2001 as a partnership between the NSPCC and Sport England. The unit was set up in response to evidence that sport can provide access for a person to abuse children. As coaches often work with children over a long period of time, trust develops between the coach and the child. Research indicates that the majority of abuse is committed by a person who the child knows and has come to trust. Therefore, the CPSU has been put in place to help create a safe sporting environment for children. This is done through the promotion of good practice and by encouraging people to confront practice that is harmful to children.

It is the responsibility of any person caring for or working with children, both parents and coaches, to ensure they are taking into account the child or children's rights and helping them to fulfil their potential. Some parents or coaches may push a child to compete and train when the child is either not interested or not physically able to cope with the regime. This would be considered a form of abuse as the adults are pushing the child into doing things that they do not want to do. It may also give the child a 'win at all costs' attitude, which could result in the child becoming aggressive and prone to foul play in their sport or even taking performance-enhancing drugs – all of which turn sports participation into a negative experience.

Safeguarding Self

Good Practice

In almost every sporting situation, children will look to their sports leader as their source of inspiration and knowledge. Children will frequently copy their instructor so it is imperative that the sports leader behaves in a suitable manner that would be appropriate for a child's role model. A sports leader should ensure that they encourage winning but do not encourage children to adopt a 'win at all costs' attitude. Children need to learn to lose with good grace and develop sportsmanship behaviour.

A person working with children should always follow these basic guidelines:

- Ensure they work within the bounds of applicable codes of practice
- Maintain safe and secure sporting environments
- Establish good working relationships with the children and their parents
- Control the behaviour of participants.

A sports leader should also be aware of the rights and needs of children; these are detailed in the section entitled 'The UN Convention on the rights of children' (on page 303) and in the following pieces of information.

Good Practice Policy

A number of laws have been passed and agencies set up to promote the safety and welfare of children. Any person working with children should be aware of the relevant acts and agencies so that they can ensure they are working within the law and know how to get help and advice should they need it.

Recruitment

Any person recruited to work with children should have a CRB check prior to any contact with children. A CRB check will find out if a person has had any prior convictions, has been cautioned, has been given a reprimand or has been given a warning for a criminal offence.

In line with 'Child Protection: Preventing Unsuitable People from Working with Children in the Education Service' (2002), any person deemed inappropriate from the CRB check should not be employed to work with children.

Recognising Signs of Neglect and Abuse

Child abuse can take many different forms, but it can basically be defined as any form of physical, emotional or sexual mistreatment or lack of care that leads to injury, harm or distress. Most people responsible for abusing a child are in a position of trust and are known by the child and the family. Abusers can be male or female adults, or other young people. Any person under the age of 18 is considered to be a child; if they are suffering from any kind of abuse, you should have an awareness of the different types of abuse and the signs to look out for – very few children will admit to suffering from some form of abuse.

The main types of child abuse are:

- Physical abuse
- Sexual abuse
- Emotional abuse
- Neglect
- Bullying.

Physical Abuse

Physical abuse is where a person physically hurts or injures a child. A syndrome called Munchausen's syndrome by proxy is classed as physical abuse.

In sports, a coach may force a child to train or compete when they are physically not up to it, or give the child drugs to enhance their sporting ability; these are both forms of physical abuse.

Sexual Abuse

Sexual abuse is where a person uses children to meet their own sexual needs. This includes any form of sexual physical contact, showing children pornography or talking to them in a sexual manner. Many coaches will make physical contact with the children they are coaching in order to help them with their techniques or ensure their safety. It is imperative that coaches do their very best to ensure that the children are happy with this handling and that all contact is entirely appropriate.

Emotional Abuse

Emotional abuse is the consistent emotional ill-treatment of a child. This may involve telling the child that they are worthless, inadequate or unloved, or shouting and taunting the child, which may well result in severe and long-lasting adverse effects on the child's emotional development. Emotional abuse can also take the form of having greater expectations for a child than are appropriate for their age and ability. In sport, a coach could be guilty of emotional abuse if they constantly criticise the child, are sarcastic to the child or bully them.

Neglect

Neglect is when a parent or carer does not meet a child's basic physical and/or psychological needs so that it could result in the child suffering from ill-health or impaired development. Examples of neglect include inadequate provision of love, affection, food, shelter, clothing and medical care. Failing to protect a child from physical harm or danger is also a form of neglect. In sport, examples of how a coach could be guilty of neglect are if they do not ensure that the children are safe or if the environment is too hot or too cold.

Bullying

Younger people are often the perpetrators of bullying. Bullying can be verbal or physical and usually takes place over a period of time. This form of abuse can have a huge impact on a child's life and there have even been cases of children taking their own lives rather than face their bullies again.

A sports leader working with a group of children should make it explicit from the start that they will not tolerate any form of bullying and that it is the responsibility of every person to ensure that bullying does not happen. If any child is aware of any bullying, they must be instructed to tell the sports leader immediately. Some sports leaders discuss with the children what they think bullying is and then draw up some conclusions so that all the children know how they are expected to behave with one another.

If bullying has taken place, a sports leader must find out the facts and individually talk to the bully(ies) and the victim(s). They should then take appropriate action – this should be detailed in the facility's policies and guidelines. If the bullying was a one-off incident and there is more than one bully, it may then be appropriate to break up the group dynamics and split the bullies into different groups – many groups of bullies lose their confidence if they are not with their friends.

Bullying should always be dealt with swiftly and effectively, otherwise the bullies may gain confidence and it could become harder to put a stop to the bullying.

Effects of Abuse

Any child who has suffered abuse in the past or is currently suffering from abuse will usually experience long-term physical and/or emotional, sometimes life-changing, effects as a direct result of that abuse. Extreme cases of child abuse may result in the death of that child. All forms of abuse usually leave a child with psychological, health and/or developmental difficulties.

Many children are left with feelings of low self-esteem and may also wet the bed and have frequent bad dreams. Some children develop a range of anti-social and/or self-destructive behaviours in an attempt to try to cope with the abuse. They may be excessively aggressive to other children or bully them; alternatively, they may be very withdrawn and avoid communication and friendships with other children.

A child that is experiencing chronic abuse can experience behavioural changes. They may be easily startled and overreact to loud noises or a person shouting and sounding cross. Some children start to harm themselves as this somehow helps them to deal with the abuse they are receiving. Others may drink excessive amounts of alcohol or take drugs in an attempt to deal with the abuse they have received.

Signs of Abuse

A sports leader can help to keep children and young people safe by watching for unexpected changes in their appearance and behaviour. A child subjected to some form of abuse may show some of the following signs.

- A change in their behaviour. For example, a bubbly happy child may suddenly or gradually become quiet and withdrawn.
- Distrust of a particular person.
- A sudden inability to concentrate or performance declines for no apparent reason.
- Refusal to attend school or club.
- Has no close friends.
- Refusal to get changed in front of other people, or wants to keep covered up even in warm weather.
- Inappropriate sexual awareness or behaviour for their age.
- Some form of injury on parts of the body that are not usually injured. For example, it is common for children to have cuts and bruises on their knees from falling over; however, it is unusual to have injuries on other parts of the body such as the stomach, chest or back.
- An unsatisfactory explanation for an injury, e.g. the child has a black eye and bruising to the chest and they say they walked into a door.
- Significant weight gain or weight loss over a short period of time.
- Poor personal hygiene.
- Constant hunger.
- Extremely passive or extremely aggressive.
- Discomfort in or near the genital area – this could be observed from an inability to perform a sporting technique because of discomfort in the genital area.

However, if a child is exhibiting some or all of these signs it does not necessarily mean that they are being abused – there may be another explanation. Alternatively, a child that is being abused or who has been abused may not show any of these signs.

Course of Action

If you are working as a sports leader and you have any reason to believe a child is being abused, you must take action. The organisation you are working in should have clear policies and guidelines on how to deal with this situation.

If the child is keen to talk to you, the best thing that you can do is to follow these guidelines.

- Give them your full attention and listen carefully.
- Tell the child that you will not be able to keep what they have said to you secret but that you will only tell people who are going to make their situation better and, if appropriate, that these people will help to stop the 'bad' things happening to them.
- Ensure that you respond to what the child says with sensitivity.
- Encourage the child to talk, e.g. ask 'Do you want to tell me about this?' Do not put any pressure on the child to talk to you.
- Keep calm and try not to appear shocked. You may find what the child is saying upsetting but you should do your best to keep listening.
- Do not attempt to make any form of contact with the alleged abuser.
- If you believe the child's safety is in imminent danger, you should alert your sports facility's child welfare person and either they or you should contact the police or social services to take further action and help to ensure the health and welfare of the child.

When the child has finished talking to you, you should write a detailed account of what was said. If your centre has incident report forms, then this would be appropriate documentation to record the discussion on. If no incident report form is available, an example of an incident report form is shown in Figure 24.10; you could copy and use this.

The report should remain confidential and only the people who need to know this information should be given access to it in order to help protect the child.

Child Protection Incident Report Form

Sports facility: ______________________

Your name: ______________________

Your position: ______________________

Contact number: ______________________

Child's name: ______________________

Child's address: ______________________

____

Child's date of birth: ______________________

Parents'/carers' names and address: ______________________

____

Date and time of any incident: ______________________

Your observations or details as reported to you: ______________________

____

What the child said and what you said: ______________________

____

If you are passing on someone else's concerns, record their name, address, position and contact number:

____

____

Action taken so far: ______________________

External agencies contacted (date and time):

Police – yes/no

If yes – which: ______________________

Name and contact number: ______________________

Details of advice received: ______________________

____

Social services – yes/no

If yes – which: ______________________

Name and contact number: ______________________

Details of advice received: ______________________

Signature: ______________________

Print name: ______________________

Date: ______________________

Source: Adapted from www.nspcc.org.uk

Key learning points 4

- The main types of child abuse are: physical abuse, sexual abuse, emotional abuse, neglect and bullying.
- People who abuse children are often people who the child and/or family trust.
- A child suffering from abuse may exhibit some or none of the typical signs of abuse.
- Any information a child discloses regarding abuse should be documented on an incident report form and reported to the appropriate people.
- If a child is deemed to be in imminent danger, immediate appropriate action should be carried out.
- Bullying should be dealt with swiftly and effectively.

Quick quiz 4

1 What are the basic needs of a child?
2 What are the rights of a child?
3 Which organisations promote the rights of a child?
4 How does sports participation develop a child's social and psychological skills?
5 What agencies have been set up to promote the health and safety of children in sport?
6 How should a person respond if an abused child confides in them?
7 What course of action should a person take if a child has told them that they are being abused?

Student activity 24.4 — 120–150mins — P7 P8 P9 M3 D2

When working with children and young people, you will need to be aware of ways that you can safeguard and promote their welfare and behave in a manner that is appropriate to the age that you are working with.

Task 1

Write a report that describes different strategies that can be used by people working with children and young people to support their safety.

Task 2

Prepare a presentation that:

- Describes the different legislation, policies and procedures in place to safeguard children and young people.
- Explains and evaluates how procedures keep children and young people and those working with them safe.

Task 3

Write a leaflet that can be handed out to people working with children and young people that describes different strategies that can be used to ensure their own protection when working with children and young people.

Further reading

Lee, M. (1997) *Coaching Children in Sport, Principles and Practice*, Spon Press.

Useful websites

www.nspcc.org.uk/inform/cpsu/resources/bullying/bullying_wda60599.html
Free access to online resource outlining how to challenge bullying in sports clubs; includes links to icebreaker exercises and other resources

www.kidsexercise.co.uk/TeamSports.html
Online article that explains the benefits of playing team sports; also links to wider site that offers advice such as sports nutrition and free exercises (downloadable) for young people

25: Sport as a Business

25.1 Introduction

As you are probably well aware, sport is a huge industry, including sports participation, spectating, clothing and equipment. This unit explores the factors that help to make a sports business successful. Organisation of sports businesses, including the structure of staffing, is examined, followed by the different types of sports business that exist. Methods of market research are then explored. The unit concludes with a look at the various different types of legislation that apply to sports businesses, and the financial influences upon them.

By the end of this unit you should:

- know how businesses in sport are organised
- know what makes a successful sports business
- know the legal and financial influences on sport as a business
- be able to use market research and marketing for a sports business.

Assessment and grading criteria

To achieve a PASS grade the evidence must show that the learner is able to:	To achieve a MERIT grade the evidence must show that, in addition to the pass criteria, the learner is able to:	To achieve a DISTINCTION grade the evidence must show that, in addition to the pass and merit criteria, the learner is able to:
P1 describe the organisation of two different sports businesses	**M1** compare and contrast the organisation of two different sports businesses	
P2 describe what makes a successful sports business	**M2** explain what makes a successful sports business	
P3 describe three legal influences on a sports business	**M3** explain three legal influences on businesses in sport	
P4 describe a basic cash flow for a selected business		
P5 plan market research related to, and appropriate for, a selected sports business		
P6 conduct market research related to, and appropriate for, a selected sports business, recording and interpreting results	**M4** conduct market research related to, and appropriate for, a selected sports business, explaining the results	**D1** analyse the results of the market research, drawing valid conclusions
P7 describe the marketing activities of a selected sports business		
P8 produce a promotional plan for a selected sports product or service, drawing on market research.	**M5** justify a promotional plan for a selected sports product or service.	**D2** evaluate the promotional plan, identifying areas for improvement.

25.2 How Businesses in Sport Are Organised

P1 M1

Organisation

There is a range of different types of business; the main differences are determined by the number of people who own the business and how much of the business they own.

Sole Trader

A sole trader business means that there is only one person in charge of the business. That person must be able to afford to set up the business or have a loan approved by a bank or building society. This person is then able to make all the decisions on how the business is to be managed. They must be able to keep records of all the money going into and out of the business, which can then be examined by an accountant to ensure that accurate books are kept on income and expenses, that correct payments of tax and VAT are made, and so on. The sole trader is then able to keep all the profits; however, they are also personally liable for any debts.

Partnerships

This is very similar to a sole trader, but, as the name suggests, in a business partnership, two or more people own the business. In this way, the partners benefit by sharing the costs and responsibilities of the business. The profits of the business are then shared out between the partners. One partner may have put more money into the business, which would result in the profits being shared out in relation to the amount of money each person has put in. In most partnerships, each partner is involved in the decision-making process and all are liable for any debts. Some sports businesses may have 'sleeping' partners. This means that the sleeping partner has no say in how the business is run, but they are a partner because they have contributed money to the business.

As with a sole trader, a partnership business must keep books on money coming in and going out of the business, and the partners are responsible for paying the correct taxes and VAT, and so on.

Limited Companies

A limited company is a business that is registered on a government list called Companies House. There are two types of limited company: private limited companies and public limited companies. Both types of business have limited liability, which means that if the business goes bankrupt, any debts are the debts of the company and not of the employees (unlike in a sole trader or partnership business). A limited company must complete a Memorandum of Association. Once this has been submitted, a Certificate of Incorporation is issued to the company, which allows it to begin trading. In a limited company, at least one director is responsible for decision-making and running the business.

A limited company must complete annual reports and an account summary and submit it to Companies House for filing. A limited company is owned by a number of people who hold 'shares'. Each person with shares in the company is called a shareholder. The profits of a limited company are divided out between the shareholders. People who own lots of shares will receive a greater percentage of the profits compared to shareholders who own a smaller number of shares.

- **Private limited companies** – only certain individuals are able to buy shares. Many family-based businesses are private limited companies, and only family members are given access to buy shares. There are other, much larger-scale companies that are private limited companies, such as Manchester United and Virgin.
- **Public limited companies** – any person from the public can buy and sell its shares on the stock market.

Franchises

A franchise is when someone (franchisee) buys a business that is already successful and sets it up in a different location. A person wishing to buy a franchise would need to buy a licence to use the name, products and services of the business. They would also be given management support in setting up and running the business. The person buying the franchise would then be required to run the business in line with the franchise agreement drawn up between the franchiser and franchisee. Most franchises will be restricted to a certain location and will be for a limited period. A franchise may then pay ongoing fees to the original business or give the franchiser a share of its profits, or both. A franchise could exist as a sole trader, a partnership or a limited company; the type of company will determine the legal structure.

Organisational Structure

Every organisation has a structure with various levels, which is often depicted as a staffing structure or organisational structure. The person at the top of the chart is in charge and ultimately responsible for the success of the sports business and the welfare of staff and customers.

A typical hierarchical structure would look like the one shown in Figure 25.1.

Most people working in a sport or leisure facility will probably need to report to a duty manager. A duty manager will monitor the progress of the employees and ensure they are keeping to the rules and regulations of the job specification. The duty managers will then report to the general manager, who is responsible for monitoring their work.

Finances are dealt with by finance managers, who are usually in charge of an accountant or a team of accountants depending on the size of the facility. Their job role covers such aspects as profits and losses made by the facility, payment of staff, tax deductions, etc.

The human resource manager is responsible for recruiting new staff and ensuring current staff are being treated fairly and in accordance with the rules and regulations that are specific to the environment.

The Finance and Human Resource Departments provide a support service to the general manager and all three department managers report to the managing director. The managing director is accountable to the board of directors. The board of directors may consist of a range of people who include councillors, elected employees, trades union representatives and elected customer representatives. The board of directors oversee the running of the organisation with the aid of reports from their managers. They hold regular meetings to review the finances of the facility and make decisions on how to improve the facility and the services it has to offer.

Sports Businesses

There are a range of different types of sports business. The majority aim to make money, although some are there to provide a service to the community and their focus is not on making a profit.

Public Sports and Leisure Clubs

These sports facilities are funded by the government and do not aim to make a profit. These types of facilities usually offer lower-priced access to a variety of physical activities, including swimming, badminton, five-a-side football, fitness classes, and so on. Any person who is receiving income support, is a senior citizen, is under the age of 16 or is a student will usually be given a discounted rate for whichever physical activity they choose to take part in.

Private Sports and Leisure Clubs

These types of clubs aim to make a profit. They are often members-only and usually charge a joining fee to become a member. Thereafter, members are usually required to pay a monthly fee in order to stay a member and use all the centre's facilities. These types of clubs frequently offer additional services compared with public sports clubs – for example, showers will often have shampoo and shower gel, towels are given out to members to use after their shower. Jacuzzis and saunas are also commonplace in these sorts of clubs, unlike many of the public clubs. Any person using these types of facilities will usually pay a lot more money than if they were to use public-sector facilities.

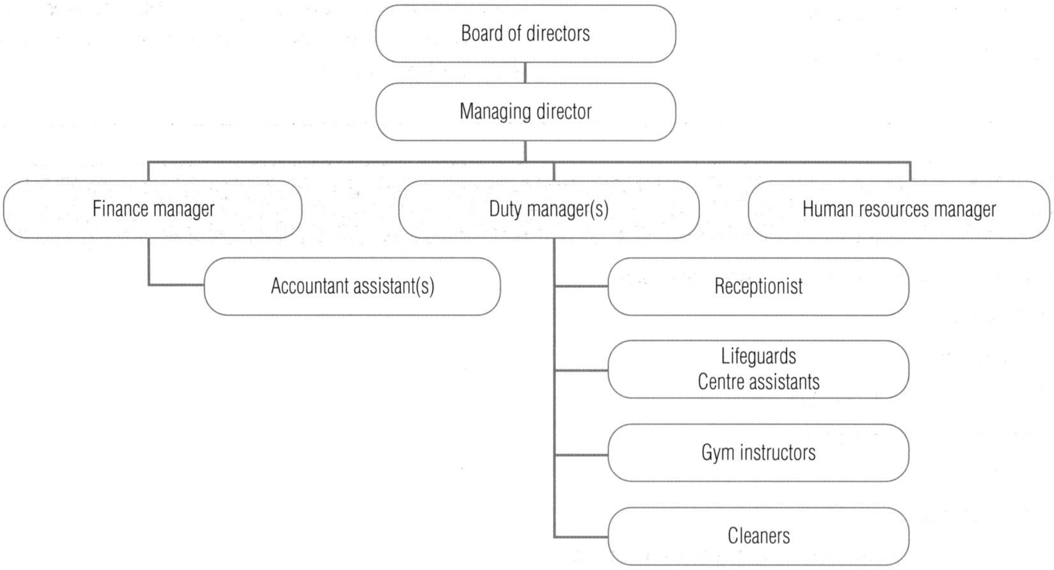

Fig 25.1 A typical hierarchical structure of a sports facility business

Professional Sports Clubs

Professional sports clubs pay their players for competing for them. Players will often receive a set salary for staying with the club, and bonuses when they play particularly well – for example, football clubs may give their players a bonus if they score a goal. Professional sports clubs will usually offer their players good playing and training facilities, and some will offer rehabilitation services too. These days, the majority of league football clubs are professional clubs.

Amateur Sports Clubs

An amateur sports club is open to the whole community and the club should offer no discriminations to membership. The cost of using the facilities should be of an affordable price so that most people are able to join and use its facilities. Many amateur sports clubs offer a range of different types of membership, and discounted rates for children, students, the unemployed and retired people. The club should not aim to make a profit, and any excess money gained should be reinvested in the club, donated to charity or given to other amateur sports clubs. The club will usually reimburse players for any travel costs when they play at away games, and it may provide or pay for its members to go on coaching courses.

Up until 1995, rugby union was an amateur sport and players did not receive payment in the same way as professional sports players. They would have received expenses and other forms of benefits in order to ensure that they remained with their club.

Key learning points 1

- The different types of business include: sole trader, partnerships, private limited companies, public limited companies and franchises.
- Every organisation has a structure with various levels: the person at the top of the hierarchy is in charge and ultimately responsible for the success of the sports business and the welfare of staff and customers.
- There is a range of sports businesses, including public sports and leisure clubs, private sports and leisure clubs, professional sports clubs and amateur sports clubs.

Student activity 25.1 — 60 minutes — P1 M1

Task 1

Using the internet and newspapers, try to find out about and list different sports businesses that are:

- Sole traders
- Partnerships
- Public limited companies
- Private limited companies
- Franchises.

If you have a newspaper such as *The Times*, it will contain details on stocks and shares, so you will be able to find out about public limited companies in this section.

Task 2

Select two different sports businesses, then describe and compare and contrast the organisation of each one.

Q Quick quiz 1

1 Give an example of a sports business that is a:
   (a) Sole trader.
   (b) Partnership.
   (c) Public limited company.
   (d) Private limited company.
   (e) Franchise.

2 Give an example of a:
   (a) Public sport and leisure club in your local area.
   (b) Private sport and leisure club in your local area.
   (c) Professional sports club in your local area.

25.3 What Makes a Successful Sports Business?

P2 M2

A number of factors will determine whether a sports business is successful; these factors are illustrated in Figure 25.2.

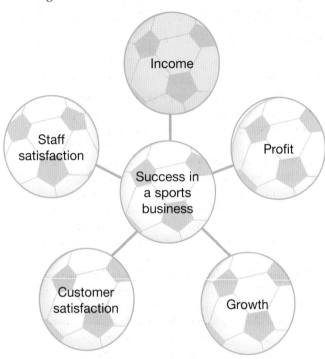

Fig 25.2 Success in a sports business

Income

This is the amount of money that the business makes. The business will then have to deduct money from its income to pay taxes and so on.

Profit

Profit literally means to make progress. If a business is not making a profit after a certain period of time, it will usually have to close down. A business will make a profit if the money coming in to the company is more than the money that is going out. The money going out of the business includes staff salaries, the cost of the product or services, tax deductions, rent, and so on.

Growth

If a business is doing well, it will usually grow in some shape or form. Many successful businesses will grow by taking on more staff to cope with greater demand for the product or service. Some businesses may open a branch in a different location so that they are able to sell to a larger market. Other businesses may grow by opening a website, either to trade their product online or to advertise their services.

Customer Satisfaction

All sports businesses require customers to buy their products and/or services. Therefore, in order for the business to succeed, it is vital that the customer is satisfied with the product or service they receive. If the customer is satisfied, the benefits your business will receive include the following:

1. **Customer loyalty** – customers will return to a business if they feel they have been treated well. If, however, they feel that they have been treated poorly, such as waiting too long for service or not having complaints dealt with effectively, they are much less likely to return to the business.
2. **New customers** – new customers can be generated through word of mouth from existing customers. If someone is happy with a business they are more than likely to recommend it to other people.
3. **Increased sales and profits** – if customers are happy, they will continue to use the products or services provided by the business, which in turn increases the amount of money a business makes.
4. **A good image** – most sports businesses want to portray a good image to the public and this can be done through providing good customer care.
5. **Employee satisfaction** – employee satisfaction can be gained through ensuring that employees are given thorough training in customer care. This training will help to ensure that employees can handle complaints rather than becoming upset by them.
6. **A competitive edge** – a competitive edge is very important in sports business as there are usually a number of facilities that provide the same services in one area. If one business provides better customer satisfaction than another, it is likely to have more customers.

Staff Satisfaction

If staff are happy in their work, they will generally do their jobs well. Therefore, if staff are satisfied, this usually has a knock-on effect which makes the customer satisfied. If staff are not satisfied, they may take time off sick or may not be very efficient at their jobs. The process of recruiting staff also costs time and money, so it is in the employer's interest to do its best to ensure that staff are happy.

Key learning points 2

- The success of a business largely depends on whether it is making a profit.
- Other factors to consider include customer satisfaction, staff satisfaction, income and growth.

Student activity 25.2

30–45 mins P2 M2

1 Draw a spider diagram that shows the factors required to make a successful sports business.
2 Write a report that describes and explains the factors that make a successful sports business.

25.4 Legal and Financial Influences on Sports Businesses

P3 M3

Legal Influences

A number of laws have been passed to help protect employees and employers while at work. Some of these are included in Unit 3: Assessing Risk in Sport.

Discrimination

A number of laws have been passed which make it illegal for an employer to discriminate against a person on the grounds of their sex or marital status, sexual orientation, race, religion or disability. Therefore, employers must recruit and pay staff in accordance with their job specification. All staff should be able to be eligible for promotion, training and benefits in accordance with their working ability, and discrimination should not occur.

The following Acts have been passed to prevent discrimination at work:

- Race Relations Act 1976 (amended and updated 2000)
- Equal Pay Act 1984
- Sex Discrimination Act 2000
- Employment Equality Regulations (Religion or Belief) 2003
- Disability Discrimination Act 1995.

Health and Safety

The Health and Safety at Work Act has already been covered in Unit 3: Assessing Risk in Sport. However, there are additional health and safety issues that any person working in a sports business should be aware of:

- **The Display Screen Equipment Regulations 1992** set out clear guidelines for any people working with visual display units (VDUs) such as a computer screen. The business is eligible to pay for all its employees who use a VDU to have an eyesight test. They must also make employees aware of the correct posture to assume when working at a computer, provide adjustable chairs for employees, ensure the screen brightness and colour on the screen is adjustable, and encourage employees to take regular breaks.
- **The Health, Safety and Welfare Regulations 1992** require every employer to provide free drinking water in the workplace, which is accessible to all employees. They should also provide proper toilet facilities and, where possible, there should be separate toilets for males and females. The number of toilets an employer should provide is determined by the number of employees it has.
- **The Management of Health and Safety at Work Regulations 1992** state that the employer must carry out risk assessments where necessary, and if the business has more than five employees, these risk assessments must be filed. The employer should take extra precautions if its employees are pregnant or under the age of 18; it must have procedures in place for dealing with emergencies, and should employ health and safety specialists to carry out training and inform employees of the health and safety issues that are relevant to them.
- Emergency procedures should be in place to evacuate a sports centre, including procedures to deal with fire, chemical release, explosion, terrorist threats, and so on. It is very important, that in the event of an evacuation, customers and staff are evacuated as quickly and safely as possible. All sports centres should have a policy that sets out clearly for customers what to do and where to go, and for staff what everyone's role is in evacuating a building, including muster points and a policy for readmission to the building. As a member of staff

you would be expected to help show customers the way to fire exits and ensure that they are congregating at a safe and correct muster point.

Treatment of Employees

- **The Employment Act 2002** provides guidelines for how employees should be treated. These guidelines include details on maternity and paternity leave entitlement, the rights of parents to request flexible working hours, disciplinary and grievance procedures and rules for fixed-term workers. Any person planning to start their own business who will be employing people to work for them should ensure that they examine this in its entirety, so that they are aware of how the law expects them to treat their employees.
- **The Working Time Regulations 1989** detail the length of time employees are expected to work. These regulations state that employees should:
  - Work an average of 48 hours per week
  - Work for no more than 8 hours on a night shift in a 24-hour period
  - Be entitled to at least one day off a week
  - Be entitled to a break if their working day is longer than 6 hours
  - Be entitled to four weeks' paid leave per year.
- **The Christmas Day Trading Act 2004** is a law that prohibits the opening of large shops on Christmas Day. It also places restrictions on the loading or unloading of goods at these shops on Christmas Day. One of the reasons this Act was passed was to help ensure that as many people as possible would be entitled to a day off on Christmas Day. This act is applicable only in England and Wales.

Consumers

- **The Fair Trading Act 1973** is there to protect consumers against businesses that continue to conduct themselves in a way that is detrimental to consumers' interests. Examples of this act include requiring businesses to give refunds for faulty goods, and ensuring that businesses provide accurate descriptions of the goods and services they are providing.
- If a business does not meet the needs of the employee as set out by the various guidelines and legislation, it may be deemed to be in 'breach of duty'. Breach of duty basically means that the business has failed to do what it 'reasonably' should be expected to do and has therefore been negligent in some way. An employee could then take their employer to court and sue them for any damages caused. The court would determine if it believed the business was indeed negligent and the extent of the damage caused, and award compensation to the employee.

Financial Skills

All business involves financial transactions, which is when money comes into the centre and when money is spent by the centre on buying products and paying wages. In order for a business to make money, the profits must be greater than the outgoings.

Money goes out of the business for a variety of reasons. Most businesses will have to pay rent or a mortgage for the site that they use. They will also have to pay their staff or themselves a suitable salary. If the company is a limited company, the cost of the shares will help to determine if the business is successful. If a business is doing well, the cost of the shares will go up and investors will need to pay more money to buy shares. However, if the business is not doing well, the cost of the shares will decrease and shareholders will lose money when they come to sell them on the stock market.

There are many different types of financial transactions within a sport and active leisure centre. These can include:

- Food and drink stock
- Sport products stock
- Customer accounts
- Staff wages
- Facility maintenance.

Many sport and leisure centres have systems in place to help with the financial skills in a business, and most will employ one or more accountants to keep records of the money transactions.

Key learning points 3

- The following Acts have been passed to prevent discrimination at work:
  - Race Relations Act 1976 (amended and updated 2000)
  - Equal Pay Act 1984
  - Sex Discrimination Act 2000
  - Employment Equality Regulations (Religion or Belief) 2003
  - Disability Discrimination Act 1995.
- The following legislation protects the health, safety and welfare of employees:
  - Display Screen Equipment Regulations 1992 are a set of guidelines for any employees working with visual display units
  - Health, Safety and Welfare Regulations 1992 require every employer to provide appropriate facilities for its workers
  - Management of Health and Safety at Work Regulations 1992 require employers to carry out risk assessments.
- The following legislation relates to the treatment of employees:
  - Employment Act 2002 provides guidelines on how employees should be treated
  - Working Time Regulations 1989 detail the length of time employees are expected to work
  - Christmas Day Trading Act 2004 is a law that prohibits the opening of large shops on Christmas Day.
- The Fair Trading Act 1973 is there to protect consumers against unfair trading.

Q Quick quiz 2

Choose a term from the following list to answer the questions below:

- Accountant
- Data Protection Act 1998
- Working Time Regulations 1989
- Profit
- Muster point
- Income
- Customers
- Christmas Day Trading Act 2004.

1. This Act prohibits the opening of large shops on Christmas Day.
2. This Act details the length of time employees are expected to work.
3. This person keeps track of money transactions in a business.
4. This Act means that it is illegal to use the information gained from individuals for anything other than its original intention.
5. This is a place where people should go when there is an emergency.
6. This literally means 'to make progress'.
7. All sports businesses require these to buy their products and/or services.
8. This is the amount of money that the business makes.

Student activity 25.3 60–90 mins P3 P4 M3

Task 1

Examine a sports business of your choice and select three legal influences on that business and write a report that describes and explains each one.

Task 2

Draw a spider diagram that illustrates cash flow for your selected sports business, then write a report that describes the cash flow for the business.

25.5 Market Research and Marketing by Sports Businesses

P5 P6 P7 M4 D1

Marketing is basically the process of a business communicating with the public to make them aware of the product or service it is selling, and to make this product or service sound as appealing as possible. It has many purposes. Figure 25.3 gives examples of the different uses of marketing.

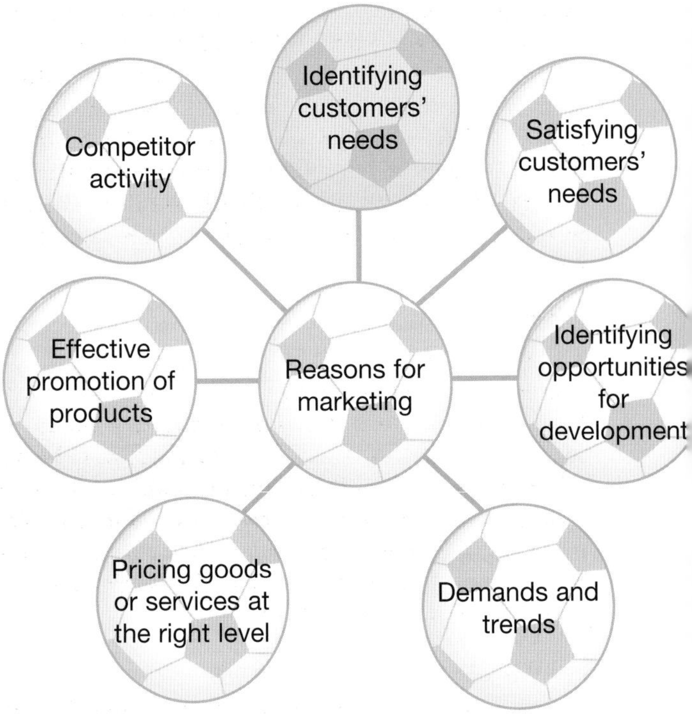

Fig 25.3 Reasons for marketing

Different Uses of Marketing

Key term

Marketing: the process responsible for identifying, anticipating and satisfying customer requirements and profitability (Institute of Marketing).

Identifying Customers' Needs

A business will want to find out what its potential customers need. Once this need has been identified, the business can produce the right products and services to meet it. For example, a leisure centre may not be offering the types of refreshments its customers would like. The customers would prefer freshly made hot drinks rather than machine-made ones, and more healthy snacks. The leisure centre could introduce a freshly made coffee stand, staffed by a person who is also able to sell fruit and other healthy snacks.

Satisfying Customers' Needs

Once a customer's needs have been identified, there need to be continual checks to ensure that the product and/or service offered has met these needs – for example, are the refreshments offered at the right price? Is there enough variety? If customers' needs are satisfied, there is much more chance that they will continue to use the facility and therefore either help to maintain or improve current levels of business.

Identifying Opportunities for Development

Research carried out to determine customers' needs may also identify opportunities for the business to develop. For example, a customer survey may not only find out that the customers want different refreshments to be supplied by their leisure centre, but that they would also like some sort of crèche facility, so that parents are able to take part in physical activity without having to take their pre-school child to a nursery, employ a childminder or make other childcare arrangements. This would then generate more income from the crèche facility and more income from the parents paying to take part in their chosen physical activity.

Demands and Trends

Many sports businesses are affected by a change in the market's demands because of new trends. This is clearly reflected in the continual new trends in exercise classes. For example, up until around six years ago, the exercise cycle was found only in the gym, but now a 'spinning' cycle is commonplace in many aerobic studios; boxing gloves and pads were used only by boxers, but now 'boxercise' classes also use this type of equipment. The different trends in exercise mean that a sports business has to determine if its customers demand this new exercise; if so, it has to buy in the new equipment and either train staff to meet the needs of the new trends or employ other staff who fit the bill. If the business does not keep in touch with demands and trends, they may lose customers to other businesses who are in touch with and are meeting customers' changing needs.

Pricing

A sports business will need to ensure that it is charging enough money to make a profit, but it will have to ensure that it is not pricing its goods or services too high so that its customers are not able to afford to use the facility. The business will also have to ensure that its pricing is competitive – for example, if a similar business offers its goods and services at a much lower price, customers may choose to go to the lower-priced business instead.

Promotion

A sports business will need to sell itself to the public so that people will choose to go there. Most businesses take a lot of time and effort in promoting a positive image of themselves and the products and services that they have to offer. Posters, leaflets and adverts in local papers are used to promote the business. Many gyms advertise themselves using photos of good-looking and toned people using their facility. This is done to encourage people to think that if they join that particular gym, they too will look like the people in the advert. Many businesses will encourage customers to use their facility by offering various promotional discounts – for example, during the first few weeks of January, when people are looking to keep to their New Year's resolution of getting fit or losing weight, many gyms will offer a 'no joining fee' promotion to encourage potential new customers to join their gym.

Competition

Virtually all sports businesses have some sort of competition – for example, think about the many different brands of sportswear: Adidas, Nike, Reebok, to name but a few. In the same way, you would rarely find one sports facility servicing the needs of a large community. Therefore, most sports business will need to keep a close eye on their competition to ensure that they are able to maintain their customer base. Some businesses will strive to make themselves different from their competition; this is called the unique selling position (USP). The business will then promote its exclusive products or services so that they appear very attractive, and therefore maintain its customers with the prospect of potentially attracting new ones. For example, if there are two leisure centres in close proximity and leisure centre A has tanning beds while leisure centre B does not, leisure centre A has the USP and could advertise to promote its tanning beds. It may further promote its USP by offering a 'swim and sun offer', whereby the customer is offered a discounted swim followed by a tanning session.

Methods of Marketing

A business may use a number of different sources of information in order to carry out market research.

Primary Sources

Any information that is gained directly from its current or potential customers is from a primary source. This type of information is usually gained from questionnaires or direct observation of customers.

Secondary Sources

This type of information is gained from studying information about customers, such as national statistics and sales records.

Selection of Appropriate Methods

The type of information used must be appropriate and relevant. The data should have been collected from a suitable time period – for example, national statistics should be the most recent ones published.

Marketing Activities

There is a huge array of different methods of marketing. Primary marketing research is very popular, and in order to ensure the data collected are relevant and appropriate, the researcher must take a number of factors into account.

Whichever method of market research you use to directly find out information about your customers, you should ensure that it will be as quick and as easy as possible for the customer to complete. Occasionally businesses will offer incentives for customers to complete their market research – for example, the name of every person who completes the questionnaire will be placed into a 'hat' and the person whose name is pulled out will win a year's free membership.

Sampling

Although it is not possible to collect data from every customer, the data collected are going to be used to represent the views of all the business's customers. Therefore, the sample of people used in the marketing activity should represent a cross-section of all the customers. For example, in a leisure centre, if the sample was taken between 10 a.m. and 11 a.m. on a Monday morning, it would probably consist mainly of retired people and mothers with young children, and therefore would not be a true representation of all the customers who use the facility. However, if the sampling took place throughout the day – for example, 6–7 a.m., 9–10 a.m., 12–1 p.m., 3–4 p.m., 6–7 p.m. and 9–10 p.m., it would give a much clearer picture of the views of all the facility's customers. Another method of sampling could be to pick every twentieth customer throughout the day. This again would give a good representation of the customers who use this facility.

Surveys

Surveys are usually in a questionnaire format. They can be carried out in writing, face to face or by telephone.

The questionnaire should be brief so that it does not put off the customer. The questions should be relevant to the topic of interest. This information can then be examined and the business could alter its services and products accordingly.

Product Testing

Most new products go through a pilot phase in which they are tested on a small scale. In this way, if there are any problems with the product, these can be brought to the business's attention and rectified. For example, many new sports drinks are tested on the public before they are sold nationwide. A market researcher would invite people to taste the new product and complete a questionnaire on its taste, proposed pricing, and so on. This research would then inform the sports drink manufacturer if the drink needed to be made sweeter, if it should be a different colour, if it is in the wrong price bracket, and so on.

Marketing Plan

A marketing plan is devised to help a business achieve its goals. The plan usually consists of four interlinked factors (see Figure 25.4).

The Product

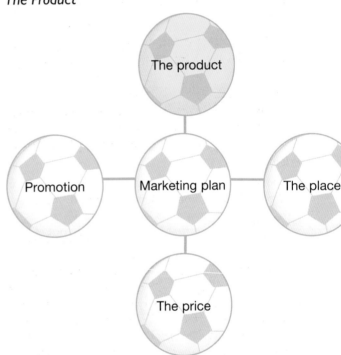

Fig 25.4 Marketing plan

The product is basically what the business has to offer its customers. Many sports businesses will develop new products or redevelop existing products in order to meet customers' needs. Many businesses will brand their products. The process of branding a product will give a business's customers a good idea as to what to expect from that product, and, if the brand is successful, customers will become loyal to

Student activity 25.4 | 45–60 mins | **P7**

For this activity you will need to visit a sports business and possibly speak to a member of staff.

Find out how the sports business carries out marketing activities. If possible, while you are at the venue, ask for customer questionnaires and interview members of staff.

You can also look in your local paper to see if the business advertises there, and check out their website if they have one.

it. For example, some people will choose to purchase sports clothing made by Adidas because they like the quality, style and cut of the clothing. Once a product is branded, various famous people can be sponsored by that brand and advertise the business's products. Customers who admire the sponsored celebrity may then choose to buy products from that particular brand, as they feel it has been endorsed by their favoured celebrity. For example, David Beckham has been sponsored by a variety of brands, including Adidas, Pepsi, Gillette, Police sunglasses and Vodafone.

The Place

Once the product has been determined, the place in which it is available to the customer has to be decided.

The location of the business is very important; there is no point having a really good product if the customer is unable to get to it. Factors to consider when determining how a product reaches its consumer are:

- Location
- Type of facility used to distribute the product.

Location

Most gyms and leisure centres will be located close to good transport links, such as roads, bus routes and possibly railway stations. They will also be placed close to where large numbers of people live and/or work. Many large gyms are located just outside town centres, in their own retail complex which contains other leisure facilities such as cinemas and restaurants. Locating outside the town centre usually means that the facility has lots of room for parking (usually free parking too, unlike in most town centres) and is not unduly affected by excess traffic, as in rush hours.

Type of facility

Factors to consider when deciding on the type of facility include the size, the layout and the cost of the premises. The size of the facility should be able to accommodate the predicted number of customers and ideally have the potential to expand if the business takes off. The layout of the facility should be planned to satisfy the needs of the business. For example, the changing rooms for the swimming pool would be placed so that a person may change and walk directly from the changing room to the swimming pool. If the facility is to have a jacuzzi and sauna, these should also be placed so that they may be accessed directly from the changing rooms.

The Price

Factors to consider when pricing a product are:

1. **The actual price of the product** – in order to make a profit, the business must charge more than the raw cost of the product.
2. **The price the competitor charges for the product** – the business should try to sell its product at a similar or cheaper price than its competitor.
3. **The demand for the product** – the number of people who want to buy the product should be monitored regularly, as demand for products will vary throughout the year (for example, many people plan to join a gym and get fit during the New Year or before their summer holidays).
4. **The aims of the business** – the majority of businesses aim to make a profit, although some businesses, such as a public-sector businesses, primarily aim to provide a service to the community.

Promotion

In order to try to make customers aware of their product and encourage them to buy it, many businesses will spend a lot of time and money promoting themselves. The main aims of promotion are to remind customers of the products they are selling, to raise the profile of a product, to try to make their product seem more attractive than a competitor's product and to offer incentives to customers if they choose to buy the product.

Businesses will place adverts in papers and magazines that they think potential customers will read. Many promotions have a short, catchy slogan, such as 'Just do it' for Nike.

Some businesses may contact potential new customers directly through letter or phone calls; they may also sponsor a well-known person to help promote the product.

Key learning points 4

- Market research is carried out in order to identify customers' needs, satisfy customers' needs, identify opportunities for development, determine demands, trends and pricing.
- A business may carry out market research by using primary or secondary sources.
- Marketing strategies should select an appropriate sample that will represent the views of all the customers.
- A marketing plan is devised to help a business achieve its goals and usually consists of four interlinked factors: product, price, promotion and place.

Student activity 25.5

2–3 hours

P5 P6 M4 D1

First of all, you will need to work out what you want to find out from your research and how you are going to get your information.

Task 1: Planning market research

Produce an action plan to demonstrate how you will plan your research. This should include:

- Your reasons
- Methods of research (e.g. questionnaires, product testing)
- Areas (e.g. customer types, customer behaviour, sales trends, market share).

Task 2: Conduct market research

Design an appropriate method of sampling, then select:

- An appropriate sample of people to conduct your research on
- Appropriate times to sample.

Conduct appropriate market research for a selected sports business and record the results.

Task 3

Write a report that interprets the market research you have carried out, then try to explain and analyse these results, drawing valid conclusions.

Quick quiz 3

1 What are the reasons for a business to use market research?
2 Give examples of the different types of sources used in market research.
3 Give examples of ways a business could carry out market research in order to gain information on the views of the majority of its customers.
4 What is a marketing plan?

Useful websites

www.jobswithballs.com
Details jobs in the sports industry and provides advice on applying for jobs

www.leisureopportunities.co.uk
Details jobs in the leisure industry and provides regularly updated news articles from the sports & leisure industries from around the UK

www.health-club.co.uk/
Online industry magazine with news and vacancies for people working in the health and fitness industry updated daily.

www.smallbusiness.co.uk/channels/business-insights
Lots of free video presentations and printable advice covering sound principles for running a business; topics include how to find and keep customers, marketing your business effectively, making presentations, and the importance of having a good website.

26: Work Experience in Sport

26.1 Introduction

There are a huge variety of jobs in this sector so it is vital for you to be aware of the range of occupations available and to gain first-hand experience of what jobs in sport entail. Not only will this give you a better picture of what is expected of you in your career of choice, it will also demonstrate your commitment to future employers.

This unit provides you with information that will allow you to plan and carry out a practical work-based experience within the sports industry. It explores the different types of sports industry organisations, sources to locate jobs, how to apply for jobs, interview skills and how to evaluate your experience.

By the end of this chapter you should:

- know about the opportunities for work-based experience in sport
- be able to prepare for a work-based experience in sport
- be able to undertake a work-based experience in sport
- be able to review a work-based experience in sport.

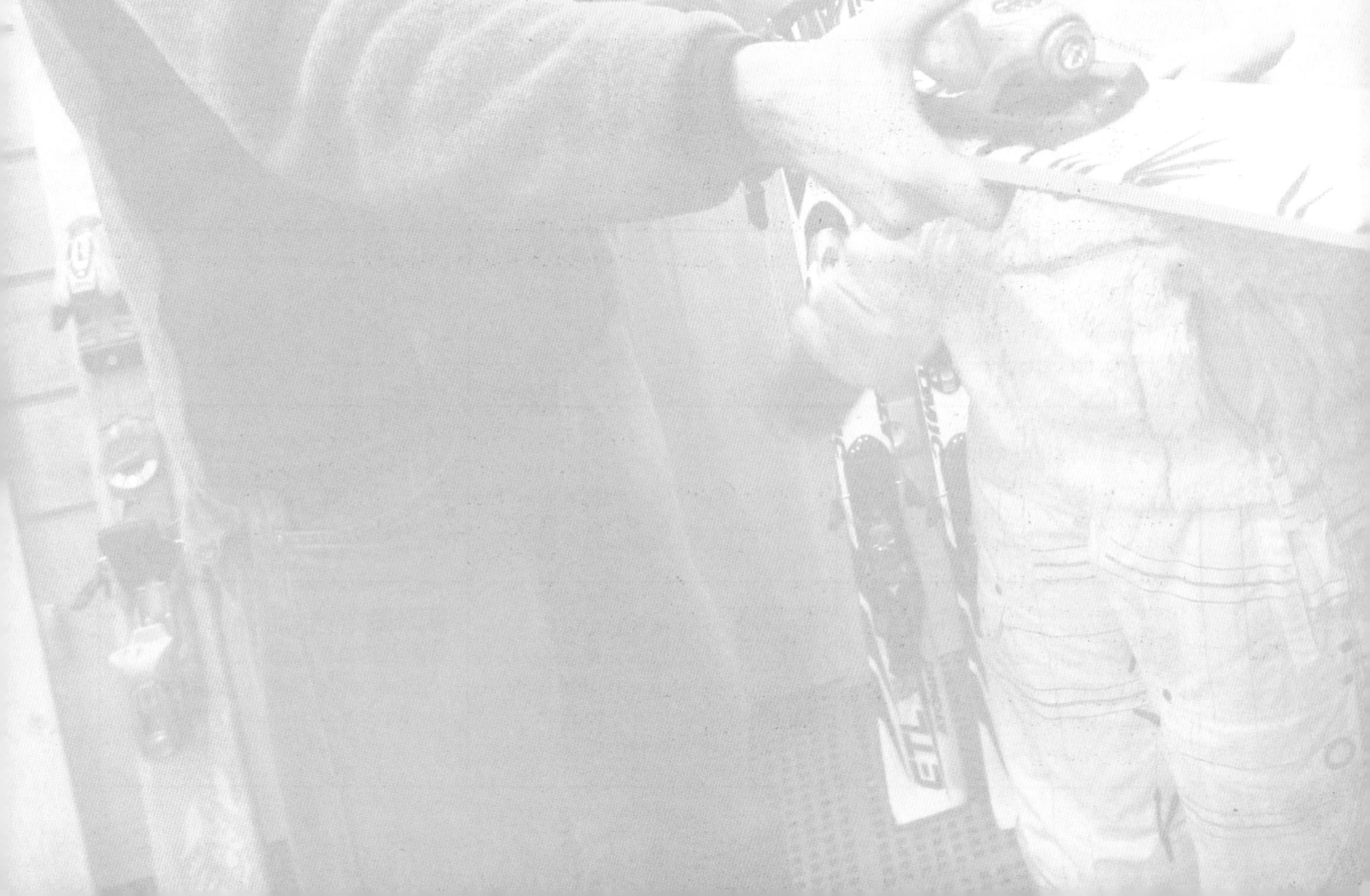

Assessment and grading criteria		
To achieve a PASS grade the evidence must show that the learner is able to:	**To achieve a MERIT grade the evidence must show that, in addition to the pass criteria, the learner is able to:**	**To achieve a DISTINCTION grade the evidence must show that, in addition to the pass and merit criteria, the learner is able to:**
P1 describe four realistic opportunities for appropriate work-based experience in sport	**M1** explain four realistic opportunities for appropriate work-based experience in sport	**D1** evaluate the opportunities for appropriate work-based experience in sport
P2 select an appropriate work-based experience in sport and complete the application process		
P3 demonstrate interview skills as an interviewee		
P4 prepare for a work-based experience in sport, identifying targets, aims and objectives	**M2** justify identified targets, aims and objectives of work-based experience in sport, suggesting how they can be achieved	
P5 undertake a selected appropriate work-based experience in sport		
P6 maintain a record of activities and achievements during a work-based experience		
P7 present evidence of activities and achievements during a work-based experience		
P8 review a work-based experience in sport, identifying strengths and areas for improvement.	**M3** explain identified strengths and areas for improvement and make suggestions relating to own further development.	**D2** justify identified strengths, areas for improvement and suggestions for further development.

26.2 Opportunities for Work-Based Experience in Sport

P1 **M1** **D1**

The various sectors that provide opportunities for work-based experience in sport include:

- health and fitness – gyms, health clubs and leisure centres
- sport and recreation – football, hockey and swimming clubs
- outdoor education – outdoor pursuit centres, water sports centres and indoor ski slopes.

The provision of sports facilities and opportunities in Britain is the result of the interaction between the public, private and voluntary sectors.

Public-Sector Provision

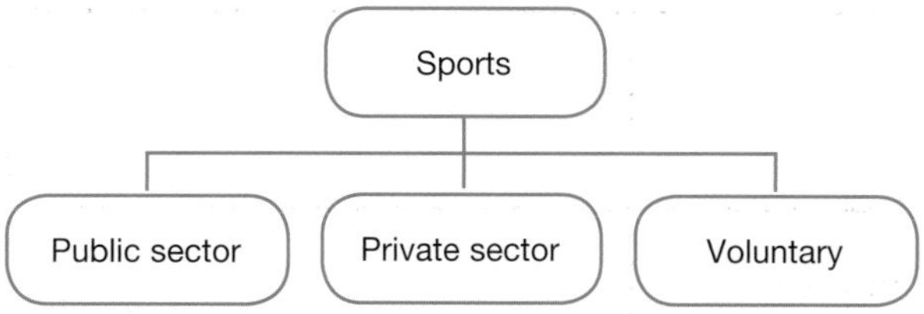

Fig 26.1 Sports provision

Key term

The public sector: institutions funded by money collected from the public in the form of direct and indirect taxes.

The public sector collects money through income tax, community charges, business taxes, valued added taxes on spending and national insurance. It then makes decisions on how to spend this money. These decisions are based on priorities and are seen as political decisions. The government may see the National Health Service and education system as priorities for spending and this position would be the basis for its decisions on spending. If the government does not see sport as being important it allocates only a relatively small amount of its budget to sports facilities, organisations and performers.

The public sector is made up of national government and local government (or local authorities), each of which has different responsibilities in sports provision.

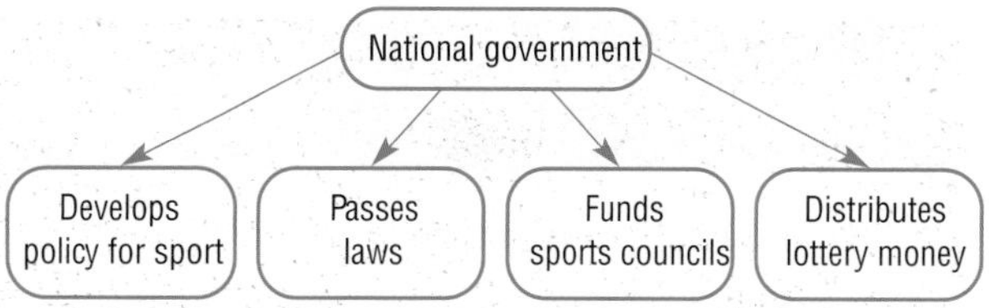

Fig 26.2 National government's responsibilities in sports provision

National government is funded by taxes (income tax, VAT, business taxes) and receives money from the National Lottery (Lotto). Its role in sport is indirect, as it does not fund buildings or the running of facilities, but provides money to other organisations to spend on sport. It has a role as an 'enabler' and the main recipient is Sport England. National government provides grants and loans to local authorities, as well as offering technical assistance. Sport is the responsibility of the Department of Culture, Media and Sport (DCMS). It has the following roles in sport:

- represents interests of sport, arts, tourism and heritage
- promotes sporting success at the highest levels
- helps develop government sporting strategy
- funds the Sports Councils in Britain and Northern Ireland
- funds other agencies involved in sports provision
- distributes money raised by the National Lottery.

Sport England is responsible for the development of sport in England, while the Sports Councils for Scotland, Northern Ireland and Wales are responsible for the development of sport in their respective countries. The main purpose of Sport England is to:

- get more people involved in sport
- provide more places to play sport
- win more medals through higher standards of performance.

Local Government

Local government or local authorities are responsible for providing facilities for sport and physical recreation. Provision is usually divided into the areas shown in Fig 26.3.

Facilities in the public sector are usually named after the town or city they are in, e.g. Colchester Leisure Centre, Watford Baths, Wimbledon Recreation Centre.

Student activity 26.1 — 20 minutes — P1 M1 D1

Find out the following information.

- Who is the Secretary of State for the Department of Culture, Media and Sport?
- Who is the Minister for Sport?
- Where is your local office of Sport England or Sports Council for Scotland, Northern Ireland or Wales?
- What is the address of your local office?

The majority of funding comes from the council tax and will go to the county council, with the rest going to the local authority and some to the county police force. Other sources include receipts from trading, such as leisure centre entry fees, rents from council housing, loans from banks and grants from national government.

Student activity 26.2 — 45 minutes — P1 M1 D1

The government (national & local) spends around £1000 million a year on sport. There are many courses to study sport in Britain and there is a huge amount of media coverage of sport. Thus, we can assume that sport is significant in British society. But why? What are the benefits of playing, watching and talking about sport?

Answer the following questions:

- List the ways you can think of that sport contributes to the British economy.
- What benefits does sport have for participants and spectators? Consider why you participate in or watch sport.
- What are the social benefits of sports participation and watching sport? How does it improve the world we live in?
- What are the international benefits of sports participation?
- What are the educational benefits of sports participation?

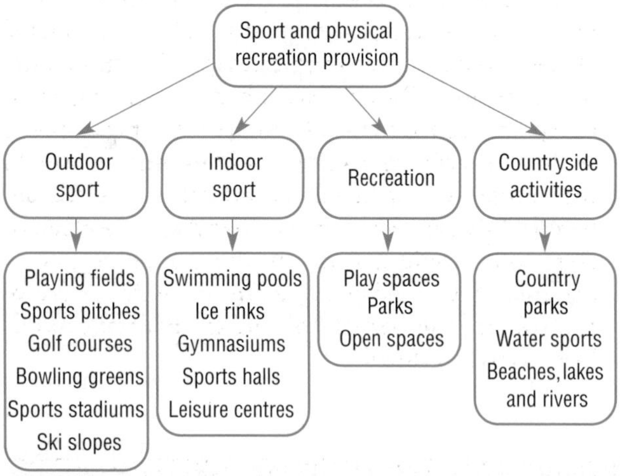

Fig 26.3 Local government's responsibilities in sports provision

Key term

Private sector: sport is provided by individuals or groups of individuals who invest their own money in the facilities with the main aim of making a profit.

Private-sector sport is provided by individuals or groups of individuals (companies) who invest their own money in facilities. As a result, these facilities are usually named after people, such as David Lloyd clubs, although some have a brand name, such as Virgin Active or Cannons.

The private sector provides sports facilities for two main reasons:

- to make a return on their investment for themselves and their shareholders
- to make a profit out of sport.

Claims are sometimes made that it is for other altruistic reasons, such as improving the standards of a sport or improving the community the facilities are in. However, these facilities would not exist unless their owners could make a profit.

The private sector provides for sports increasing in demand. It is able to respond quickly to new trends or to instigate new trends. It provides facilities where it can attract large numbers of customers, or more exclusive facilities where it can attract fewer customers but charge more. It is involved in the following areas:

- **active sports** – tennis, golf, health and fitness suites, snooker and pool, water sports and ten-pin bowling
- **spectator sport** – stadiums for football, rugby, cricket, tennis, golf (football is by far the most popular spectator sport)
- **sponsorship** – this has risen dramatically over the last 15 years.

The role of the private sector can be summarised by this quote from George Torkildsen (1991):

> 'The major difference between the commercial operator and the public or voluntary operator is the raison d'être of the business, the primary objective of the commercial operator being that of financial profit or adequate return on investment.'

The Voluntary Sector

Key term

Voluntary sector: clubs that operate as non-profit-making organisations and which are essentially managed by and for amateur sportsmen and women.

Most amateur clubs are run on a voluntary basis. Some voluntary clubs own facilities, but the majority hire facilities, usually provided by the public sector. In the main, the clubs that most people tend to join to enable them to participate in competitive sport are in the voluntary sector. Voluntary-sector clubs often work in partnership with the private or public sector. They might use public-sector facilities or gain sponsorship from the private sector. In the evening you may find the swimming pool at your leisure centre being used for swimming club or kayaking club training.

Funding of Voluntary Clubs

The voluntary sector is funded primarily by its members in the form of subscriptions. Every club will have an annual subscription fee and match fees. This is to cover the costs of playing, travel and equipment. The club may try to raise some money in the form of sponsorship. This is often by a local company or by one of the players. Some clubs have local benefactors who put money into a club as a gesture of goodwill. Clubs also run fundraising events such as discos, race nights or jumble sales, particularly if they are trying to raise money for a tour or special event.

Clubs can apply for other sources of funding:

- National Lottery grants
- grants from national governing bodies
- grants from government
- grants from the local authority.

These types of grants are usually to enable clubs to build or improve their facilities.

Partnerships

Partnerships occur when two or more of the sectors come together to provide opportunities for sport. We have already seen how the public sector rents out its facilities to the voluntary sector to give them an opportunity to play sports. Sponsorship, which is primarily provided by the private sector, is given to the public and voluntary sectors.

Sports facilities are also built as partnerships. The new English National Stadium at Wembley is a private-sector initiative by Wembley plc, but it has received a National Lottery grant from the public sector. It will also go into partnership with other private-sector organisations to raise finance and gain sponsorship.

Compulsory competitive tendering (CCT), introduced to the leisure industry in 1990, was aimed at developing partnerships between the public and private sectors. The aim was to hand the management of sports centres to private-sector organisations while the ownership of the centres remained with the public sector (local authorities). The theory behind this arrangement was that the private-sector companies would aim to run the centres for profit and thus they would be run more efficiently. Today we can still see the benefits of this arrangement in our local sports facilities.

Student activity 26.3 — 30 minutes — P1 M1 D1

Go to your college library and find out the names of voluntary clubs in your area for the following sports:

- athletics
- ice skating
- rugby union
- rugby league
- hockey.

26.3 Types of Occupation

There is a huge range of jobs available in the sports industry, from sports massage therapist to mountain leader. In order to gain the skills and qualifications you require, you may need to continue your studies to a higher level or complete a part-time course. The following list gives a range of different jobs available in the sports industry but is by no means exhaustive:

- fitness instructor
- leisure attendant
- sports centre manager
- kayak instructor
- sports coach
- sports development officer
- sports/PE teacher or lecturer
- mountain leader
- professional sports performer
- sports massage therapist
- sport and exercise scientist
- sports nutritionist
- sport psychologist
- sports groundsman
- sports retailer.

Fitness Instructor

This involves assessing people's fitness levels, designing their exercise programmes and instructing these programmes in the gym. Fitness instructors may also teach aerobics classes and circuit classes, and supervise people in the gym.

Instructors need sound anatomy and physiology knowledge gained from a sport science course, and also a recognised fitness instructor's award from a training organisation such as Premier Training International, YMCA or Focus. To teach specific skills, such as aerobics, circuits or stability ball work, extra qualifications are required. First aid and CPR qualifications are also essential. Instructors must have good communication skills, be friendly and able to remain calm under pressure.

Leisure Attendant

Leisure attendants are responsible for preparing and supervising the sports hall, swimming pool and changing rooms in a leisure facility. Most leisure attendants are also involved in coaching or supervising sports sessions in their sports hall.

A sports qualification is desirable but not essential. The National Pool Lifeguard Qualification is compulsory in order to work in a swimming pool. To coach sports, leisure attendants need specific national governing body coaching awards.

Leisure attendants need to be outgoing and people-orientated. Communication skills are important as you may have to deal with a range of people.

Sports Centre Manager

Managing a sports centre involves some of the following activities:

- managing and motivating staff
- programming facilities and organising activities
- establishing systems and procedures
- preparing and managing budgets
- monitoring sales and usage
- marketing and promoting the centre
- dealing with members and any complaints or incidents.

Managers may have been promoted into this position having qualified with a BTEC First or National Diploma or GNVQ. Most managers will hold higher-level qualifications such as a degree or HND in leisure management or business studies.

To be an effective manager you need the following personal qualities: confidence, enthusiasm, assertiveness, communication skills, self-motivation, presence and professionalism.

Kayak Instructor

A kayak instructor is usually qualified in a range of outdoor pursuits and works at an outdoor pursuits centre. The role involves checking equipment, ensuring weather conditions are appropriate and then teaching a range of skills to kayak safely and effectively.

You will have to have a high level of personal proficiency (three-star minimum) and then attend an instructor training course. You also need to be qualified in rescue skills and first aid. You must have good communication skills, be able to withstand cold and wet working conditions, and also have very good safety awareness.

Sports Coach

Sports coaches are usually former or current competitors in their sport. They are responsible for developing the physical fitness and skills of their athletes. They need to be able to evaluate their athletes' performances and offer feedback to improve these. As a result, they require knowledge of many aspects of sport science, such as anatomy and physiology, biomechanics, nutrition, psychology and sports injury.

Every sport has its own system for awarding coaching qualifications, and coaches must hold the relevant award. Many coaches also hold qualifications in sport or sport science.

Coaches need to be able to motivate athletes and have their trust. They need to be good communicators and listeners, and able to show patience and empathy towards their athletes.

Sports Development Officer

A sports development officer works to increase participation rates in sport and provide opportunities for people to play sport in a local area. They work for local authorities and may have responsibility for specific groups of people, such as ethnic minorities, women or disabled people.

Most sports development officers have at least a BTEC National in sport or sports science, and usually also hold a degree or HND in sport, sport science or leisure management, along with a range of coaching qualifications. You need an interest and knowledge in a range of sports and the needs of a community. You have to be able to communicate with people from different backgrounds and be sensitive to their needs. Good leadership, motivational skills and an organised approach to work are also necessary.

Sports/PE Teacher or Lecturer

You can teach PE in schools to children from the age of four to eighteen years. If you choose the younger-aged children you also usually have to teach a range of other subjects from the National Curriculum. If you teach PE in a secondary school this is usually the only subject you will be required to teach. A lecturer teaches in a college or university and usually specialises in a few subject areas, such as physiology or psychology.

A teacher needs to be educated to degree level and to be qualified as a teacher. There are two ways to do this:

- take a four-year teaching degree such as a Bachelor of Education (BEd) or a Batchelor of Arts with Qualified Teaching Status (BA (QTS))
- take a three-year degree in sport science or sport studies and then complete a one-year Postgraduate Certificate in Education (PGCE).

To study to become a teacher you must have passed GCSE English and maths (at grade C or above and a science if you wish to teach primary or key stages 2/3), and at least two A levels.

Teaching is a very demanding profession and you need to be patient and able to deal with young people and their various needs. Teachers need to be organised, and able to maintain discipline and adapt their communication skills to the group they are teaching. You should also have a good level of personal fitness and enjoy working with young people.

Mountain Leader

A mountain leader may work in an outdoor pursuits centre and lead mountain walks or they may be involved in leading a venture scouting group and instruct the group on how to carry out an expedition.

A mountain leader must have gained a great deal of personal experience walking and navigating in the outdoors. They must then attend a mountain leader instructor course, which involves mountain walks, night walks and camping overnight. They must keep a logbook and then complete a mountain leader assessment to ensure they are proficient in all the skills required for mountain leading. They can then carry out a mountain leader course for winter conditions and undergo another assessment. A mountain leader must be able to withstand cold and wet conditions, have excellent navigational skills, a first aid qualification, good communication skills, and excellent health and safety knowledge.

Professional Sports Performer

Ultimately the goal of every sports performer would be to play their sport full-time at a professional level. However, it is only the most talented who get this opportunity and there are only a limited number of sports where you can play professionally. Football, cricket, rugby league, rugby union and golf have the largest number professional players. However, most professional players have a second job to ensure their income.

No formal qualifications are needed, although you need to investigate the best route into a sport as every sport will be slightly different in how it recruits young players.

Technical efficiency at the chosen sport, along with physical fitness, are the most important assets, as well as self-motivation, commitment and determination.

Sports Massage Therapist

A sports massage therapist has a varied job, using their massage skills to prepare athletes for competition, helping them to warm down after competition and then dealing with any injuries or soreness they may suffer. They can also treat the public who have injured themselves during non-sporting activities such as gardening.

A sports massage therapist needs to hold a sports therapy diploma. These courses are accredited by the Vocational Training and Charitable Trust (VTCT) and can be studied at most colleges of further education. Private training organisations, such as Premier Training International, also offer these courses in an intensive 12-week format. It is possible to do a degree

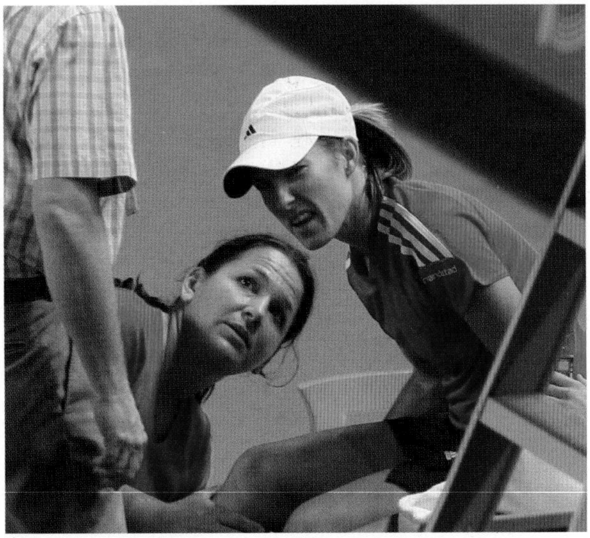

Fig 26.4 A sports massage therapist at work

in sports therapy or sports rehabilitation at a limited number of universities.

A sports massage therapist always needs to adopt a professional approach, as their job involves physical contact with people. They should be patient, caring and sensitive to an individual's needs. A high standard of personal hygiene and good communication skills will be important to be successful.

Sport and Exercise Scientist

The aim of the sport and exercise scientist is to maximise the performance of an individual in their care. This will involve applying their knowledge and skills in the subjects of physiology, biomechanics and psychology to give the performers any possible advantage. Physiology will involve fitness testing and monitoring physical condition; biomechanics will involve examining the performer's technique and equipment to analyse where improvements can be made; psychology will be applied to ensure the performer is correctly prepared mentally.

A sport scientist will hold a degree in sport science and possibly a master's degree or a PhD in their chosen field of expertise.

Sports Nutritionist

A sports nutritionist gives an athlete advice about how to organise their diet to ensure they maximise the effects of their training and reach competition in the best possible shape. They may also provide advice on the use of supplements.

A sports nutritionist needs to be qualified as a dietician first. This will involve completing a three-year degree to become recognised as a state registered dietician. To specialise in sports nutrition you need at least one year's experience before completing a sports dietetics course run by the Sports Nutrition Foundation.

Sport Psychologist

A sport psychologist is involved in mentally preparing athletes for competition. It is a varied job which will differ depending on the individual needs of performers. A psychologist is involved in helping teams and individuals set goals for the short and long term, learn strategies to control arousal levels and stay relaxed in stressful situations. They are also often involved in lecturing and conducting research, as well as actually practising their skills.

A sport psychologist would usually be a graduate or sport scientist who had then completed postgraduate training. This would involve a master's degree or a PhD in sport psychology.

Psychologists need to have good listening and interviewing skills in order to assess the needs of their athletes and to develop strategies to help them. A psychologist should be able to build up a relationship of trust and be seen as someone who the athlete can talk to confidentially.

Sports Groundsman

A groundsman is responsible for preparing and maintaining the condition of outdoor facilities, such as golf courses, cricket pitches, football pitches and tennis courts.

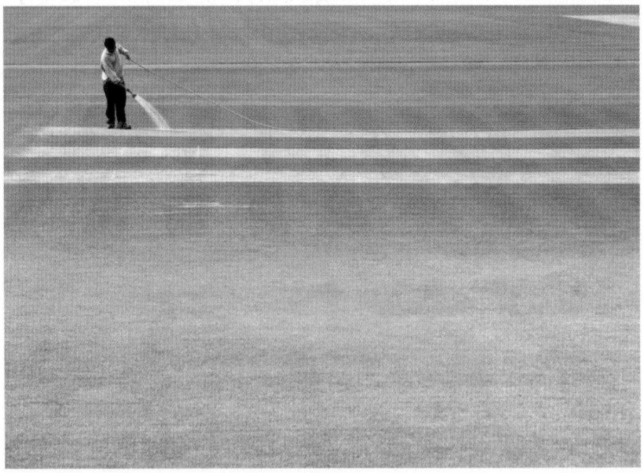

Fig 26.5 Sports groundsman

Entrance qualifications are not essential. You can study for an NVQ in turf management, or go on to HND or degree level. These courses need to be recognised by the Institute of Groundsmanship (IOG).

Sports Retailer

Sports retail involves working in a sports shop selling sports goods. This can involve using your knowledge of sport and matching a client's needs to specific products. Different types of runners require different types of running shoes and you need to be able to identify which shoes they need.

A knowledge of sport is needed, but many people working in retail need business skills and customer care skills. A qualification in business studies or leisure studies would be appropriate. If you have aspirations to run a sports shop, it may be necessary to hold an HND or degree in a management-based subject.

An ability to deal with members of the public and a willingness to meet their needs is necessary. You must be good at communicating and be able to stay calm under pressure.

26.4 Work Placement Considerations

Before choosing your work placement, you will need to bear in mind a number of factors to ensure the location and the actual placement are suitable for you.

Location

While deciding where you would like to carry out your project you should also include in your decision-making the locality of the placement. If the sports facility is not within walking distance how are you going to get there? You will need to investigate methods of public transport and look at the cost and travel times. If the facility is too far away from home for you to travel in to every day you will have to see if the facility provides staff accommodation and if it would be available to you. Alternatively, you may have family living near to your chosen facility and be able to stay with them for the duration of the placement.

Placement Requirements

You need to speak to your supervisor prior to the placement in order to see if you need to provide your own clothing and, if so, what is required. Most leisure centres provide their staff with a uniform but outdoor pursuit centres staff usually provide their own clothing. This could be quite expensive if you do not have any of your own already, so it may be worth asking your supervisor if they have any kit you could borrow for the duration of the placement.

Any equipment you require will usually be provided, such as a whistle for a lifeguard. Again, it is worth asking your supervisor if you need to buy anything and check that you can afford it prior to your placement.

Occupation Information

The purpose of a work placement is to help you determine if the job you have chosen to undertake or observe is suitable for you. Therefore, once you have thought of a job you would like to perform you will need to find out if you have or are going to have the right qualifications to be accepted on this job.

If you would like to work in outdoor pursuits, you will need to have a good level of personal proficiency and/or be working towards water-based or land-based outdoor pursuits qualifications – mountain leader, kayak instructor, etc.

On top of the qualifications required, every job has a different set of roles and responsibilities that you must examine and check to see you are capable of carrying them out. Working in the sports industry often entails working unsociable hours. If you want to work only in the daytime you may have to consider a different job.

Regulations

There are a number of regulations in place to help protect employees, employers and customers whilst at work:

- Health and Safety at Work Act 1974
- Control of Substances Hazardous to Health Regulations (COSHH) 1994
- Health and Safety (First Aid) 1981
- Safety at Sports Ground Act 1975
- Fire Safety & Safety of Places of Sport Act 1987
- Children Act 1989.

Skills

While on your work placement you will probably realise that you already have a number of skills that are appropriate. You may realise that you have good interpersonal skills and find it easy to deal with customer's questions and/or complaints. But you will no doubt also find that there are some skills that need to be developed. You may find it difficult to meet deadlines or that you are always rushing to get to work on time. You would need to improve your time-management skills.

You will be taught a number of new practical skills such as putting up and taking down equipment. You will no doubt have some knowledge of this from practical units you have covered and find that you just need to adapt these skills to meet the requirements of the new apparatus.

Key learning points 1

- The three different sectors that provide sports facilities are **public**, **private** and **voluntary**.
- Dual and joint use is where organisations share the facilities.
- There are many different occupations in the sports industry – it is important to find out the skills required for each job to find out if it would be suitable for you.

Quick quiz 1

Public	Private	Voluntary	Sports Massage Therapist	Sports Psychologist
PE Teacher	Wembley	Virgin Active	Sport & Exercise Scientist	Dietician

Select the word or words from the table above to answer the following questions:

1 This type of sector tries to make a profit out of sport.
2 Institutions in this sector are funded by taxes and indirect taxes.
3 This is the non profit sector.
4 This is an example of a sports centre in the private sector.
5 This is an example of a facility that has been funded by both the private and the public sector.
6 You would need a degree to go into this profession.
7 For this profession you would need a therapy diploma.
8 The aim of this job role is to maximise the performance of sports performers.
9 In order to become a sports nutritionist you would need to qualify in this profession first.
10 This job requires a person to mentally prepare athletes for competition and training.

Student activity 26.4 — 10 minutes

The sport and leisure industry has a whole host of possible job opportunities and career paths and you may find a variety of them appeal to you.

Task 1

Investigate and list four possible jobs or careers in sport that you feel you would be interested in pursuing.

Task 2

First, find out if the job that you are interested in offers the opportunity for a work-based experience for you to find out more first-hand. For example, if you were interested in sports medicine it would be very difficult to find a work-based experience observing and carrying out the tasks of a highly trained medical professional! However, if you were interested in becoming a gym instructor then this job role is relatively easy to observe and shadow.

Then, research where you may carry out your work-based experience for each of your selected jobs or careers in your local area.

Task 3

Write a report that describes, explains and evaluates your selected opportunities for work-based experience in sport.

26.5 Application Process

P2

After having read a job specification for a particular role, you can then decide if you would like to apply for this role. To apply for work you need to use a suitable method to approach a prospective employer. Most job advertisements will specify which method you should use. There are three main methods that you may be asked for.

- **Curriculum vitae (CV)** – a concise written document that summarises your skills, qualifications and experience to date for a prospective employer; should be accompanied by a covering letter.
- **Application form** – some jobs will not accept a CV and will, instead, ask you to complete a pre-designed application form asking you to show why you are suitable for the job; should also be accompanied by a covering letter.
- **Letter of application** – some jobs will require you to apply in writing; the information required will be similar to that of a CV, but will be presented in a different format.

Curriculum Vitae

A CV is used for a range of reasons:

- to demonstrate your value to the employer
- as a marketing tool to get an interview
- to sell yourself to the employer.

There are three main styles of CV.

- **Chronological** – this is the most common format and involves you presenting your experiences of education and work in date order.
- **Functional** – this type highlights your skills and is directed towards a certain career. You may be qualified in more than one subject, but you would highlight only the skills that are relevant for the type of work you are trying to gain.
- **Targeted** – this type of CV emphasises skills and abilities relevant to a specific job or company. It is tailor-made for one job. You would examine the job specification and then adapt your CV to show how you meet it.

Preparing a CV

A CV needs to be prepared meticulously and you should spend time deciding what your main selling features are. If you are still a student, you may not have been involved in full-time work, but you will still have important features to highlight. You must include any work experiences, part-time and voluntary work you have undertaken. You will need to start by compiling a biography of your life with dates and events. You will also need to consider what skills you have at present, and which ones are transferable to the type of work you are seeking.

A CV should include the following information.

- **Personal details** – full name and address, home telephone number and mobile number, email address and date of birth.
- **Current position and employment** –your position and main responsibilities if you are employed.
- **Key personal skills** – highlight your main personal skills, attributes and abilities.
- **Education and qualifications** – the names and dates of all academic qualifications received, with the most recent first.
- **Training or work-related courses** – any additional vocational or on-the-job training you have received.
- **Previous employment** – all the past employment you have had with the following information: name of employer, job title and a brief summary of responsibilities. Also include any periods of work placement.
- **Leisure interests** – the interests you have outside the academic environment; the sports you play and at what level (it may be appropriate to list some of your achievements in sport), and other hobbies and activities in which you are involved. It is particularly good to state any positions of responsibility you have held, such as club captain, scout leader or cadet force rank.
- **Other relevant information** – anything else you feel may be of value to the employer, such as an ability to drive.
- **References** – the name, addresses and phone numbers of two people (referees) who can vouch for you. If you have a current employer, they should be the first; if not, a past employer or someone else in a position of responsibility, such as a teacher, would be appropriate. It is important that you ask them before using them as a reference in case they are not willing to write you a reference.

Sample CV

An example CV is shown on pages 334 to 335.

Curriculum vitae

Name:	Rebecca Sewell
Date of birth:	17 October 1982
Address:	125 Mill Crescent, Reading, Berks RG6 3JS
Nationality:	British
Tel:	01345 245131 (home); 01345 684877 (work); 07754 759868 (mob)
Email:	racsewell@aol.com

Current employment

Fitness instructor at the Premier Gym in Reading (2004–6)

A graduate in Sport Science (BSc Hons) with specialist skills in fitness instruction, teaching circuits and aerobics and core conditioning training.

Main responsibilities

- teaching aerobics and circuits
- conducting fitness assessments, designing exercise programmes and instructing workouts
- selling memberships and sports clothing.

Key skills include:

- fitness testing, programme design and instructional skills
- ability to teach exercise to music
- good communication skills
- good motivator of people
- financial management skills of budgeting and monitoring budgets
- computer and internet literate
- first aid and CPR competent
- selling and marketing skills.

Education & qualifications

2000–3	Thames University. BSc (Hons) Sport and Exercise Science (2:1 gained)
1998–2000	Reading College of Sport. BTEC ND Sport Science: 8 distinctions, 8 merits, 2 passes
1995–9	Campbell School, Reading. 10 GCSEs: PE (A), English Lang (A), English Lit (A), French (A), Biology (B), Maths (B), Chemistry (B), German (B), Geography (B), Physics (D)

Work-related courses

Fitness Trainers Award (2003)

NVQ RSA Exercise to Music (2002)

NPLQ (2004)

First aid at work (2005)

Stability ball training (2006)

Previous employment

2003–4	Leisure attendant at Springfield Baths Main duties included pool supervision and life-guarding, laying out equipment in the sports hall, coaching and teaching children's sport at weekends and during holidays.

Previous work experience

1999	Three-week placement at Hills Spa Health and Fitness Centre This involved shadowing the fitness trainers and duty manager, serving the members and advising them in the gym.

Hobbies & interests

I am involved in local athletics and am captain of the ladies' team. I run the 800m and 1500m and am currently the Berkshire county champion at 800m.

I enjoy travelling overseas, particularly to Australia and New Zealand.

My hobbies are reading and going to the cinema.

Other relevant information

Full driving licence and own car.

Referees

Mr W. Samways	Miss J. Gatehouse
Fitness Manager	Head of Sport Science
Premier Gym	Thames University
Garfield Road	Stratton Way
Reading	Easthampton
Berks RG16 4LP	Bucks BK34 7BJ
Tel. 01345 874098	Tel. 0152 854339

Student activity 26.5 45 minutes P2

Using the example provided, prepare a CV for yourself which you could send to a prospective employer.

Completing an application form

Many employers will produce their own application form, which you need to fill in when applying for a position. They will use this form to select the candidates they wish to interview. It is important to give yourself plenty of time to complete the form. Forms that are completed incorrectly or untidily will probably be discarded without being read. If you complete the form properly, you will already have an advantage over your rivals. Remember, you get only one chance to make a first impression. Here are some useful tips on completing the form.

- Photocopy the form first and use the copy to practise on. Check over what you have written and, when you are satisfied, copy it on to the original.
- Read the instructions on the form carefully and follow them exactly. For example, it may ask you to use black ink or block capitals. This is important because the form may need to be photocopied and will copy well only in black ink.
- Even if some of the information on the form is given in the covering letter, you must still include it on the form. Never write 'refer to CV', as the reader may not bother.
- Think about answers very carefully and plan your responses. For example, questions such as 'Why do you want to work for this company?' need to be researched and responded to appropriately.
- Check that your referees are willing to provide a reference for you before you put in their details.
- Take a photocopy of your form so that you can remind yourself what you wrote before an interview.
- Make sure you do not miss the closing date, and post the form well in advance.
- Include a covering letter with your application form.

Letter of application

A letter of application relates your experience to a specific company or job vacancy. It should always be sent with a CV and perhaps an application form. It should be businesslike and complement the information in your CV. If you are writing in response to an advertisement, make reference to the job title and where you saw the vacancy advertised, and ensure the letter is addressed to the correct person. Indicate why you are attracted to the position advertised, and highlight why you think you are suitable and what key personal skills and experiences you have that are

(Your name) ______________________

(Your address) ______________________

(Name of person applying to) ______________________

(Address of company writing to) ______________________

Date ______________________

Dear ______________________ (person's name)

(First paragraph to explain why you are writing, i.e. for which job and where you saw the vacancy)

(Next paragraph to explain what you are currently doing, i.e. employment or education)

(Next paragraph to discuss why you are applying for the job and what you like about it)

(Next paragraph to justify why you are suitable for the position – relevant experience or skills)

(End your letter by saying that you can attend an interview and hope to hear from them soon)

Yours sincerely*

______________________ (Sign your name)

______________________ (Type your name)

* If you do not have a person's name and addressed the letter to 'Dear Sir or Madam', you should end with 'Yours faithfully'.

Fig 26.6 How to write a letter of application

relevant to the vacancy. Finish the letter by stating that you look forward to hearing from them soon and would be delighted to attend an interview at their convenience.

Student activity 26.6 30 minutes P2

Use the template above to draft a letter of application.

Student activity 26.7 60 minutes P2

From the previous learner activities, preparing a CV and writing a letter of application, you should now have the skills and resources to apply for a suitable work-based experience in sport.

Task 1

Select an appropriate work-based experience in sport – it should be one that:

- you can access easily
- is suitable for a student to go on a work-based experience
- is in the sports industry!

Task 2

Ensure that your CV and letter of application are suitable for your selected work-based experience in sport and send them off to the most appropriate person at your selected facility/organisation.

26.6 Preparation for Interview

P3

One of the most important parts of the interview is the preparation that takes place beforehand. Learn all you can about the company and the job role. This can be done via the internet – it would be even better if you actually visited the workplace. During the visit not only will you have worked out how to get there, you will also be able to see how the people who work there dress, find out exactly what facilities are available and may even be able to ask some of the staff questions that could help you in your interview.

Questions

You should think about which questions you are likely to be asked. For example:

- Why are you interested in this job?
- What are your strengths?
- What are your weaknesses?
- What do you think this job entails?
- Why do you think you will be good at this job?

Once you have worked out suitable answers, practise answering them out loud either with a friend or in front of a mirror. You may wish to record yourself with a camcorder or tape recorder and then see or hear yourself 'in action' and make improvements where necessary. You should also study your body language, which includes your facial expressions, mannerisms and gestures. If you smile and look enthusiastic this will portray the right image. You may find that you slouch or have a blank facial expression without even being aware of it while answering questions.

Be prepared to discuss anything you have written on your CV or letter of application. You may be asked why you decided to study a BTEC qualification or to explain your choice of work placement, etc.

You should also prepare questions to ask the interviewers as this will show them that you are interested and want to know more about the company or job role. Be sure not to ask questions that have already been answered within the job role specifications or during the course of the interview.

Dress

You will need to decide what you are going to wear well in advance of the interview. If you are not sure what to wear, it is best to choose smart, dark-coloured clothes such as a suit or smart trousers or skirt and a shirt/blouse. Clothing that is too tight or revealing is rarely acceptable attire for an interview. Ensure that your clothes are clean and ironed and also comfortable. Ensure that your hair is clean and you have a suitable haircut or style for the interview. If you have lots of visible body piercings, you may wish to take some out in order to portray the image you think the company is looking for.

Location

If possible, go and visit the place you are going to for interview beforehand. Travel at the same time of day you will be leaving for your interview time so that you can see if there are any issues with rush hour traffic, etc. You should always plan to arrive at your interview location at least ten minutes in advance to allow time to compose yourself.

Interview Skills

Body Language

Body language can say an awful lot about how we feel, how confident we are and how enthusiastic we are. People will often make a first impression about someone based upon their body language alone. Therefore, it is important to convey the right message by using appropriate body language.

- Greet your interviewer with a firm handshake.
- Maintain eye contact as this shows that you are interested in what the person has to say. You should not overdo the eye contact, though, as this can sometimes look threatening.
- When answering questions, emphasise key points by leaning forward and using expressive gestures.
- Speak with an expressive voice to convey your enthusiasm and interest rather than a monotone voice which suggests a lack of interest and boredom.
- You should sit with your back up straight as this communicates self-assurance and eagerness. Do not slouch as this gives the impression that you are not interested or are lacking in confidence.
- Do not fidget or twiddle your fingers while the interviewer is talking as this shows you are not paying attention.
- When the interviewer is talking, nod your head and smile in relevant places to demonstrate your interest in what they are saying.

Answering Questions

You will have rehearsed many of the answers that you give during the interview and therefore know what you need to say and how to say it. However, you will undoubtedly be faced with a few questions that you have not prepared for. Give yourself a few seconds to sit and think about your answer and then respond honestly and as positively as possible. If you do not understand the question, ask the interviewer to repeat it. If you still do not understand the question you can respond in a variety of ways.

- Ask 'Do you mean . . .?', which shows that you understand some of what they said but need clarity.
- Ask them to explain their question in more detail.

Student activity 26.8 — 30 minutes — P3

Name: David Oldham

Age: 38

Position: Leisure Centre Manager

What annoys you the most from job applications and interviews?

I don't like it when you interview people who haven't bothered to find out anything about the organisation. I also get very annoyed by interviewees who arrive late without a good reason. How people dress is very important too, if I have an interviewee turn up in jeans it shows that they are not too bothered about making a first good impression – the whole aim of an interview is so that interviewee can try to show me that they want the job!!

What is your top tip for people who are applying for a job?

Make sure your CV is up to date and not too long – two sides of A4 is usually the maximum that I would expect. If a person does have an invitation to an interview then it is a good idea to try to learn around four to five things about the organisation and job role and dress smartly.

What is your favourite interview question?

I've interviewed many people for this role, why should I choose you?

What sort of things do you want your interviewee to discuss in an interview?

I want to hear about their personal skills and qualities and then evidence to show how they have put these skills and qualities to good use! There's not much point telling me that they are good communicators or good at working as a member of a team if they have no way of showing me that they have done this in the past and done well at it.

Questions

1 From reading the case study above, list five ways in which you could prepare yourself for an interview.

2 How would you answer the interview question 'I've interviewed many people for this role, why should I choose you'?

3 List four of your skills and four of your qualities. Now write a sentence for each to describe where each skill or quality has been used in a real life situation.

4 What would you plan to wear for an interview?

5 What sort of body language should you use in an interview and why?

Student activity 26.9 30 minutes P3

There are a number of skills that you can practise before going into a real life interview situation. You will need to ensure you are able to verbally communicate your interest in the job, your skills and qualities that are appropriate for the job as well as actively portray your interest and enthusiasm through your body language.

It is always a good idea to practise your interview skills prior to the real thing.

Task 1

With a friend, role play a situation where you are the interviewee and your friend is the interviewer. Ensure your friend has a range of different questions to ask about your skills and qualities that are suitable for a job that you are interested in.

If possible, try to video record the interview process.

Task 2

Ask your friend for feedback at the end of the interview and observe the video footage. From this information, make a mental note of your strengths and also the areas that need to be improved upon.

26.7 Preparing for a Work-Based Experience

P4 M2

You will need to consider what your aims and objectives are prior to your work-based experience in sport.

Personal Skills

A work placement is an opportunity to try out a job and start to understand what knowledge and skills are needed for that position. Answering the questions below will start to give you an idea of what your next step should be. You can discuss this audit with your tutor or work placement officer when you have a meeting with them to arrange your industrial placement. This will help you to gain a placement which is fulfilling, worthwhile and develops your skills and personal qualities.

Ask yourself the following questions.

- **What skills do have I now?** Look at practical skills of coaching and teaching, key skills such as written and verbal communication, problem-solving and application of number, IT and skills gained from previous work experiences such as clerical and administrative skills.
- **What skills would I like to acquire?** This is difficult because there may be skills you have not gained because you haven't been in a situation to gain them. As a result, you may not be aware that you need them. However, try to be realistic and think what skills you may need in a job, such as communicating with the general public.
- **What qualifications have I gained?** This is just a list of all the qualifications you currently hold. Also list here any qualifications you are hoping to gain.
- **What personal qualities do I have?** Think about personal qualities in the following areas.
  - **Working with other people**: are there particular people you would not like to work with? Do you prefer to work in large or small groups? How do you feel about working as part of a team? Are you happy dealing with the public?
  - **Leadership**: how good are you at leading groups? Do you prefer to lead large or small groups? How do you feel about selling to people?
  - **Responsibility:** how do you feel about responsibility in the following areas – cash, equipment, other people's work, meeting deadlines, other people's safety and welfare.
- **What do you want from a job?** Split this up into what you would want and what you would not want. Consider the following areas.
  - **Pay**: do you want enough to get by on or is getting a high wage important to you? Would you like to be paid by results? Would you like to be paid extra for extra work you have done?
  - **Hours**: do you want to work fixed hours (9 to 5), or do you not mind doing shift work? How do you feel about overtime?
  - **Prospects**: how important are the opportunities for promotion and the presence of a career structure?
  - **Location**: do you have a fixed idea of where you want to work, or are you willing to relocate to find the right job? How important is an easy journey to work to you?

- **Working with others**: is it important for you to work as a part of a group, or would you rather work alone? How do you feel about managers and supervisors, and are you looking for a certain style of leadership?
- **What the job entails**: are you looking for job satisfaction or a job that pays well? Are you keen to utilise certain skills and abilities? Do you want to help other people?

Targets

Once a decision has been made about your future career it is an appropriate time to think about setting targets. Remember, you may not be able to walk into your dream job immediately and while this remains your long-term goal it is important to set realistic short-term targets to lay the pathway to achieving your dream job.

When targets are set you need to use the SMART principle to make them workable. SMART stands for:

- **S**pecific
- **M**easurable
- **A**chievable
- **R**ealistic
- **T**ime-constrained.

Specific: the target must be specific to what you want to achieve. You may need to improve your lifesaving leg kick in order to pass your pool lifeguard award.

Measurable: targets must be stated in a way that is measurable, so they need to state figures. For example, I want to be able to tow a person 25 m in one minute.

Achievable: it must be possible to actually achieve the target.

Realistic: we need to be realistic in our setting and look at what factors may stop us achieving the target.

Time-constrained: there must be a timescale or deadline on the target. This means you can review your success. It is best to state a date by which you wish to achieve the goal.

Key learning points 2

- Ensure that your CV is well presented and runs to no more than two pages.
- Ensure that you fully prepare yourself for an interview, taking into account how you will get there, what sort of questions you may be asked and ensuring you speak clearly and use appropriate body language.
- Make sure you have some clear aims, objectives and targets that you hope to and can realistically achieve whilst on your work-based experience in sport.

Student activity 26.10 — 60 minutes — P4 M2

You are now ready to start preparing for your work-based experience in sport. Before starting on your work-based experience though, you will need to consider what you are hoping to achieve during your placement period.

Task 1

Prepare an action plan for your work-based experience in sport which identifies your:

- targets
- aims
- objectives.

Task 2

Write a few paragraphs to justify the targets, aims and objectives you are hoping to achieve whilst on your work-based experience in sport. At the end of each justification, write a few sentences to suggest ways in which you think you can achieve your targets, aims and objectives.

Undertake a Work-Based Experience

P5

While undertaking your work-based experience there are a number of situations and considerations you will need to think about prior to and during the experience.

Planned Activities

While on your work-based experience you will probably participate in planned activities. These may include testing chlorine levels in the swimming pool, staff meetings, cleaning duties, setting up and checking equipment, etc. Ensure you know the timing of these events, have been shown exactly what needs to be done and have a supervisor where necessary to ensure you are carrying out these planned activities safely and effectively.

Wherever you work you are part of a team that is responsible for running a safe and secure environment. Most working environments have a manual that covers details on how every part of the facility should operate under normal conditions and what to do in an emergency situation. These are usually referred to as Normal Operating Procedures (NOP) and Emergency Operating Procedures (EOP).

The NOP gives instructions on how to deal with everyday situations, whereas the EOP gives instructions on how to deal with minor and major emergency situations such as disorderly behaviour from customers or dealing with a drowning incident.

Working in the sports industry usually means you deal with customers on a regular basis. You therefore need skills in dealing with the public. These skills are very important so that you can be sure you are giving the customers the treatment they deserve to ensure they keep coming back to your leisure facility. You will need to learn what the customers' needs are and how you can meet these requirements or even exceed them.

> **Key term**
>
> **Customer service:** This refers to the level of assistance and courtesy given to those who use the facility.

26.7 Customer Service

The leisure industry is very competitive and customer service plays an important role in ensuring the facility you work in keeps its customers (after all, with no customers there would be no leisure facility!). If customers are happy with the services you provide, the facility in which you work will experience a number of benefits, including:

1. **Customer loyalty** – customers will return to a facility if they feel they have been treated well. If, however, they feel that they have been treated poorly, such as waiting too long for service or not having complaints dealt with effectively, then they are much less likely to return to the facility.
2. **New customers** – new customers can be generated through word of mouth from existing customers. If someone is happy with a facility, they are more than likely to recommend it to other people.
3. **Increased sales and profits** – if customers are happy, they will continue to use the facility, which, in turn, increases the amount of money an organisation makes.
4. **A good image** – most leisure and recreational facilities want to portray a good image to the public and this can be done through providing good customer care.
5. **Employee satisfaction** – can be gained through ensuring the employees are given thorough training in customer care. This training will help to ensure the employees can handle complaints rather than becoming upset.
6. **A competitive edge over other facilities which provide the same service** – a competitive edge is very important in the leisure industry as there is usually a number of facilities that provide the same services in one area. If one facility provides better customer service than another one, they are likely to have more customers than the other.

Equal Opportunities

Every person should ensure that they deal with the people that they meet in an unbiased and equal way whether it is at work, home or school. This means that you should not discriminate for reasons of race or ethnic origin, gender, culture, disability, sexual orientation or social differences.

Different Age Groups

In the leisure industry you can expect to deal with people of all ages, from babies and toddlers right through to the over-sixties. Therefore, you should

Day & date	
Hours worked	
Description of work/ activities	
Achievements & skills gained	
Concluding comments	

Fig 26.7 Record-keeping is important – use your log!

be able to have an understanding of their needs – be aware of where the baby-changing facilities are, ensure you know about reduced prices for the over-sixties, be aware of special swimming sessions for different groups, etc.

Different Cultural Backgrounds

You need to be aware of different cultural needs and be able to cater for them accordingly. Some cultures will not allow males to see females in their swimsuits. Therefore, you must be able to give these females details of when there are female-only swimming sessions. These sessions would also have to have only female lifeguards on duty too. You should be aware of people who use the facility who do not have English as their first language and ensure there are signs and promotional materials that they can understand.

Special Needs

A good leisure facility is able to cater for every person in its local area, including people who have specific needs. An example of a person with a special need is someone with restricted mobility. These people may require the use of a walking stick or wheelchair. In these cases the facility should have appropriate access so that they may enter the building unaided. If the building is on two storeys there must be a lift or ramps to allow the person to move up to the next floor. If the facility has a swimming pool there must be some form of access available for people with disabilities, such as a chair hoist.

Record-Keeping

P6 **P7**

You will need to record your activities while on placement so that you are able to assess exactly what you have done and how well you have performed these activities.

The best method of recording this information is to keep a daily diary of activities.

An example of the format you could use for your daily diary is shown below:

Other information that you may wish to include in your diary is as follows.

- Interview a member of staff and find out what the roles and responsibilities of their job are, and how they have come to be in their position. Also find out what qualifications they have and what skills they need to do their job effectively.
- Find out the organisation's operating procedures for a range of tasks. An operating procedure is how a company completes certain tasks. This will depend upon the type of organisation you work for, but try to find out how it deals with new customers, how it manages the work it does in the gym, how it deals with cash and cashing up, how it manages the pool, and so on.
- It is of utmost importance that you are inducted in health & safety procedures on your first day. Take a note of the following: what the evacuation

procedure is, where the fire exits are, where the assembly point is, where the first-aid kit is, who is a trained first aider, where the phone for emergencies is, where the fire extinguishers are, what safety equipment is available and when you need to use it.

- Make a record of what you did each day in the workplace and any new skills you gained.
- Every day ensure that you record the objectives you have met or are close to meeting, and check them off against the SMART targets you have set for yourself prior to starting the work-based experience. You may find that you need to review the timescales or other factors in your SMART targets as you may be achieving some of your targets faster or slower than expected.

26.8 Evaluate a Work-Based Experience

P8 M3 D2

So that you and your tutor(s) are able to assess how well you have performed on your work-based experience, you should carry out a full review of your placement and present your evaluation to these people.

Monitor and Review

In order to be able to assess your work placement project you should review your work periodically to ensure it is all going to plan. Try to evaluate your strengths – are you working well with the team? Then assess which areas you need to improve. For example, do your customer service skills need attention?

Always be vigilant to see if any opportunities arise that may improve your experience. This could be something as simple as asking to sit in on a staff meeting which may give you additional information for your job role.

Make a note of the skills you have acquired and developed while on the placement. You may wish to record this evidence on your CV as they will probably be transferable skills and therefore relevant for future employment.

From your time on the work placement you should have a good idea of what you need to do to develop your career in the sports industry. You may find that some organisations will pay for you to carry out any further training needs you require, while others will expect you to fund the training yourself.

You should also try to gain feedback from a variety of sources, including your supervisor, colleagues and possibly a customer or two that you have had regular contact with. Through interviews or questionnaires try to gauge their assessment of your performance. You can then use this information to determine the areas in which you excel and the areas in which you need to improve.

Presentation

Try to work out the best way of presenting your evaluation. Here are a few ideas:

- poster presentation
- oral presentation
- diary/logbook
- written assignment
- video presentation.

You may wish to use one form of presentation or a combination. This will depend on a variety of factors, including who you are delivering the presentation to and the facilities you have to use.

Key learning points 3

- Ensure that you are aware of the facility's normal operating procedures and emergency operating procedures.
- Ensure that you have learned some basic customer care skills.
- Keep a daily written record of everything that you have done whilst on work experience.
- Review your strengths and areas for improvement both during and after the work-based experience.

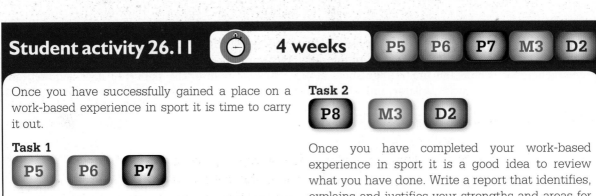

Student activity 26.11 4 weeks P5 P6 P7 M3 D2

Once you have successfully gained a place on a work-based experience in sport it is time to carry it out.

Task 1

P5 P6 P7

Carry out your work-based experience in sport. To evidence that you have carried out this work-based experience, keep a diary to record all other activities and achievements that you have gained whilst on your placement.

Task 2

P8 M3 D2

Once you have completed your work-based experience in sport it is a good idea to review what you have done. Write a report that identifies, explains and justifies your strengths and areas for improvement.

From this review think about what you could do in order to develop your skills and abilities and write a report that provides suggestions on how you could fulfil this development.

Useful websites

www.sportactivensa.co.uk/howwecanhelpyou/students/iminhigherfurthereducation.ashx

Career advice from the National Skills Academy, including links to sports and active leisure-related degrees and other qualifications.

www.uksport.gov.uk/vacancies/

Jobs bulletin board that is regularly updated with details of vacancies from grassroots to elite level sport in the UK.

http://careersadvice.direct.gov.uk/helpwithyourcareer/jobprofiles/

Specific careers advice for anyone thinking of becoming a fitness instructor, sports coach, sport psychologist, or sport scientist, with quick links to job descriptions, person specifications, and advice on how to get started.

42: Research investigation in sport & exercise sciences

42.1 Introduction

This unit will explore the skills, knowledge and understanding required for you to be able to undertake a major research investigation. The first part of this unit examines how you can identify a research problem that you are interested in investigating. Ways in which to conduct a literature review are then examined so that you can gain information from research conducted by other people to help formulate your own research. Methods of implementing and interpreting the results of your investigation will be examined followed by ways in which you can review your investigation. The last part of the unit covers the scientific format required for you to be able to present your project in the appropriate format.

By the end of this unit you should be able to:

- design a research investigation
- implement the investigation and interpret results
- review the results of the research investigation
- present the research investigation successfully.

Assessment and grading criteria		
To achieve a PASS grade the evidence must show that the learner is able to:	**To achieve a MERIT grade the evidence must show that, in addition to the pass criteria, the learner is able to:**	**To achieve a DISTINCTION grade the evidence must show that, in addition to the pass and merit criteria, the learner is able to:**
P1 produce a valid research proposal for a sport and exercise sciences-based research investigation, with tutor support	**M1** produce a valid research proposal for a sport and exercise sciences-based research investigation, with limited tutor support	**D1** independently produce a valid research proposal for a sport and exercise sciences-based research investigation
P2 describe the research design for a sport and exercise sciences-based research investigation	**M2** explain the research design for a sport and exercise sciences-based research investigation	**D2** justify the research design for a sport and exercise sciences-based research investigation
P3 implement the research investigation, describing data collection techniques	**M3** implement the research investigation, explaining data collection techniques	**D3** present and interpret collected data, analysing the research results.
P4 present and interpret collected data, applying statistical techniques to describe the research results	**M4** present and interpret collected data, explaining the research results	
P5 review the investigation results, explaining areas for future consideration	**M5** critically analyse the investigation results, justifying areas for future consideration.	
P6 produce the research investigation, following standard scientific format.		

42.1 Designing a Research Investigation

P1 P2 M1 M2 D1 D2

Research Proposal

P1 M1 D1

Often the hardest part of the plan is getting started. Thinking of a good idea takes time. It is useful to have a number of topics you hope to look at and then, if one idea proves impractical or too hard to test, you have an alternative. A good research proposal contains a question that you can answer, such as 'are netball players fitter than football players?' A good research proposal also needs to be practical so you can test it. You need to think about the time available, what resources and equipment you have and the subjects you can use. It needs to be of importance so that your conclusions have an implication for somebody or something. How will your research help an athlete, coach, official, teacher, administrator or manager? Finally, your research should be interesting so that others will read it and you will stay focused enough on it to complete it. It could take more than six months for you to finish the whole project.

What is to be the focus of your study? If you do not already have an idea in mind, you need to come up with one. A good way to start is to think about a sport or type of exercise that you know a lot about or that takes your interest. If, for example, you are a keen cyclist, you may wish to do a project on some aspect of cycling. Another way to narrow the area is to do it by a discipline within sport and exercise science. For example, you may decide to do a project involving biomechanics. You could even combine the two areas to arrive at a project that incorporates the biomechanics of cycling.

Therefore, the main factors that you need to consider include:

- Is the focus of your study interesting to you?
- Is the focus of your study interesting to others?
- Is it worthwhile?
- Has it been done before?
- Is it possible and within your limitations?

Review of Associated Literature

A literature review is where you carry out research to find out about other sports scientists experiments related to your area of interest. There are three main objectives of a literature review:

- presents and examines the current literature in your chosen area of interest
- summarises the relevant and appropriate information
- critically analyses the information gathered; including identifying gaps in current knowledge; showing limitations of theories and points of view and by formulating areas for further research

The literature review will show you what researchers have already done and help you to avoid repeating research that has already been undertaken. When carrying out your literature review, make sure you record the details of all of the sources that you use as these will be required in the reference section within your presentation of your project. The information that you need includes:

- author
- year of publication
- title of book or article
- edition (or volume)
- place of publication
- publisher
- page numbers for a journal article.

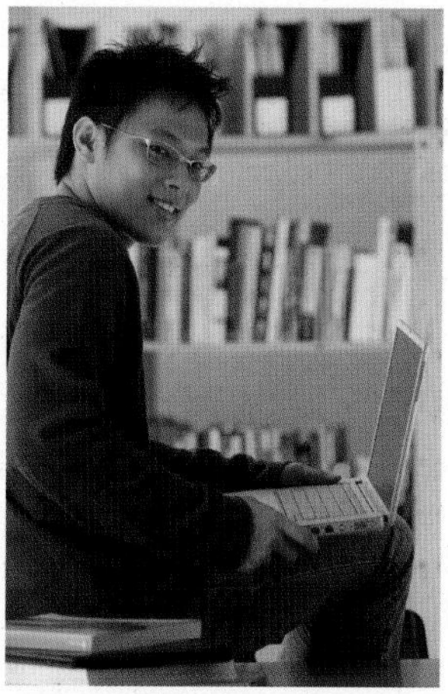

Fig 42.1 Your local library can be a good source of information for your research

You should include in your literature review your opinions and personal response to the information that you find so that it is in fact a critical summary of the literature.

When you are researching the different types of information you will need to consider the validity of the information and consider if the information is from a valid and trustworthy source. This can be done by checking key factors, which are:

- Who?
- What?
- When?
- Why?

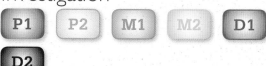

This will allow you to determine if the information produced is likely to be valid and relevant for your research investigation.

- **Who?** This examines who has carried out the research and authored the work. You are attempting to determine if they are qualified and experienced in this particular field. Where you have found the information will also have an impact on the validity of who has written the information.
- **Textbooks** Textbooks are a reliable source of information, which means that you can be certain that the information they contain is accurate because textbooks have usually been written by subject specialists and are then reviewed by experts to ensure the work is accurate.

More and more people are using electronic sources of information. Many libraries subscribe to e-books and e-journals so the material can be read on the computer screen. There are also searchable databases, which have been developed in certain subject areas. 'SPORTSDiscus' is one example. This is a database of information from across the globe in the area of sport and exercise science. It can be accessed via the internet and a subscription is required.

Websites

Information presented on the internet should be treated with some caution. Information can be posted on a website by anybody. It does not have to be reviewed or checked in any way. Having said that, the internet does contain some very useful websites from valid sources, e.g. British Nutrition Foundation, British Association of Sport and Exercise Sciences, etc.

Journals

Journals are written by subject specialists, reviewed by subject experts and come out at regular intervals throughout the year. As they are published so frequently, the information they contain is up to date with current facts and trends relating to specific subject areas. Most libraries will stock a range of relevant journals and you can also access some journals via the internet (however, some journals charge a subscription cost in order for you to access articles so check to see if your centre has a subscription with the journal you are interested in).

- **Why?** If you take into account the reason why the work has been carried out it will provide insight into whether there may be any bias in the reported results. For this you will need to consider who the information is intended for and how easily you can determine if the information is based on fact or opinion. For example, if the information is produced by an organisation which produces consumer products such as a sports drink manufacturer, the research may have some bias to show the organisation's product in a positive light.
- **When?** In some areas of sport and exercise sciences concepts and theories are continually being updated from ongoing research. It is therefore important to check that you are using the most appropriate and up-to-date information to ensure that the information you are using is as accurate as possible.
- **What?** This refers to the information that you find: not all of it will be relevant for your research investigation. Make sure you read the abstract or summary at the start of the article so that you can check that the resource is appropriate for you.

Your literature review should be a critical analysis of the research that you have discovered. This means that you should question what has been said, compare and contrast the information from the different sources and produce an evaluation based on your ideas and conclusions based on the information that you have presented.

Primary & Secondary Research Sources

In your literature review you will probably use both primary and secondary resources. What are these?

A **primary** resource is information gained directly from the researcher carrying out the investigation. Examples include:

- original data from physiological testing, e.g. heart rates

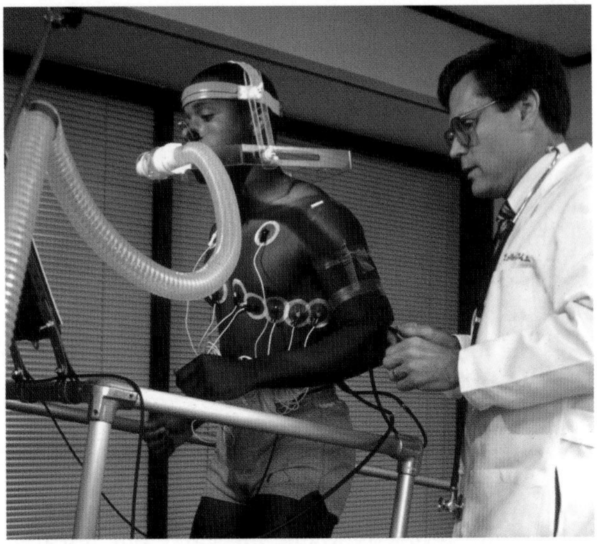

Fig 42.2 Carrying out primary research

- photographs
- film footage
- interviews
- government documents.

A **secondary** source is one step removed from the original source and is based on primary source materials. If you were examining the number of yellow and red cards for the teams competing in the last three football World Cups, you would need to collect the data from all these competitions. This might involve looking up information on the internet, for example. This data would therefore be secondary data, which was originally recorded by somebody other than you.

Investigation Aim

The aim of the investigation must be clear. Along with finding a good title, this is an area that people find hard to get right at first. You may have a general idea for a project (e.g. fitness in football players), but not a specific aim. Using fitness in football players as an example, what would you test and who would you test? The topic is too general. It needs to be focused on one particular aspect of fitness in football players.

Contrast this with the following topic: the anaerobic fitness levels of college male first-team and second-team football players. This project is far clearer. What is to be measured is specific – anaerobic fitness. But you would still need to decide how to measure this and justify your chosen method. The people you are going to investigate are clearly stated. The objective is very clear. Therefore you have something that you can test. You might suggest that first-team players will have a higher level of anaerobic fitness than second-team players. This would be easy to test, by measuring it in both sets of players and then comparing the values.

Having a good question to test helps make your research clear. It helps you to think about how you intend to collect the data. The aim will define the scope of your project. If you are looking at fitness in young male footballers, this is what your conclusions should be about. You might like to generalise to older footballers, or females or rugby players, but you would be speculating. So remember, keep the research focused on one area. For example:

Title: Do isotonic sports drinks increase cycling endurance performance?
Aim: To assess whether isotonic sports drinks increase the time that a person can perform endurance cycling.

Hypothesis

Your investigation should also have some sort of hypothesis. A hypothesis is basically a theory that you plan to prove or disprove through your research. A hypothesis will include two variables and a prediction of what you think will happen. For example, drinking sports drinks while cycling will improve endurance performance.

A **null hypothesis** is where it is expected that there will be no relationship between the two variables. For example, there will be no difference in cycling endurance performance if a cyclist drinks a sports drink.

Hypotheses are usually used when you are carrying out **quantitative** research. However, when you are using **qualitative** research, it is not always necessary or appropriate to include a hypothesis in your project; instead, you would state what you think you will find out from the research.

Research Method

The most common type of research method is to have two groups: one that undertakes some form of training or treatment and one that does not. You would then test both groups at the start of the research and both groups at the end of the research and see if there is a difference. This is termed a 'pre-test post-test' research design.

Another method of research is to use a **comparative study**. You might wish to examine how much sport and physical education children do in schools and the effect this has on the sport they take part in outside school. In this case, what you are measuring is how much sport is played outside school by children. What you would change would be the amount of sport and physical education played in school, but this cannot be done. Therefore, you could compare one school with another, where one school provides more sport during normal school hours and compare it with one that provides less sport during school hours, or even compare countries' provision (France and England).

A **longitudinal study** allows you to compare evidence or information over time. For example, how the amount of physical education in schools has changed over the years. If you can access the information from some time ago, you can compare this to current statistics. You may have to start the study up by taking current statistics and then comparing these to data produced in a period of a few months or a year. This type of research method is often used in the study of health and disease. It requires time; some longitudinal research can last for many years.

Scope

The scope of your project is basically who the results of the project would be applicable to. For example, if you were to carry out your research on eight people, the results would probably only be applicable to similar people. So, if you selected eight male club cyclists to test if sports drinks affect their endurance, the results would really only be applicable to males who are at the same club level.

Limitations

In this section of your research proposal you will need to explain any limitations to your investigation. Limitations are possible shortcomings or influences that either cannot be controlled or are the results of the restrictions imposed by the researcher.

Some limitations refer to the scope of the study, which is usually set by the researcher. An example of a limitation may be that you will only be able to sample a small population of participants such as Caucasian males between 18 and 25 years old.

Implications

The implications for your research investigation will include such factors as what sort of resources and equipment you need in order to carry out the investigation.

Student activity 42.1 120–180 Mins P1 M1 D1

The first part of designing a research investigation is to carry out research in your selected subject area and produce a research proposal.

Task 1

Produce a written valid research proposal for a sport and exercise-based investigation. Your proposal should contain the following information:

- area of study
- statement of problem
- review of literature
- investigation aim
- research hypotheses
- research method
- scope
- limitations
- implications.

42.3 Research design

P2 M2 D2

Health & Safety

It is very important to ensure the health and safety of participants in your investigation and also to consider the legal implication of your actions. You must ensure that your testing procedures meet certain considerations deemed necessary to minimise any risks to the subject. This will involve following strict procedures, which are usually outlined in the protocol that you are following, and carrying out a risk assessment prior to any testing. Where risks have been identified, ways to eliminate or reduce the risk to the subject should be included, such as having a medically trained person present during the testing process.

Ethical considerations

Ethical considerations respect the rights of subjects who are involved in the investigation in order to ensure they are not negatively affected by your tests or work.

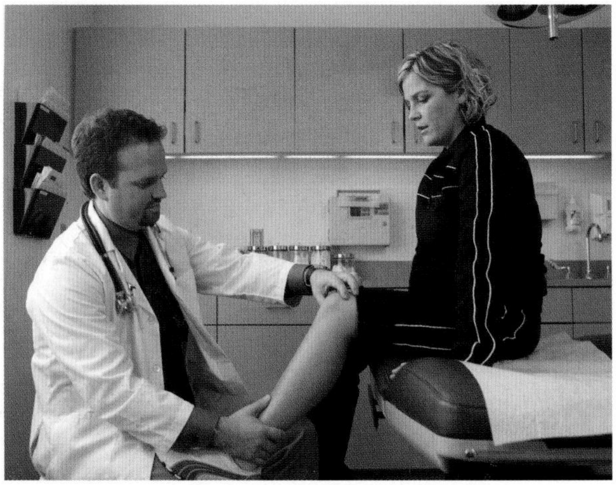

Fig 42.3 You must respect the rights of your subjects

As most of the studies in sport and exercise sciences involve carrying out tests on humans, it is necessary for you as the researcher to ensure that your research setting or activity does not frighten, embarrass or negatively affect the participants (Tuckman, 1978).

The design of the research investigation should ensure that all participants take part voluntarily, complete an informed consent form, are not harmed in the process of the investigation, and that participants' results are anonymous and kept confidential (de Vaus, 1996).

Your subjects should be made aware of their right to withdraw from a test or programme of exercise at any time during the study. The decision to undertake a test or exercise programme rests with the individual; if they decide they do not want to continue, you must stop the test. You should explain the full procedures and programmes that any individual will be following, give them details of the group they will be in, if any, and tell them who will be testing them. This is an important part of testing, as it allows you to be sure that the subject is clear about what they are doing. You do not want the results to be affected by a lack of understanding on the subject's part.

An informed consent form should be produced and signed by the subjects who are involved in the investigation. An informed consent form should contain the following information:

- a fair explanation of the procedures that the participant will be expected to follow
- a description of the possible discomforts and risks to the participant
- a description of the benefits to be expected from carrying out the research
- an offer to answer any enquiries concerning the procedures
- an instruction that the participant is free to withdraw consent at any time and terminate the testing process.

Anonymity

Participants should be referred to by a method that ensures that they remain anonymous so other people

1 Explanation of the tests

You will perform a series of tests which will vary in its demands on your body. Your progress will be observed during the tests and stopped if you show signs of undue fatigue. You may stop the test at any time if you feel unduly uncomfortable.

2 Risks of exercise testing

During exercise certain changes can occur, such as raised blood pressure, fainting, raised heart rate, and in a very small number of cases heart attacks or even death. Every effort is made through screening to minimise the risk of these occurring during testing. Emergency equipment and relevantly trained personnel are available to deal with any extreme situation which occurs.

3 Responsibility of the participant

You must disclose all information in your possession regarding the state of your health or previous experiences of exercise as this will affect the safety of the tests. If you experience any discomfort or unusual sensations it is your responsibility to inform your trainer.

4 Benefits to expect

The results gained during testing will be used to identify any illnesses and the types of activities that are relevant for you.

5 Freedom of consent

Your participation in these tests is voluntary and you are free to deny consent or stop a test at any point.
I have read this form and understand what is expected of me and the tests I will perform. I give my consent to participate.

Client's signature
Print name
Date
Trainer's signature
Print name
Date

Fig 42.4 An example of an informed consent form

reading the information who have not directly been involved will not know exactly who the subjects are or their experimental results.

Anonymity can be preserved by giving the subjects an identification number, which is used instead of their names.

Confidentiality

The Data Protection Act (1998) states that any information collected from a subject must be kept confidential. Therefore, when information is kept, only authorised people should be able to access this (for example, password-protected computer programmes, locked storage facilities etc.). When reporting results to people not directly involved in the investigation, personal details of the subjects should be omitted. However, it is possible to allow third parties to access information relating to the general background details of the subjects, such as age, gender, ability level etc. so that they can determine the demographics of the population that the information refers to.

You must also ensure that you have permission to carry out the testing from the centre in which you are carrying out the investigation. Your research proposal will usually have to be submitted to your Ethical Advisory Committee, which will examine your proposal to ensure that full consideration is given to the health and safety of the participants taking part and that the rights of the participants are protected.

Sample

As it is not possible to carry out your intended investigation on every appropriate person, it is necessary to select a sample. A sample is a subset of a population. Samples are studied, data is collected and statistics are calculated from the samples so that one can make inferences or extrapolations from the sample to the population. A population can be defined as including all people or items with the characteristic one wishes to understand. Therefore, when deciding upon your sample, you will need to ensure you have access to a representative sample (or subset) of the population you are wishing to study.

The determination of sample size is often limited to the number of people who are willing to take part in your investigation that fit into the parameters of the population that you are investigating. On the whole, the larger your sample size the more reliable the statistical inferences.

Type of Research

You will need to determine if you are going to carry out research that uses qualitative or quantitative data.

Qualitative research focuses on investigating subjective data, including the perceptions of the people involved. Qualitative research is usually carried out in the form of interviews, observations and questionnaires, and examines the why and how of human behaviour.

Interviews, focus groups and observations are all methods of qualitative research.

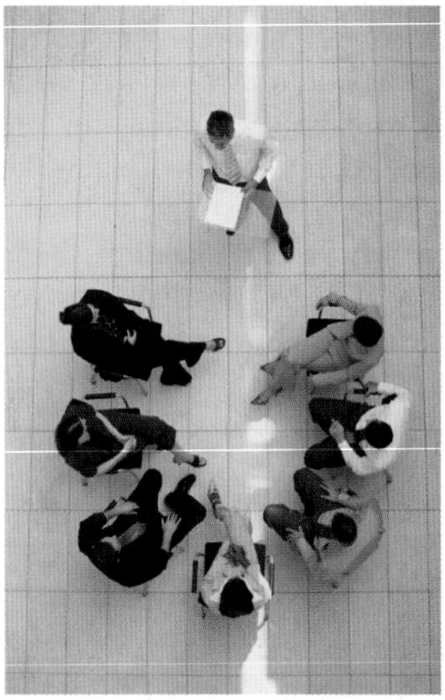

Fig 42.5 A focus group

Quantitative research concentrates on what can be measured and involves collecting and analysing objective (often numerical) data that can be organised into statistics. Quantitative research differs from qualitative research in the following ways:

- data is usually gathered using more structured research instruments
- results provide less detail on behaviour, attitudes and motivation
- results are based on larger sample sizes that are representative of the population
- research can usually be replicated or repeated, giving it high reliability
- analysis of the results is more objective.

However, quantitative research is often resource-intensive and can take several weeks to many months to design, implement, and analyse.

Resources and Equipment

You will need to consider what sort of equipment you need to carry out your investigation and whether your centre has access to it. Your centre may have a sport and exercise science lab or have access to one at another institute. Talk with your supervisor to find out exactly what is available and whether this will meet your planned needs; if not you will have to adjust your research design.

Statistical analyses

Your results section will require some statistical analysis to make sense of the data collected and draw conclusions from it. You can carry out some statistical analyses with a calculator if you know the statistical equation. However, there is also available a range of statistical packages that can carry out the statistical analyses for you once you have learned how to use the software. SPSS is an example of one that is used in sport and exercise sciences.

Reliability

The reliability of the tests you are planning to form should also be taken into account.

> **Key term**
>
> **Reliability:** if a test is repeated, it will give the same results.

If you recorded the same thing on two separate occasions, would you expect the value to be the same? Imagine you were coaching a cyclist, and to monitor his training and recovery you had to record his resting heart rate each morning. Assuming that your cyclist was not overtraining or suffering from an illness, you would expect the resting heart rate to remain fairly constant over a number of weeks. If you measured similar values each morning, this would display good reliability. You would then be assured that your measuring technique was reliable. If the values did change, you could then be sure it was due to something other than your measuring. Your subject might be suffering from a cold, which may have elevated his or her resting heart rate.

Validity

The validity of the tests used also needs to be considered.

> **Key term**
>
> **Validity:** whether the test actually measures what it is supposed to measure.

Many fitness tests are available to measure different aspects of fitness. Therefore, you need to be sure that the test you are using does actually measure the component of fitness that you are investigating. For example, if you want to measure the flexibility of a person and choose the sit-and-reach test, you are actually only measuring the flexibility of their back and hamstrings. This may not be a true representation of their overall flexibility, as they may have very flexible shoulders and hips.

Key learning points 1

- A **research proposal** should outline:
  - statement of the problem
  - review of literature
  - critique of literature
  - investigation aim
  - hypotheses (null and alternative)
  - research method
  - scope
  - limitations
  - resources.
- A **research design** should outline the:
  - ethical considerations
  - health and safety
  - type of research
  - sample
  - methodology
  - resources
  - statistical analyses
  - validity
  - reliability of the investigation.

Student activity 42.2

4–5 hours

P2 M2 D2

Task 1

Prepare a written report that describes, explains and justifies the research design for a sport and exercise sciences-based research investigation. You should include the following in your report:

- ethical considerations
- health and safety
- type of research
- sample
- methodology
- resources
- statistical analyses
- validity
- reliability.

Implementing the Investigation & Interpreting the Results

P3 M3

This part of your investigation can take some time. Where you are carrying out physical testing on subjects it is a good idea to have practised the protocol with people who are not your subjects so that you:

- are familiar with the process
- can use the equipment appropriately
- can record data accurately.

Data-Collection Techniques

If you are using specialist equipment, it is essential that you can use it correctly. Your major consideration will be how true the data is that you collect. Data should be accurate and precise, and for this to be the case, a certain level of knowledge and skill on the part of the tester will be required. The data can be only as precise as the measuring system. If a metre rule has only centimetre increments, you will be able to record only to the nearest centimetre (i.e. 1.75m, not 1.755m). The accuracy of the data relates to how close your measurement is to what you actually intend to measure. Checking that equipment is calibrated correctly will help ensure accuracy.

An example of calibrating a piece of equipment would be to pass a sample of a known percentage of oxygen through a gas analyser and check that it is giving the correct reading. If it is not, the piece of equipment should be adjusted until it is producing an accurate reading. Some pieces of equipment should be calibrated prior to every use, such as an online gas analyser, but other equipment, like weighing scales, rarely needs calibration.

Key term

Calibration: the process of checking and adjusting equipment to ensure that it is providing accurate readings.

Laboratory & Field-based Data Collection

Data collection is generally divided into laboratory-based tests and field-based tests. Laboratory tests are performed in a closed environment.

Key term

Closed environment: a situation that is tightly controlled, where things do not change.

In a closed environment, things are closely controlled and maintained. The advantage of this is that there are fewer factors that will affect the results. Let's say you wanted to perform a fitness test on one of your athletes. In a laboratory-based test, the room temperature would be constant, the amount of exercise can be measured exactly and there will be no effects from spectators or fellow players. These conditions make the results reliable. That means you could reproduce the test conditions easily and be able to compare results from one test to another.

It would seem, therefore, that laboratory tests are very useful – and they are. But sport is not played in a lab! This is the reason for field-based tests, or tests that are performed in a real-life setting. If you were a football coach and you wished to measure your players' fitness, you could do this out on the football pitch, on grass, where players play their games. You could organise the bleep test on the pitch. The results will be affected by the weather, the state of the pitch, your players' footwear, etc., but at least the results can be related to football (i.e. running on grass).

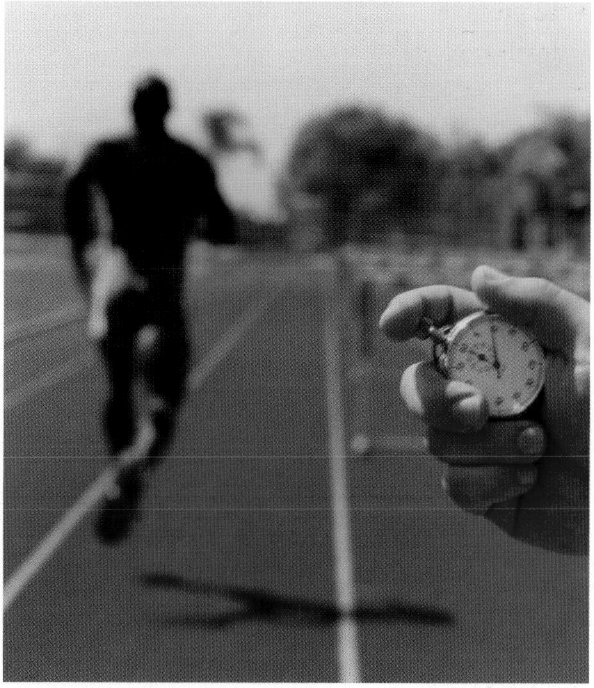

Fig 42.6 Field-based fitness testing

Most projects will involve recruiting a group of people to test. The group you choose is called the **sample.** If you were examining the amount of exercise undertaken by college students, it would not be practical to question all students, so you would just question a sample. The sample you use should not be biased in any way. They would not all be the same age, or all from one course, unless you specifically state '18-year-old college students'. Your sample will be made up of volunteers or those who are available at the time, such as your classmates. You should try to avoid any bias in your research, as this limits any conclusions that you make.

Key term

Bias: influence in an unfair way.

You may be a keen netball player and want to prove that netball players have higher VO_2max compared to hockey players.

Your choice of subjects could bias your results in favour of this being proved correct. For example, you might choose netball players who play at a higher level than the hockey players. Or you might choose netball players who play in positions that require

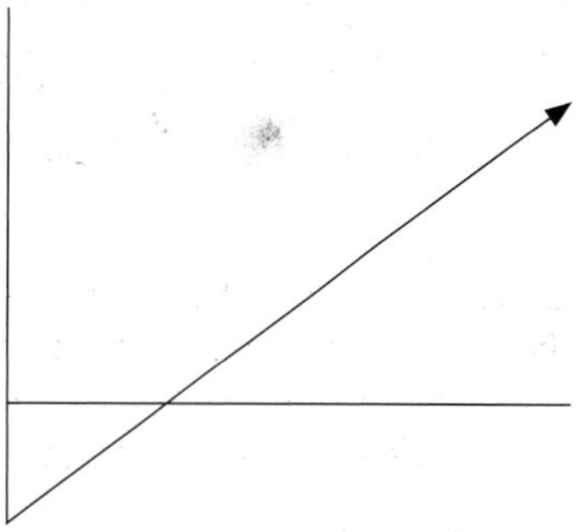

Fig 42.7 Graphical representation of data

high levels of aerobic fitness, such as the centre and the wings, and then choose hockey players who play in positions that require low levels of aerobic fitness, such as the goalkeeper. This would bias your sample and probably prove your theory to be correct.

You may wish to conduct your test in a realistic environment. This is called a **field-based test**. If you use specialist facilities, this is termed a **laboratory test**. The advantages of doing laboratory tests are that they are more controlled, as you do not have to worry about external factors like the weather. But remember, sport is not played in a lab, so field tests, although difficult, may give you a truer picture of what is actually happening.

Questionnaires

Not all research involves collecting and analysing numbers. Some research requires information on a person's behaviour or attitude towards something. This is common in qualitative research.

Questionnaires, interviews and observations are used to gather evidence and, although the data or information is in a different format to quantitative research, the question of truthfulness or exactness is just as important. Is the information you obtain valid? If you set out to measure anxiety levels and do so using a questionnaire, are the answers you receive accurate? Does your questionnaire actually measure anxiety? Do people tell the truth? All these issues need to be addressed.

What about reliability? If you repeated your questionnaire in similar situations, would you obtain similar results?

The design of the questionnaire, the type of questions and the way they are worded can all affect the validity and reliability of your results. This will also be the case if you decide to conduct individual interviews rather than administer questionnaires.

Recording Results

A clear data sheet can save both time and confusion when recording results. Imagine you have designed a questionnaire to investigate the amount of sport and exercise undertaken by college students. Once all the completed questionnaires have been returned, you need to record all the results in a clear and effective format. Putting them in one table will allow you to see all the results together and will be better for subsequent analysis.

There are many ways of recording data. For example, you could record the most common answer. This is called **frequency analysis** – looking at how often something occurs. You could even list things as the most frequent, the second most frequent, the third most frequent, and so on. This is called putting things in rank order. It is important to do this sort of analysis with your data so that you can start to make sense of it.

You may have used a questionnaire asking a series of questions and then coded the answers. For example, the possible answers may be: Strongly agree, Agree, Disagree, Strongly disagree. By giving these answers numbers from 1 to 4, you can more easily carry out data analysis (e.g. what is the average reply?). Remember to indicate which number is at which end of the scale of agreement/disagreement.

You could convert your answers to percentages and work out what percentage agrees or what percentage answered 'yes' to a question. If you have a long list of answers or a lot of possible answers, you can examine the range of responses. If you were measuring heart rates of a group during a fitness test, you could use all these methods. Who has the highest heart rate (rank order)? How many had heart rates between 131 and 140 beats per minute (b.p.m.) compared with 141 and 150 bpm? What was the average? What percentage was below a certain figure (frequency analysis)? Even what the difference was between the highest and the lowest (range). The list of options is almost endless.

Presenting the Data

Using graphs to illustrate your data helps to show trends and relationships in a more obvious way than by simply using tables of information. For example, look at the data in Table 42.1.

When this data is shown in the form of a graph, it can be clearly seen that as exercise intensity increases so does heart rate.

For numbers, one method of presenting the values is to chart them as a frequency distribution. One type of frequency distribution is a scatter plot. This type of plot records a point for each time a certain value occurs. Instead of showing a series of points, vertical bars can be used; this is called a histogram.

The most important consideration when displaying data is the presentation. Data should be displayed in the most effective format (there is no need to include raw data). Tables of data should contain units and must have a suitable title. Graphs should also incorporate units and labels and contain a title. Any picture, photograph or diagram, including graphs and histograms, but not tables, is referred to as a figure.

Exercise Intensity (W)	Heart rate (bpm)
20	72
40	85
60	94
80	102
100	110

Table 42.1 The heart rate of a subject at different exercise intensities

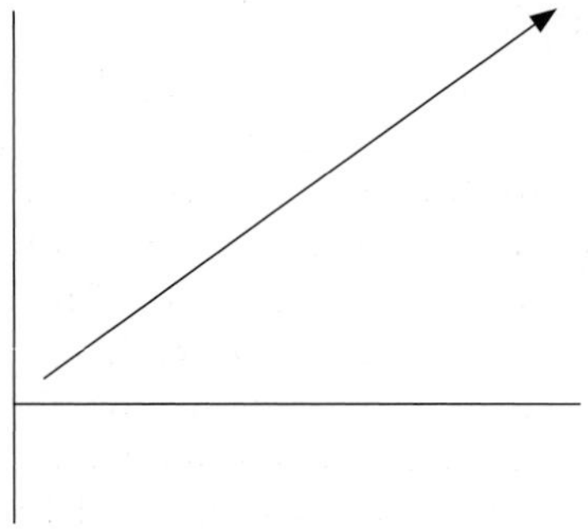

Fig 42.8 A graph showing a positive correlation

Data Interpretation

Qualitative Data Interpretation

With qualitative data, there tends to be lots of information (e.g. long lists of answers to questions or descriptions of behaviour). This information needs to be reduced into a manageable amount. This process of data reduction is called **coding**, i.e. grouping the data into meaningful segments.

In qualitative analysis, there are no right and wrong answers. You interpret the data as you see fit. Coding can be time-consuming, especially if the amount of data is large. To this end, computer software has been written to analyse the data. Currently, the most popular qualitative data analysis packages are NUD-IST, ATLAS and Ethnograph.

It is important in any form of research to verify that the data you have is accurate and that the conclusions you reach are valid. In qualitative research, this is done via **triangulation**. This is a method of cross-checking information using different sources or different methods of data collection. It is a common technique used by detectives and journalists. If two people say the same thing independently of each other, it is more likely to be true.

Quantitative Data Interpretation

Numerical analysis of data is called **statistics**. Descriptive statistics are about describing data (i.e. the average value or the range of numbers). Inferential statistics are more detailed. They examine things like relationships or differences in data. They can be used to determine the answer to your research question or your hypothesis. Relationships look at how one thing affects another and can be analysed using correlations. Differences decide if one group is different from another.

Correlations

To measure if two things are related, a **correlation** can be performed. Correlation means association or relationship. For example, the question 'is heart rate related to environmental temperature?' can be answered with a test of correlation. The correlation will give an exact level of the relationship between the two things: this value or number is called the **correlation coefficient** and is normally given by the letter 'r'. If two things are in an exact relation with one another (i.e. as one goes up, so does the other), they have a **positive** correlation.

The correlation coefficient (r) to represent this is $\leqslant 1$. If there is no relationship, r is 0. However, if the relationship is the other way round, i.e. one goes up as the other goes down, this is a **negative** correlation. In this case, r would be -1. Therefore, you can see that r can be between $\leqslant 1$ and -1. A high correlation, association or relationship is just that; it does not necessarily mean that one thing causes the other.

Once you have measured r, what does it mean? When a correlation is calculated, a probability or significance value is also given, in addition to the r value. This significance value is a number (e.g. 0.10). The value gives the likelihood of what you are testing being true. For example, if you were testing a relationship and you had a significance value of 0.10, this would mean that 10 times in 100 you would be wrong if you said there was a relationship. The good side of this is that 90 times in 100 you would be correct. In social science (i.e. sports science, psychology), the customary significance value is 0.05 (being wrong 5 times in 100). If the significance value is higher than 0.05, then there is no relationship (or at least, it is not significant). Statistically, the specific significance value of 0.05 is written as $p < .05$.

A **Pearson product–moment correlation** is one type of test that can be performed. In order to do this, a number of criteria must be met. The main assumptions are as follows:

- Data must be from related pairs; data should be collected from the same subject (e.g. height and mass from the same person).
- Data should be interval or ratio (explained previously).
- Each variable should be normally distributed (normality).

If the assumptions for a Pearson product–moment correlation are not met, a **Spearman rank–order correlation** is performed.

If the relationship were significant, the statistics would be reported as ($r = .931$, $p < .05$). The significance value is less than 0.05. This means the relationship is meaningful.

Difference Tests

Difference tests can be divided into two types: **parametric** and **non-parametric**. Parametric statistics should be used when the data are normally distributed and interval or ratio level. Non-parametric statistics are used when the data is not normally distributed.

Difference tests are used for studying the effect of something on a group of individuals. For example, how training affects fitness levels. The outcome of difference tests is reported in the same way as a correlation, but, rather than a relationship, a significant difference is referred to. For example, there is a significant difference ($t = 1.352$, $p < .05$) in heart rate between a group that does exercise and a group that does not.

With parametric statistics, the most frequent difference tests are t-tests. An independent t-test is used when investigating differences among groups. A dependent t-test is used when you are investigating a difference inside the group. If the data is not parametric, t-tests cannot be performed and alternative tests are used. The **Mann-Whitney U test** is a non-parametric difference test that can be used with different groups. The **Wilcoxon matched-pairs** test is a non-parametric test that can be used within the same group. Another non-parametric test is the **chi-square test**. This looks at the frequency of occurrence of something.

Outliers

Outliers are unusual data measurements. They can be the result of error or they may be correct readings caused by a strange event (e.g. where a subject has an abrupt change in heart rate). The trouble with outliers is that some information (like the average) can be greatly affected. If this is the case, the median could be used instead of the mean, as the outlier would not affect it. Many people try to ignore outliers, but you need to think long and hard about doing this. Was the data point a mistake or is it a genuine reading? If you have any uncertainty, you can include results both with and without outliers, to see how much they differ.

Key learning points 2

- Data collection techniques will vary depending upon whether you are carrying out quantitative or qualitative research.
- All data should be collected using appropriate units.
- Ensure that the data you collect is valid, reliable and free from bias.
- Data should be presented using graphs and tables.
- Statistical tests include *t*-tests, Pearson's Moment Correlation Coefficient, Analysis of Variance, Correlation Coefficient.
- SPSS is a statistical package used by sport and exercise scientists.

Student activity 42.3 — 2–6 weeks — P3 P4 M3 M4 D2

Once you have completed your research proposal and design you can make a start on carrying out your investigation.

Task 1

Implement your research investigation, making sure that you adhere to your research design. With your supervisor, describe and explain your data collection techniques for your investigation.

Task 2

Produce a written report that presents the data that you have collected from your investigation. Ensure that you have used appropriate statistical tests on the data collected so that you can describe, explain and analyse the research results in your written report.

42.4 Presenting & Reviewing a Research Investigation

P5 P6 M5

Use scientific format for the research investigation

Your project will be reported in writing. The general structure of a written project is given below. On the front will be the title page, followed by the preliminary pages, which comprise:

- **i.** Abstract
- **ii.** General contents
- **iii.** Contents page for figures and tables
- **iv.** Contents page for appendices
- **v.** Acknowledgements

Introduction
Literature review
Method
Results
Discussion
Conclusion
References
Appendix

Title page

This should have on it the title of the study, the person who wrote it and the year. You may wish to include the name of your college.

Abstract

A summary of all sections of the report, it is a review of the entire project. The abstract must be clearly separated from the main body of the report. Normally in the region of 250 words, it will contain information on the aim, research plan, outcomes and overall conclusions. This summary of the research appears as the first page of the report, but is usually written last since you cannot summarise until the end.

Contents page

This will list the units or the sections of the report, together with the number of the page on which each begins. Have separate contents sections for figures and tables and appendices.

Acknowledgements

The part of the project where you can write something personal to thank those people who may have helped you during the project. It could also include thanks to your supervisor for support, plus others you would like to mention.

Introduction

The purpose of this is to give an outline of the research area. It should address the question why you are doing the project. The introduction sets the tone of the project. What is the project all about? How did you become interested in it? It should make the objective of the project clear. It should be interesting so that anyone reading this would want to find out more. The end of the introduction should be the aim of the research.

Literature review

An in-depth analysis of the research, this will be a detailed look at all areas within the project. Key terms need to be defined. You should explain why your research is needed and how athletes, coaches and physical educators will benefit. Try to evaluate what is already known about your research topic. You can use many sources of information for your literature review. Conclude the review with a statement of what it is you are going to test.

Method

This should be relatively simple to write, as it explains what you did. It can be divided into sub-sections. In the first part explain about the subjects, how many, what groups, give details on the average age, what sports they play or their current fitness level. This will give a good indication of the subjects that you have in your project. Next include your research design: how you collected your information. After the research design, give a list of the equipment you needed to use. The final part of the method is to report the protocol and procedures of the tests that you undertook. Give enough information so that anybody reading would be able to reproduce exactly what you did.

Results

This section contains the actual data collected by you. Data should be presented in as clear a format as possible so that it is easy to read what you found. You do not need to include lists of numbers or piles of questionnaires unless you are specifically asked for this. Results can be summarised using descriptive statistics. Patterns that you see in the data do need to be described (e.g. heart rate increases with time). Tables and graphs are the best way of presenting lots of data but you will need to write about what is in the table or graph. What was the average heart rate? What did heart rate go up to? What time did heart rate start to decrease? These are the sorts of areas you need to be looking for. Besides describing results, statistics are used to analyse results to allow conclusions to be made. These are called **inferential statistics**. They allow you to make accurate statements about your results. Consider an investigation to see if a given training programme lowered the resting heart rate of a group of individuals. Your results might show that the average resting heart rate of the training group is 58 b.p.m, while that of a control group (a group of subjects who did no training) is 61 b.p.m. There is a difference of 3 b.p.m, but is this meaningful or is the difference just due to chance? A statistical difference test (e.g. *t*-test) would be able to establish if the difference in the values was significant, i.e. large enough to mean something. Where calculations are performed in analysing data, a sample calculation is helpful to explain the analysis. This can be included in the main text or in an appendix.

Discussion

This is the most central part of your research as it is your chance to explain what has happened and why. This section should include an analysis of the results. Do not merely repeat the results that you have just described. Try to give a summary of what you found.

Relate your results to the main theory and previous studies and always refer back to the aim of your project and to what you said in the literature review. Why do you think your results ended up the way that they did? Was it because of time? How much time did other studies use? Consider your subjects: were they homogeneous or different? For example, were they a mixture of amateurs and pros? What effect would this have? If they are all amateurs, do they have more room for improvement (training status)?

Read the discussions from studies that you used in your literature review. Did your idea of what was going to happen come true, and if not,why not? Also, explain what went wrong and why. What could you have done better, or were there elements beyond your control? Explain how the project could be improved. What changes would you make to methodology (look at your limitations)? Could any other physiological factors have had an effect on your results? How would you like to develop research in this area in the future? What factors would you now take into account?

Conclusion

This should be statements of fact. What are your main findings? These should relate back to the aim of your research. Your conclusion does not need to be too long or detailed. Just list the findings by summing up the results and how the results could be used more practically. For example; this study suggests that using weights that strengthen the arms has an affect on swimming performance and it is recommended that this type of training is used within the training schedule of male club swimmers aged between 16 and 18 years.

References

This section will list the references used in the report. In the text you will have quotes or citations referring to other people's work and then at the end of the report you will have a detailed list. The Harvard system of referencing is commonly used in academic work. You need to report the reference in the text itself by giving the author of the work and also the year of publication. The full title of the work is given in the references section. If work is transferred into your own words, this is called paraphrasing and quotation marks are not needed. If a quote is included in the text, you should use single quotation marks.

In your report a reference would appear like this:

> 'Recovery for athletes is essential (Child, 2004)'.

If you are referencing more than one book you can name them all, in order of date of publication:

> 'The stresses imposed by training can be harmful (Child, 1999; Tyzack, 2002; Watt, 2003)'.

If more than one author was involved in the work you would reference them all:

> '(Ball, Brees, Chance & Stokes, 1989)'.

You do not need to consistently list all authors. Once you have listed them once you can then refer to the first author followed by *et al.* This is only the case if there are more than three authors. For example:

> 'Ball *et al.* (1989) have shown that . . .' .

You may come across two authors with the same surname. If this is the case use initials, for example:

> 'A report (Barton, R., 2006) has indicated . . .' .

If you need to reference more than one article by the same author in the same year add letters to the different references:

> 'Thomas (2000a, 2000b) showed that . . .'

Sometimes it may be necessary to refer to letters, emails or conversations. These are called 'personal communications' and would be referenced as follows:

> 'In a telephone conversation on 10 August 2005 Mr J. A. Gilbert pointed out that . . .' or 'Mr D. Goodchild's letter dated 1 May 1998 claimed that . . .'

You may need to refer to work with no author's name:

> 'A recent report by the American College of Sports Medicine (2001) states . . .' or 'the *Teesside Times* (15 July 2007, p. 4) reported that . . .'

There are guidelines for entries in the list of references, depending on what you are referring to. Books are referenced as follows:

> Thomas, J. R. and Nelson, J. K. (2005) *Research Methods in Physical Activity*, 5th edn, Illinois: Human Kinetics.

Journals and periodicals are referenced as follows:

> Morris, T. (2000) 'Psychological characteristics and talent identification in soccer', *Journal of Sports Sciences*, **18**, 715–26.

In this case, the volume number of the journal appears in bold, followed by the page numbers of the article you are referencing (not bold).

Material that has appeared online (i.e. on the internet) is a little different as it has not been published in the traditional way. Sometimes the date it was posted on the internet is given. Whether it is or not, the date you accessed it *should* be given. Therefore, an online reference would appear as follows:

> Sport England (2006) 'Equity and Inclusion'. www.sportengland.org/index/about_sport_england/equality_standard_for_sport.htm [accessed 24 April 2006].

Appendix

After the reference section comes the **appendix**. Here you can include any information that does not readily fit into the rest of your report. This is where you would put your raw data (which would otherwise just fill up the results section), and data collection sheets. You can refer to any of the appendix in the main body of the report. Multiple appendices should be labelled as Appendix A, B and C, etc. If you refer to an appendix in your report you could do it like this: 'Appendix A shows that . . .' or 'Crowd attendances are on the increase (see Appendix A)'.

Reviewing your investigation

Reviewing your investigation is useful to you as a learning experience and to anyone who might listen to, read or hear what you have done. You could evaluate your project by performing a SWOT analysis. This relates to your strengths, weaknesses, opportunities and threats.

- **Strengths**: what you have learned from the project. This could be personal, such as how to collect data, how to present information, or more general, such as the results of your study.
- **Weaknesses**: these will be your limitations or the limitations of your research. You may have been limited in the people you could test or you may not have been able to measure what you first set out to measure. Being clear in your limitations shows you have a good understanding of your research, so do not think of this as something negative.
- **Opportunities**: if you were to do the study all over again, what would you do the same, what would you do differently? What could somebody else do if they were to follow up your study? How could they improve on what you did?
- **Threats**: is there anything that questions the validity of your information? Are you sure the conclusions you arrived at are true? Is the information all your own?

Be specific and give examples. If you think your data presentation was one of your strong points, where is the evidence? Include an example of one of your graphs.

Future Considerations

This is the reflective part of the research. Use the information from the SWOT analysis. What would you change? What did not work as expected? If you could go back several months, what would you do differently? Even more importantly, what advice can you give to somebody who wants to do research in the same area? What things could they investigate that would add to what you have found? You can always improve on things, so do not be afraid to say what went wrong in your own study, as it shows you have an understanding of the research that you undertook.

Student activity 42.4 — 10–12 hours — P5 P6 M5

Once you have completed your investigation it is time to present your findings and carry out a review of what you have found.

Task 1

Present your investigation in a scientific format. In the discussion section of your write-up, review and critically analyse the results that you found. In your conclusion explain and justify areas for future consideration.

Key learning points 3

- A research project should consist of the **preliminary pages**, **main text** and **endmatter**:
- Preliminary pages should comprise:
  - abstract
  - general contents
  - contents page for figures and tables
  - contents page for appendices
  - acknowledgements.
- Main text should comprise:
  - introduction
  - literature review
  - method
  - results
  - discussion
  - conclusion.
- Endmatter should comprise:
  - references
  - appendix.

References

Bartlett, J.E., II, Kotrlik, J.W. and Higgins, C. (2001) Organisational research: determining appropriate sample size for survey research, *Information Technology, Learning, and Performance Journal*, 19(1), 43–50.

Davis, S.F. and R.A. Smith (2003) *The Psychologist as Detective: An Introduction to Conducting Research in Psychology*, Third Edition.

de Vaus, D.A. (1996) *Surveys in Social Research*, UCL Press.

Thomas, J.R. and Nelson, J.K. (2001) *Research methods in Physical Activity*. Human Kinetics.

Tuckman, B.W. (1978) *Conducting Educational Research*, second edition, Harcourt Brace Jovanovich.

Further reading

Allen, M.B. (2005) *Sports, Exercise, and Fitness: A Guide to Reference and Information Sources*, Libraries Unlimited Inc.

Bell, J. (2005) *Doing Your Research Investigation: A Guide for First-time Researchers in Social Science, Education and Health*, Open University Press.

Clarke, G.M. and Cooke, D. (2004) *A Basic Course in Statistics*, Hodder Arnold.

Cohen, L. and Holliday, K.M.E. (1996) *Practical Statistics for Learners*, Paul Chapman Publishing.

Coolican, H. (1996) *Introduction to Research Methods and Statistics in Psychology*, Hodder Arnold.

Heyes, S., Hardy, M., Humphreys, P. and Rookes, P. (1996) *Starting Statistics in Psychology and Education: A Student Handbook*, Oxford University Press.

Hyllegard, D. (2000) *Interpreting Research in Sport and Exercise Science*, Primis.

Kane, E. and O'Reilly De Brun, M. (2001), *Doing Your Own Research: In the Field and on the Net*, Marion Boyars.

Malim, T. and Birch, A. (1996) *Research Methods and Statistics*, Palgrave MacMillan.

Morrow, J.R., Jackson, A., Disch, J. and Mood, D. (2006) *Measurement and Evaluation in Human Performance*, Human Kinetics.

Owen, F. and Jones, R. (1994) *Statistics*, Prentice Hall.

Rees, D.G. (2000) *Essential Statistics*, Chapman & Hall.

Robson, C. (2002) *Real World Research*, Blackwell.

SPSS (2007) *Base 16.0 SPSS User's Guide*, SPSS Inc.

Thomas, J.R., Nelson, K. and Silverman, S. (2005) *Research Methods in Physical Activity*, Human Kinetics.

Vincent, W.J. (2004) *Statistics in Kinesiology*, Human Kinetics.

Wragg, C. and Williams C. (2003) *Data Analysis and Research for Sport and Exercise Science: A Student Guide*, Routledge.

Useful websites

www.bases.org.uk

Membership website for sports professionals, providing details of job vacancies, careers advice, forums for coaching and sports science-related topics; limited access to non-members

www.pponline.co.uk/encyc/sports-performance-analysis-coaching-and-training-39

Article detailing how sports analysis can help coaching and training

Index